Revels in Madness

Corporealities: Discourses of Disability

David T. Mitchell and Sharon L. Snyder, editors

Books available in the series:

"Defects": Engendering the Modern Body
  edited by Helen Deutsch and Felicity Nussbaum

Revels in Madness: Insanity in Medicine and Literature
  by Allen Thiher

Points of Contact: Disability, Art, and Culture
  edited by Susan Crutchfield and Marcy Epstein

A History of Disability
  by Henri-Jacques Stiker

Disabled Veterans in History
  edited by David A. Gerber

Narrative Prosthesis: Disability and the Dependencies of Discourse
  by David T. Mitchell and Sharon L. Snyder

Backlash Against the ADA: Reinterpreting Disability Rights
  edited by Linda Hamilton Krieger

The Staff of Oedipus: Transforming Disability in Ancient Greece
  by Martha L. Rose

Fictions of Affliction: Physical Disability in Victorian Culture
  by Martha Stoddard Holmes

Foucault and the Government of Disability
  edited by Shelley Tremain

Revels in Madness

Insanity in Medicine and Literature

Allen Thiher

Ann Arbor

The University of Michigan Press

First paperback edition 2004
Copyright © by the University of Michigan 1999
All rights reserved
Published in the United States of America by
The University of Michigan Press
Manufactured in the United States of America
⊗ Printed on acid-free paper

2007   2006   2005   2004   5   4   3   2

A CIP catalog record for this book is available
from the British Library.

Library of Congress Cataloging-in-Publication Data

Thiher, Allen, 1941–
    Revels in madness : insanity in medicine and literature / Allen
  Thiher.
        p.   cm. — (Corporealities)
    Includes bibliographical references (p.   ) and index.
    ISBN 0-472-11035-7 (alk. paper)
    1. Literature and mental illness.   2. Mental illness in
literature.   3. Mental illness—History.   4. Psychiatry—History.   I.
Title.   II. Series.
PN56.M45   T53   1999   99-6460
809'.93353—dc21   CIP

ISBN 0-472-08999-4 (pbk. : alk. paper)

Acknowledgments

My first thanks must go to students and colleagues in the Department of Romance Languages at the University of Missouri who have suffered having my ideas tried out upon them or who have read chapters and made valuable suggestions. Many thanks for much patience. The same thanks must go to colleagues in Romanistik at the Universität des Saarlandes, whose help was most useful while I was teaching there.

I must also thank the Research Council at the University of Missouri, whose generous grant of a year's research leave allowed time for systematic research for this book.

Additional thanks go to the Camargo Foundation in Cassis, France, for providing an apartment and a library, as well as a forum, where some of these ideas could be developed. By the same token I wish to recognize the help that I received from the Bibliothèque Méjanes in Aix-en-Provence, whose staff helped me exploit their extraordinary historical collection of medical works. Additional thanks are due to the staff of Ellis Library at the University of Missouri for hunting down materials that, it must be said, are not always easy to find.

Finally, thanks to LeAnn Fields at the University of Michigan Press for sticking with this project!

Contents

Part 1. **Madness from Hippocrates to Hölderlin**   1

Chapter 1. Discourses on Madness in the Greco-Roman World   13

Chapter 2. Continuities and Ruptures in Medieval Folly   44

Chapter 3. Madness and Early Modernity in Shakespeare,
            Cervantes, and Descartes   73

Chapter 4. The Iatro-Mechanical Era and the Madness
            of Machines   102

Chapter 5. Neoclassicism, the Rise of Singularity, and
            Moral Treatment   131

Part 2. **The Modernity of Madness**   159

Chapter 6. The German Romantics and the Invention
            of Psychiatry   167

Chapter 7. Pathological Anatomy and the Poetics of Madness   195

Chapter 8. Modern Determinations of Insanity: Psychiatry
            and Psychoanalysis   224

Chapter 9. Modernist Poetic Discourses in Madness   250

Chapter 10. The Contemporary Scene's Affirmation of and
             Rebellion against Logos   282

            Postscript: Madness between History and Neurology   316

            Notes   325

            Index   337

Part 1

Madness from Hippocrates to Hölderlin

Introduction: Historical Considerations

Our first cases of the insane were probably the owners of those trepanned skulls frequently found in archeological digs from the Stone Age. If we are allowed to interpret these skulls in the light of much later iconography depicting surgeons removing the stone of madness through a hole they have perforated in the head, then we might read these skulls to show that madness has been localized in the head from time immemorial. Boring a hole in the skull of the mad would be the beginning of a medical history of madness, for we can imagine that the hole was drilled to bring about some therapeutic effect, or perhaps a change in conduct. From this perspective the holes are also the beginning of a legal and philosophical history of madness, since we can see, in these perforated containers of the soul, that legal and religious power had accrued to some priestly or medical group that had the power and authority to exercise force over the body of the insane, the sick, and the possessed. The power to bore into another person's skull is the power to dispose of the mad person's body in the most literal sense—and this power presupposes medical, philosophical, religious, and legal theories that we can only guess about.

This power must also presuppose the operation of some literary dimension in culture, for some power of the fictional imagination was at work in creating the worldview that imagined perforating heads to be a way to remove stones, demons, or whatever was supposed to be contained within. Later folk myths and archaic practices allow us to project back on these silent skulls a world of imaginative creation that can quite properly be called protoliterary. Of course one can also imagine that, were these Stone Age Yoricks afflicted with tumors, these trephinations might also have brought some relief to them. Conjuring imaginary beings and effecting a cure are not mutually exclusive practices. On the contrary.[1]

However intriguing these skulls may be, they are not part of a history—as opposed to an archaeology—of madness. For a history, we must turn from their silent perforations to the world of texts and writings that are the grounds for history. What I want to do in this study is explore how doctors and writers have historically made madness the center of their writing, this in view of a historical phenomenology of how the Western imagination has represented madness to itself. Literature can bridge the gap between the medical mind and the insane mind because the literary imagination has historically shared certain features with the insane imagination, as well as traits with the medical imagination that has tried to explain madness. From the outset we can theorize that the human capacity to create literature springs from the mind's potential or capacity to entertain certain kinds of insanity: not all forms of madness, but many are related to literature, especially insofar as both madness and literature enable us to believe in and be moved by what in a sense does not exist, by fictions, imaginations, hallucinations, inner voices. Madness, literature, and theory or knowledge about madness and literature all overlap, which more than justifies a study of the intertwining discourses that purport to represent madness in some sense. Madness and theories about madness have nourished literature from antiquity, and conversely literature has provided the stuff upon which theory has worked. This relationship has a history. Homer's world had relatively little commerce with madness. Perhaps it required the more self-reflexive world of Athenian theater and philosophy for madness and theories of madness to be reflected in literary works, and for literary works in turn to become myths capable of nourishing the creation of mad fantasies. These questions about the emergence of madness in Greece will occupy us in the first chapter of this study.

Throughout this study my interest is in theories about madness and in the way theory informs literature—and vice versa—and I also want to listen to voices of madness as they are molded by theory and literature. I want to let literature and theory, especially theory found in medical thought, and also philosophical thought, reflect back and forth on each other, in the hope of marking off intersections where literature, medical thought, and philosophy have defined madness in crucial ways for our history. I do this in hope of advancing our understanding of what we have made of madness in our culture, and with some hope of showing that literature has always been a dominant way by which we have attempted to know what madness is. In this study of literature, theory, and mad voices, then, it is taken as axiomatic that literature is a psychic activity that often overlaps with madness and that literature also coincides with science insofar as literary texts also propose models of experience. And, as I hope to show, these models have epistemological consequences for science.

This study is the work of a literary scholar, not a clinician. But I hope that my approach has something to say to the medical scientist as well as to the historian. This hope is underpinned by the following considerations. Both literature and medicine can be described as discourse. By discourse I mean something analogous to what Wittgenstein called language games, or organized practices of language. Although I do not follow Wittgenstein in affirming the ungrounded nature of our worldview, I find it helpful to use his view that language is essential for articulating our worldview. We use language to gain purchase on the real, and the real in turn informs the way we formulate and use language games. Language does not always determine what we take to be reality, but it codifies the rules for gaining access to reality once we have annexed a realm of experience into what can be articulated in language. (Or to give one of Wittgenstein's examples, language does not make water boil at 100 degrees centigrade, but, once that statement enters a scientific language game, that statement defines what is water.) Language games are discursive practices, with implicit and explicit rules governing the way the practice is conducted. Taking the form of literary practices or scientific disciplines, language games are used to order knowledge; they create models and systems; and, taken globally, they articulate our worldview itself.

Literature, philosophy, medical psychology, and psychiatry are in this sense language games, all of which attempt, at various times and places, to talk about the dysfunctional nature of human minds deemed to be mad. These discourses frame ways of speaking about madness, often presupposing certain public rules and practices. My point in this study is that largely through these language games does madness come to light. One can point to the symptoms of madness, to behavior, actions, gestures, and the like. But only in language is found and identified the being to whom these symptoms belong, which is to say that madness exists only when one can speak of a mad person, hence a being located through a language game or a discourse. The center of our discourses on madness has had many names: *thymos*, *anima*, soul, spirit, self, the unconscious, the subject, the person. Whatever be the accent given by the central concept, access to the entity afflicted with madness is obtained through a language game in which these concepts or names play a role, organizing our experience of the world even as the world vouchsafes criteria for correct usage of these notions. *Psyche* and *self*, for example, are parts of a discourse about mental entities for which these "concepts" are necessary if we are to make sense of how we experience mental entities in the world as we now live in it. And, as such, as concepts that orient us toward experiencing the world, psyche and soul do not present themselves as entities to be placed under the microscope. Microbes that may induce madness are, to be sure, to be seen disrupting the brain, but the full articulation of madness can only occur when we can use a language game that brings the afflicted self to light, and not simply the cerebral cortex.

In saying this I do not mean to imply that the psyche occupies a metaphysical space or that it is not amenable to scientific understanding. On the contrary the psyche—or self or person—is accessible through the multiple language games in which the empirical self manifests itself, and this can be studied scientifically from a number of viewpoints. Nor do I wish to imply that the self or soul or *thymos* is only a position in language. This is a reductionist ploy that has regularly been abused by many recent thinkers. For example, after the linguist Jakobson defined the first person pronoun "I" as a shifter or a linguistic function whose meaning is only found in the act of enunciation, it became common for structuralists and poststructuralists to reduce subjectivity to an effect of language. This kind of structuralist reductionism is typical of metaphysicians wanting to find one universal principle to explain all phenomena—and consequently, Jakobson's description of a grammatical function became a transpsychological catchall. No single grammatical description can account for the riches of the self and of real language games that express and define the self and its heterogeneous relations with the world—or multiple worlds it lives in. Outside of language lie multiple realms. But *access* to a human self and to its world is largely a matter of language. This is true of access to any human world—and explains why the study of language, literature, and medicine is a necessary project for a full understanding of our human possibilities, including the possibility of going mad.

The history of the emergence of the self is the history of the development of those language games or discursive practices that allow us to situate a self. From Homer's *thymos*, or sense of innerness, to the Cartesian thinking subject, the Lockean person, the Freudian ego, the neurological subject, or, some would argue, recently the Lacanian subject, we can trace a history of relations in which science and literature overlap in articulating these language games. This claim is not exactly a scientific point of view: rather this viewpoint provides a framework for ordering evidence. Probably no experimentation can prove or disprove the framework itself. But my point of view is not based on pure philosophical rationalism, since my "model" is meaningless without empirical demonstration. Pragmatically, then, I hope to show here that my historical viewpoint about science, literature, and self integrates great areas of culture that are often looked upon as disparate. But once we agree with the neurologist Gerald Edelman that there is no human self without language, then we have affirmed a premise from which we may deduce that language provides the common basis for understanding the human subject, scientifically and historically, as an imaginative being capable of dream, literature, and madness.[2]

There are today great differences between science and literature, though, historically, those differences are not as always as clear as one might expect. In ancient economies of discourse these differences often do not exist. From a modern viewpoint an essential difference between literature and science appears to be that what is accepted as science can lose its status because it has to define the rational and the real, whereas what are obviously literary language games cannot lose this capacity, at least today. Thus scientific models fall into oblivion, but literary texts, at least some literary texts, perennially remain an articulation of human possibilities. (It is hard at least for me to imagine a world in which Homer, Dante, Shakespeare, or Goethe would not be of current interest.) But even this difference between scientific models and literature needs qualification. For older literary myths functioning as the founding myths of a culture can lose their status as originating texts that defined the real—and then they become objects of scientific or historical scrutiny, much like some ancient medical theory explaining disease. And scientific models can lose their validity, by contemporary standards, and yet retain a tremendous fascination for us as examples of what Borges would have called fantastic literature, as examples of physiological and physical cosmologies generated by the unfettered imagination. To the modern mind, Galen's humors theory may appear as imaginative as any creation of the poetic imagination. Who can deny the grandiose poetry of Lucretius's atoms? And one can imagine that, when new paradigms have come to replace modern physics, neutrinos and muons will be viewed as fantastic characters in a contemporary *On the Nature of Things* created by mathematical geniuses (with apologies to believers in final theories).

The present study springs from the intersection of a number of concerns. I call upon the history of medicine for its theories and determinations of the causes of madness; and upon the history of philosophy for its attempts to fix the boundaries of the rational and the irrational. Paralleling these discourses is literature as a form of knowledge that defines, in conjunction with medicine and philosophy, what are the contours of the self and its relation to the world. And with that knowledge comes a desire to know what is on the other side of those contours—madness, deviance, insanity.

The reasons why I have written this study are many. They are partly personal—insanity impinges upon all of us throughout our lives—and partly intellectual in a broad sense. I want to continue the investigation into madness that Michel Foucault began in his brilliant, influential, but, I think, misguided history of madness, *Histoire de la folie*.[3] Foucault's contribution to this project is probably greater than I realize. To avoid any misunderstanding, however, I want to state from the outset that I neither endorse his view of the discontinuities that characterize intellectual history, nor subscribe to his belief in the autonomy of language and discursive systems. I will argue here, in fact, for great historical continuity, often unseen continuity, in our ways of speaking about madness.

If I am inclined to agree that without some concept like madness, there would be no recognition of the phenomenon of madness, I am also quite convinced, unlike Foucault, that our invention and use of such concepts are grounded in a reality that in some sense justifies them. For example, the concept of love provides a normative concept that allows us to entertain a psychological state. It can be argued that love would not exist without the concept of love (to borrow from Daniel Dennett an argument to which I shall return in the conclusion). This recognition of the necessity of language to articulate psychological states does not mean, however, that language is the basis for ungrounded systems of cognition. On the contrary, language often comes to articulate, in language games, what reality demands that we articulate. Poets invented love so that we might transform our sexuality, and scientists articulated organic chemistry so that a great part of the world around us could enter discourse (to borrow an example from Wittgenstein). Medical writers, philosophers, and poets have articulated madness so that we might live in a world in which the recognition of madness is incumbent upon us when something in human reality goes askew. Finally, to complete my outline of disagreement with Foucault, madness is not simply the outgrowth of a conspiracy of bourgeois reason against utopian forces of liberation. It is occasionally utopian in its urges, but insanity is many other things, as we shall presently see.

Another impetus to write this book came from my readings in the history of science. It came in fact from the realization that the history of European medicine and the history of literature are often characterized by basically the same categories for periodization: early Greek, classical Greek, Roman, medieval and Renaissance, neoclassical and Enlightenment, post-Enlightenment and romantic, modern, and, perhaps, postmodern. It struck me that this rather extraordinary fact needed more investigation. Since my initial interest in the history of science was part of a concern with how we have come to understand madness as we do, it then appeared to me that a study of the common axioms of medical theory and literature, focusing on their views of madness, might bring to light our historical determinations of the rational and the irrational, the healthy and the deviant. Then I might come to understand how we have represented madness to ourselves, first in those discourses known as early medicine as well as literature. Today these may both appear to be imaginative discourses; but both also existed in the service of knowledge. As Hippocrates put it, medicine begins as a knowledge of mankind—and so, I maintain, does literature.

I conceive of this investigation as history, which is to say that it is an attempt to offer knowledge of the past that is relevant and useful to the present. Therefore, it is not an exhaustive history, a complete list as it were, of everything in which something has been said about madness, for such a complete listing could only result in redundant demonstrations. Rather, my choice of examples for discussion throughout this study has been dictated, in part because of the importance of the examples, in part because they allow me to build an argument that I believe reflects the dominant historical reality. Virtually every example here could be replaced by another without changing the thrust of my argument (with two or three obvious exceptions). There has been nonetheless more archival research here than may meet the eye, but the arguments here do not depend on discovering new sources. I hope historians will find that this kind of research can be of interest to them.

To justify this lack of exhaustiveness, perhaps I might make a few additional comments about the philosophical framework of this work, or historical studies in general. Any historical work entails, I suppose, the minimal belief that the past in some sense exists, if only as a series of textual inscriptions that must be interpreted. But there are many approaches to this task. Historians of literature often try to use literary texts, for example, to prove theses about the nature of social reality, or they may accumulate vast amounts of erudition to demonstrate the referential character of a given text. They may choose to interpret a literary text as an extension of the psychic life of a writer, and beyond that of the writer's class, nation, or era. This plurality of approaches reflects the floating status of literary discourse in our culture. We do not assign a single purpose to discourses whose use value seems to range from pornographic wish fulfillment, or idle pleasure, to the most august functions of revealing the sacred, informing our worldview, or defending our ideology and ethics. The recent demise of the idea of a literary canon has been brought about by this pluralist view of literary history, and the idea of an exhaustive study of important literary texts now seems rather implausible.

By contrast, most historians of science do not conceive of their task in so varied a manner. Until recently at least, like most historians of a given scientific discipline, traditional historians of medicine or psychiatry have for the most part looked upon their task as one of narrating the development of a greater and greater rationality. This development would find its culminating moment in the present state of the scientific discipline that the historian was studying. In a Hegelian spirit, the goal of the history of science has been, and often still is, to demonstrate greater and greater self-fulfillment—though, unlike Hegel, most historians of science do not believe their discipline comes to an end in the last chapter of their book. (Of course, we occasionally hear talk of the completion of discipline: for example, the "end of physics" is periodically in the air, which might lead the skeptic to suggest a relation of inverse proportion between the number of claims for completion and the problems that remain to be solved.) A variant of this type of history in which science follows a linear development toward its perfection is what Nietzsche called monumental history. Here the historian engages in a celebration of the great names of the past that, taken as a symbolic display of the capacities of human reason, make up a pantheon. This exercise in hagiography, once favored by literary as well as medical historians, has been somewhat abandoned in recent times, for it also demands an exhaustive approach to its subject. Moreover, monumental history is often a form of teleological history that erects its completed pantheon by listing all those names that are synonymous with the unfolding of rationality or the creative possibilities of a discipline or a medium. At the risk of appearing reactionary I might add that the pragmatic value of monumental history is not to be underestimated. Its main failure is to see the full matrix in which the "great" individual elaborates his work (and "his" indicates the chauvinism that has traditionally been inherent to this approach).

Teleological history emphasizes the continuities of historical development by celebrating those elements in an individual's work that lead to the contemporary state of a discipline. It not only fails, as I suggested, to appreciate the full context of an individual's theory, but especially the irrational elements that are often embedded in it. For example, Newton's obsessive mysticism or Paracelsus's demented cosmology are left aside in writing the history of physics, mechanics, medicine, chemistry, or pharmacology. The erroneous and the irrational have been excluded from the pantheon. There is of course some sense to this procedure. One can reasonably ask what difference does it make that, once Harvey had shown that blood circulated, he continued to propagate the erroneous view that the function of the heart is to heat the blood. But one can also answer this question by pointing out that it is important to see that Harvey's theories are embedded in system of beliefs or a worldview that is in part foreign to us today. There is discontinuity as well as continuity between Harvey's world and ours. And historians can, sometimes with equal justification, emphasize the discontinuities as much·as the continuities. Michel Foucault preferred, in his first works, to stress absolute discontinuity between the cognitive and epistemological practices of different eras. This perspective leads to the dramatic view that history is a series of ruptures. Such a viewpoint is partially correct, and partially wrong: Harvey's discovery of the circulation of blood is and, most probably, will continue to be part of our worldview after all.

Continuity and rupture are organizational categories used by the historian. As such they are more intrinsic to the organization of discourse than to any inherent nature of things. They are categories used to order evidence, but hardly the only ones. Recurrence, reprise, circularity, and the like are also categories that we can use to make sense of cultural history. With regard to the history of medicine, for example, a continuous linear model of progress hardly seems adequate, nor is a model based upon a series of ruptures. Repetition and recycling are equally useful as categories that allow us to follow the development of medicine from century to century—at least until the revolutions in physiology, pathological anatomy, and microbiology. However, the changes or revolutions produced by these disciplines have not necessarily transformed the discourse used to analyze madness and psychic disturbances. For the clinical entities identified by doctors, scientists, and folklore in their respective descriptions of madness are often situated in language games that have lasted: Hippocrates' description of epilepsy seems to be our epilepsy, though our notions about its etiology are totally different. The clinical entity has existed historically for two millennia—even if it was nearly lost in the Middle Ages. To be sure, it is often difficult to sort out what is a clinical entity and what belongs to ordinary language. Purely medical descriptions can become, with perduring continuity, part of the ordinary language games that organize our everyday worldview. Harvey's description of the circulation of the blood became a way to organize our ordinary language games about the body. The color of blood and its rate of flow are articulated today in different terms, in ordinary language, since Harvey's work. And this transformation of everyday language is as much part of our basic cultural history as is the history of medical paradigms.

With regard to madness the historical questions are especially vexing and, I shall argue, especially crucial, for we often think that we speak of madness today in new terms. But that is not certain. Do we speak today of the same madness Aristotle spoke of in the Athens of the fourth century or Willis in the London of the seventeenth century? Faced with the difficulty of empirically deciding such a question, the historian may be tempted to accept the view that the history of science is a series of ruptures and to agree with a philosopher of science like Thomas Kuhn that our forebears lived in a world different from ours.[4] But rupture can only be read against the backdrop of continuity. Or, to offer an example familiar to most, we know that Dante knew the world was a globe, even if Dante's geography is not ours. Dante's worldview is partly ours, partly not, and the breaks between his world and ours are read against the continuity we share with him. It seems clear to me that we share enough features with Dante's worldview so that we can enter into Dante's world, through his language, with comprehension. I think the same can be argued about more obviously scientific thinkers of the past. If we shared none of the features making up the thinker's past worldview, we would understand little—which in fact is the case with regard to many of the mythic worldviews anthropologists have collected. Myths are often incomprehensible because they share no commonalities with our worldview, they play no role in articulating our world, the world of modern Westerners for whom the scientific revolution and the Enlightenment have, for the most part, determined what we take to be reality (whether we like it or not).

I am thus arguing that historical understanding means that we have to deal with the presence of continuity and rupture within different historical worldviews that, considered in their diachronic development, share some or perhaps many features. This is exemplified by the history of the self that is the self we find in ourselves. If the self exists as articulated by various language games that have unfolded historically, then the self exists as a historical project within which we can expect to find both continuities and ruptures, circularities and recurrences, in terms of its historical development. Indeed, a history of madness and its articulations can be written in terms of the development of those discourses that have defined the self. And, I suggest, it may well be that today's clinical tableaux have roots in the history of those varied discourses that have allowed us to understand what the normal self and, hence, the mad self is.

Looking at the history of our notions about madness, I find it hard to subscribe to the idea that the history of medical psychology has been a progressive weeding out of the irrational. This is not to say that we have not made some improvements in our practical dealings with the mad—relative to the worst practices in our history. (However, the next time you avoid contact with the visibly mad who are left to inhabit our city streets today, you may well wonder if we are superior to the Middle Ages with its doctrine of charity.) When one compares psychiatry to other sciences, medical or otherwise, one simply cannot speak of a break with the past with regard to our knowledge of madness (relative to virtually any historical period). New theories in neurology could change this situation. However, what we have mainly seen in this regard is that neurology's great service to date has been to reduce the number of clinical entities we consider to be madness. In part, neurology does this by describing syndromes that, once recognized as a neurological disease or dysfunction, are no longer considered to be part of madness. With regard to forms of insanity for which no organic cause is known, however, it does not seem to me that psychiatry can propose a knowledge of madness that represents any great historical advance. I make this statement, not as a criticism of psychiatry, but rather to mark out a historical framework that is neither teleological nor overlooks the obvious continuities linking our ideas about madness today with those of the past.

Until recently, most histories of psychiatry have been teleological, for they have accepted the success model to be the proper model for writing the history of a scientific discipline—and psychiatry has by and large considered itself a successful discipline. If greater rationality is the goal of science, then it follows that the currently accepted model must be more rational that what preceded. However, unlike the case of physics or chemistry, there really are no victorious models of rationality that are broadly accepted by all in order to explain what madness is. Or, succinctly put, physics is physics in Tokyo or Paris; psychiatry varies from culture to culture. To repeat: it is only when one can assign a clear organic explanation to a clear syndrome does a model become victorious—and then the syndrome ceases to be considered madness. Epilepsy, general paralysis, Parkinson's disease, and other syndromes of this type are cases in point. Or, once we know that spirochetes are making a trip through a person's brain, we are no longer inclined to call the sufferer mad, however insane the fellow's behavior may be. For the time being at least, psychotics and schizophrenics do not enjoy this advantage, if it is an advantage.

I invite you to begin a historical study that is also a work of critical analysis. This study will go from madness as represented in Athens by doctors and thespians to madness as we conceive it today. My point of departure is the historical stage when madness emerges on the Athenian *skene* at roughly the same time the Hippocratic writers are making madness into an object of medical discourse. This is the moment when it appears that logos—or reason and language as conceived by the Greeks—first reflects back upon itself and discovers alterity, or that otherness that seems incommensurate with logos. Reason makes unreason an object of representation. The following chapters of the first part of this study then continue this history of representations of madness, in literature, philosophy, and medicine, through the

Enlightenment when the neoclassical revival of the late eighteenth century brings us full square back to the Greek origins of our thought about madness. In the second half of this study I then deal with the modernity of madness, beginning with the German romantics and tracing out a history that goes through positivism, the invention of psychiatry and psychoanalysis, to conclude with some considerations of what is called our postmodern era.

My study of this development is not, however, guided by some ordering telos. Hegel is self-consciously absent here—if the *Geist* will allow such a paradox. Moreover, history conceived as the demonstration of a single thesis is usually false. I propose several theses, one of which is that the history of the development of self is better understood as a history of continuity, rather than rupture. Indeed, I maintain that in our ongoing attempts to work out discourses that define self, reason, and world, we have never fully broken with our Greek origins. Other major themes that guide this study can be quickly adumbrated. Discourses in madness are not only theoretically important, they are important for articulating the ways that madness can be experienced, lived as it were, in its alterity. In its understanding of itself and in its attempts to communicate, madness relies upon the understanding that reason offers unreason. To this end literature and medicine are equally important, as are at times theology and philosophy. These discourses allow mediation that the community can share. Moreover, literature can mediate madness from within, for the very mimetic nature of literature allows it to know madness by speaking it. Perhaps this commonality accounts for the constant theatricalization of madness that is typical of our culture. Both medicine and literature have had constant recourse to theater and to theatrical metaphors to describe, in various ways, the dynamics of insanity. Madness and literature share at least one other commonality, which is, as I have suggested, the imaginative acceptance of the unreal as real. In this shared imaginative capacity to negate the real, literature and madness have always had a tacit alliance, from the Greeks to the present, when a putative science of madness, psychoanalysis, tells us that a Greek tragic hero inhabits each of us when we come to grips with our destiny. I shall deal with that theme in the second part of this study when I turn to the tale of the enshrinement of the Greek Oedipus. But especially in the first half of this study, going from the Greeks to the Enlightenment, we shall find ample material to demonstrate the cultural unity that I see going from the Greek beginnings of our Western discourses on madness, and culminating in Pinel's psychiatric clinic as well as the prophetic madness of that would-be Greek hero, the greatest of our mad poets, Hölderlin.

Chapter 1

Discourses on Madness in the Greco-Roman World

Logos and Madness in Early Greek Literature

European literature begins with Homer, whoever Homer may have been. For several centuries Homer's work stood for the Greek world as the summation of what we call knowledge, myth, and religion. Thus one might expect some view of madness in Homer. However, this is not the case. The presence of madness is only dimly sensed in the Homeric world, though later Greek antiquity found madness in Homer in its interpretation of the character Bellerophon. This legendary hero of the *Iliad* destroyed the Chimaera, defeated the Amazons, but, at the end of his life, as Fitzgerald translates it, he was cursed and

> incurred the gods' wrath—and alone he moped
> on Aleion plain, eating his heart out,
> shunning the beaten track of men.
>
> (6.201–3)

There is nothing that plainly says this Homeric hero is mad. Most of later antiquity, as for example in the *Thirtieth Problem* attributed to Aristotle, agreed that Bellerophon was a mad melancholic. What else could explain his behavior? The Greek mind could conceive the refusal of social bonds and the ties to a common world only as a sign of madness. And madness in a hero, entailing his loss of a shared social world, was caused by the gods, by causal agents outside the world of humanity. This view of madness is not quite mythic and not quite scientific. Part mythic, part philosophical, this interpretation of madness as rupture is the basis for our later views of madness: it presents madness as a break with the social world and the community whose worldview we share through language—or what the Greeks called logos. Outside of these shared social bonds and the language that mediates these bonds lies the plains upon which the mad person wanders, without communication, lost in melancholia.

Early Greek myth and literature granted the gods a determining role in madness, especially with regard to heroes. Only a god could drive a hero from the social bonds he shared with his community and thus drive him outside of logos. The Greek concept of logos should be taken in a larger sense than the usual biblical translation "word." Logos means language, reason, harmony, proportion, all notions that apply to the relation of the individual and the cosmos. When the hero is driven from reason or logos, he, and sometimes she in Greek theater, is locked within what we call pure subjectivity. However, modern notions, such as subjectivity, are likely to mislead us when speaking of the Greeks. Logos is prior to subjectivity and is a dimension of selfhood in which all participate. It is more like a fluid in which all are encapsulated and is constitutive of the psyche. Thus the inner world is always objective insofar as it is constituted by the bonds of logos. In Homer, however, Bellerophon's example suggests an intuition of the separation of self and logos that, for the later Greeks, is the condition of madness.

Three centuries or so after Homer, fifth-century Athens created the stage on which was first enacted a portrayal of self that separated out world and ego. In Aeschylus (525–456 B.C.) the rupture between logos and self is more prominent that in Homer's exterior portrayal of a loss of shared logos. Most historians would agree that the sense of a self separate from world is, however, not yet fully developed in Aeschylus, the earliest extant tragedian. His theater remained essentially religious, though it is also true that in Aeschylus's work the gods do not intervene as in Homer. It is *ate* or fate that destroys reason and leads to madness. However, an inner self is not involved in this destruction. This seems to me to be the sense of the scene in which the ghost of Darius in *The Persians* laments about his son Xeres, whose lack of measure, or hubris, has caused the Persian defeat at the hands of the Greeks. Darius wonders if his son is afflicted with mental illness. This is not a reflection on his son's inner state. Rather it is Darius's way of characterizing the disequilibrium that marks Xeres' ambition (cf. l. 734). A clearer sense of inner world emerges in the tragedy *The Libation Bearers*. In this play Orestes, having killed his mother, claims that he can see the Eumenides, the Furies that have come to persecute him, though nobody else in the play can see them. But he believes so much in their presence that he must flee them. Orestes is entertaining an hallucination born of guilt—or so the modern reader interprets it. The gods are given a causal role in this tragedy, for the hero is driven from society by them. They drive him mad because he has committed sacrilege. Orestes has broken his relation to the gods, much like Xeres has lost his sense of proportion, and hence has broken with logos. In

The Libation Bearers this break transforms Orestes' vision and removes him from the community of shared perception. In modern terms this produces the radical change in the vision of a world perceived by a single subject.

This "modernity" should not mislead us, for, in the sequel to *The Libation Bearers, The Eumenides,* the persecuting Furies are presented as an objective presence, and, as such, they cannot be taken as a projection of psychic or inner reality. In this play Aeschylus does not seem concerned with a clear line of demarcation between self and world. In religious terms the self portrayed therein is still immersed in an objective world of logos for which there is little distinction between the inner and the outer. Logos is also part of a relation to the sacred; and as long as the sacred was perceived through logos, the metaphysical distinction of an inner self and an outer world had little meaning. The sacred is a visible harmony. And, as the obscure Heraclitus put it, logos belongs to psyche. Thus madness, like the Furies, could be visible to all—without necessarily being madness. Only when the self could be totally lost to logos could madness become the opaque otherness that we find in later Greek thought and literature.

Hippocrates and the Rationalist World of the Pre-Socratics

A transformation of the meaning of the sacred was essential for the development of a self that sees itself as separate from the world and logos. Preeminently responsible for this development was the advent of medicine. Medicine was invented as a consequence of the revolution in thought undertaken by the pre-Socratic thinkers, the first protoscientists to think in terms of rational causality. This philosophical milieu formed Hippocrates, the legendary doctor who was quite famous by Plato's time, and the other writers whom posterity has identified with him.[1] In the writings called the Hippocratic corpus emerges the view of self as a *psyche* that is something separate from the world, a world that includes the body as a unified entity set against the psyche. The development of a somatic sense perceiving the body as a unified entity seems to have developed when the psyche opposed the body as something other than itself. There is, for example, no notion for body as an unified entity in Homer. Homeric characters can speak of the parts of the body, but there is no unifying concept tying together those parts that Greek heroes cut off with such dexterity. So it is a reasonable conjecture that somatic unity could exist only once it could be opposed to some other unified concept, such as the soul or the psyche, that granted a human being a permanent identity made up of the dialectic between somatic and psychic entities. This may be the grounds for our later dualisms, but it is not the same as the subjective and objective distinctions of Cartesian and Kantian metaphysics. Greek identity is a dialectic of oppositions unified in logos.

The somatic-psychic distinction that we find in later Greek thought represents the attempt to speak rationally about what cannot be seen. From our perspective this can be viewed as a language game that posits a self that is different from the world and the body, which is part of a necessary step in differentiating what must be the case if we are to speak self-reflexively about a self—that is, about what is necessarily other than what is entertained nonreflexively. All that is other than self—gods, bodies, forces, things— these can be named, classified, and studied. For these relations and categories to be sorted out, there must be a self that exists as that place that is other than the world where these relations and categories are perceived. Once this distinction is made, then it is possible to perceive madness as that disturbance of the relation—the logos—between self and world, including the body. Only with this separation could the Greeks speak of a harmonious relation, or a state of rationality as we find in Plato, and, by contrast, a disturbed or irrational relation as in insanity.

Some medical historians have judged that little of lasting value is found in the various writings preserved as the Hippocratic corpus. This judgment implies that, before microbiology, there is no medicine. I think that it is more accurate to affirm that the pre-Socratic axioms of these writings are the foundations for some of our basic notions about self and madness. Along with the later Greek tragedies, the Hippocratic writings are among the inaugural discourses that make it possible to speak of the irrational in nonreligious terms. They contributed to the way the Greeks first spoke rationally of the self as a form of logos. We exist rationally when we exist with a shared language, which means that we have a socially guaranteed set of assumptions about the world. And these assumptions make it possible for us to exist as the social animals that we are, in our shared social world, the encapsulating world of logos.

Without this development of Greek thought, it is difficult to see how we would know madness at all, for madness would have no meaning without this view that the sane self is defined by its participation in logos. Moreover, this Greek sense of rationality precedes the development of ethical notions—such as the belief in temperance—that many take to be the acme of Greek thought. And, to return to my earlier point about the separation of self and world, it is clear that the emergence of scientific rationality occurs at that historical moment when the pre-Socratic Anaxagoras, before Aristotle, declared mind or intelligence—*nous*—to be separate from all that it entertains. When this philosopher made mind into a self-motivated principle of change, he undertook the fundamental step toward conceptualizing our relation to the world. The future development of scientific thought is bound up with the idea that *psyche* or self exists separate from *physis* or unfolding nature, and yet is subject to nature—as the Hippocratic view of mental illness shows. Mental space is at once separate from language, for it can lose its relation to logos in madness, and at the same time mind, the sane mind, exists as part of logos in its relation to being. Pre-Socratic thought seems to provide the grounds for much contemporary theory, say, for contemporary neurological theory for which nature is the ultimate ground of consciousness; or for deconstructive theories of language for which mind is a part of the linguistic system.[2]

The pre-Socratic thinkers elaborated the axioms underlying the earliest Hippocratic writings. To understand these writings one needs to imagine a social space in which logos is understood at once as language, reason, the bond of intersubjective relations, and, finally, as a form of vision. Through logos one enters the world of *phenomena,* the Greek term expressing the making present of being through vision. For the Hippocratic physician the lack of proportion in illness is perceived as an absence of logos, or a break in equilibrium. There is something circular about this reasoning, since the observed state of rupture is explained by what it is, that is, a break in equilibrium. But this circularity allows the explanation of the break in logos in terms of a natural causality—in contradistinction to Aristotle's later fourfold metaphysical causality. And with this circularity occurs the first scientific revolution in the form of Hippocrates' basic axiom that there is nothing without a cause. In this single dictum, underwritten by the Greek understanding of logos and its relational nature, the Greek "miracle" took place. There is really nothing in the preceding history of medicine, philosophy, or science to prepare us for this axiom. But there is no medicine, philosophy, or science before this dictum.

The axiom of natural causality relates the mad, through their bodies, to the world of phenomena. Vision shows that the body is subject to causal influences like heat and wind, air and diet, and these are the influences that the Hippocratic corpus sees causing sickness. Excretions, somatic regularities, external agents, all can be causes that relate to the phenomena of illness. There are no magical determinations of disease, nor are there simplifying single causal agents, such as simply fire or air. The Hippocratic texts present a series of descriptive language games in which the self or *thymos* interacts with visible or potentially visible phenomena; or specifically in the case of humors, it interacts with those humoral causal agents that inhabit the body's inner space.

There are at least two specific explanations of madness in the Hippocratic texts, one dealing with its relation to wind, heat, and other natural influences; and the better-known explanation, the humors theory that dominated Western medicine for many centuries. The humors theory was sketched out in the text called *On Human Nature* (also called *On the Nature of Man*), but was imposed on the Western tradition in later elaboration by the Greek physician Galen (ca. 120–200 A.D.). To these two views stands opposed the tragedians' older view of madness: madness in Greek tragedy is a matter of divine intervention. However, the opposition should not obscure a commonality, for both the doctors and the tragedians' views of madness are predicated on the same notion that madness is a rupture with logos. The concept of self we shall find in Sophocles shares much with what we find in Hippocrates, even if the doctor bans the gods from medicine with sarcasm. Medical naturalism is one result of the Greek view of logos; the tragic understanding of madness is another. To pursue these parallelisms, let us first examine some specific Hippocratic texts before looking at the tragic view of madness in Sophocles and Euripides—and then the knowledge of madness proposed by comedy, a genre whose existence also depends upon the Greek understanding of madness.

In a key Hippocratic work such as *On Regimen,* written in the fifth century B.C., health in all senses is, as slightly later in Plato, a matter of equilibrium, of a logos maintained between diet and exercise. This balance is part of the harmony that must exist, for the sake of health, between water and fire, heat and moisture, since these are the basic components of the body. At the end of Book 1 the writer sketches out the relations between heat and moisture and the *psyche,* a term I would translate as "self," but which has also been translated as "soul" and "intelligence."[3] All these meanings accrue, though we should also bear in mind the suggestion of "breath." In this pre-Socratic text on regimen, the self is described as partly separate from the world, and as partly tied to the phenomenal world; and it appears as the manifestation of breath, hence it is part of such observable phenomena as heat and moisture.

The logic that regulates this discourse is the pre-Socratic dialectic of contraries. Opposites unite to produce effects that are not contained within the oppositions. According to *On Regimen* "wet fire" and "dry water" combine to produce the greatest intelligence in a human being. The contrary combination of these opposites results in idiocy. And madness results when fire is dominated by the water present in the soul. The dominance of water produces what sounds like classic melancholia: people cry for no reason, they fear where there is nothing to fear, and they are forever afflicted with suffering. The mad feel nothing in the same way reasonable people do.

Madness is a condition awaiting those who do not maintain the equilibrium of heat and moisture that the harmony of diet and exercise can provide. The health-conscious will manage these contraries. When moisture risks being dominated by heat, or water by fire, the endangered patient should attempt to reduce his or her weight. Our contemporary obsession with flab finds a dialectical antecedent, if not a justification, in the Hippocratic text: reducing can in effect reduce the inflammation of the blood and prevent madness. This dialectic may seem arbitrary, but it is an attempt at rationalizing causality, partly in terms of phenomena, partly in terms of semantic guides to what phenomena are about. For the Greek logos dictates what are "opposites," even if for us there is nothing intrinsic in fire that makes it "opposite" to water. Opposition seems to be a linguistic operation. But it also easy to see that, for the Greek doctor, empirical observation buttressed the semantic reasoning by pointing to a physical causal relation between, say, diet and exercise, weight and activity. We are at the beginnings of rationality, understood as the ordering relations of logos, even if the relations between world and word have not been entirely sorted out.

In *The Sacred Disease* the physician states the brain is the source of madness. This is not a localization in a modern sense, for there was no empirical reason for the Greeks to localize mental functions in the brain. (Many did not, and the heart also gets credit in other Hippocratic texts.) The brain serves to situate somatically the source of alterity that changes the mad person's relation with logos—such as can also occur in dreams. The brain is "the seat of madness and delirium, of the fears and frights which assail us often by night, but sometimes even by day."[4] In effect the brain is an inner organ within the body and a space where the dialectic of contraries works itself out. Madness results when heat dominates the brain, or cold; or when the brain is too moist or drier than it should be in order to be in a state of equilibrium: "Moistness is the cause of madness for when the brain is abnormally moist it is necessarily agitated and this agitation prevents sight or hearing being steady" (*Hippocratic Writings*, p. 249). Unfolding under the sign of plus and minus, the dialectic of opposites has a rational plausibility, for human relations with the world do involve heat and cold, dryness and moisture. The Hippocratic theory of madness thus combines observation with a dialectic of opposites that imposes itself through the power of a coherent semantic matrix.

The structure of this drama of opposites still underlies much thought about madness, for it derives its cogency as much from its dramatic appeal as from its semantic necessity. We still define madness as a loss in equilibrium, which is a definition whose cogency seems undeniable. Greek metaphors—often geometric metaphors—rarely seem out of date, for there is often a mathematical plausibility to their dynamics. From the pre-Socratic texts also emerges the theatrical view that the self must strive for equilibrium in the midst of agonistic or conflicting forces, forces that subject the self to a constant drama of hostile opponents. So we see that the theatricalization of the self is present in Greek medicine at the same time the dramatization of madness evolves on the Greek stage. And we shall see that the drama of madness is a theme that will hardly be exhausted in the course of this study: agonistic opposites can be constantly construed as theater, as dynamics, and always as the essential dilemma of the passionate self falling victim to madness.

The humors theory of madness offers another variant on this agonistic view of the self. The drama of conflicting humors presents a parallel with the agon or conflict central to tragedy, for the dramatization of the forces of madness seems imposed by the logic of conflicting contraries. Humors are agents that explain the alterity that affects both the body and the psyche. In *On Ancient Medicine* the writer says there are an indefinite number of humors that can beset the body. That is a bit daunting, and tradition preferred, as did Galen, the most famous doctor of later antiquity, the more limited doctrine found in the Hippocratic text called *The Nature of Man*. This text limits the dramatis personae to a mere four humors that are the determinants of disease and, for later medicine, of personality: phlegm, yellow and black bile, and blood. The logos of health demands an equilibrium among them, and the doctor's task is to regulate the balance. The doctrine of four humors is probably rooted in a belief in a relation between the body and the cycle of the seasons, such as the pre-Socratic thinker Empedocles had postulated.

The pre-Socratic dialectic of opposites underlies Galen's later formulation of humors theory, a formulation elaborated with an anti-Platonic twist. In anticipation of our conclusion to this chapter, I note that, according to Galen, the soul cannot easily realize the good, as Plato seemed to think, since the soul can be so easily dominated by antagonistic somatic forces, as in melancholy, phrenetis, and mania.[5] In these three clinical entities, essentially pre-Socratic oppositions came, after Galen and through Arabic translations of the Greeks, to dominate Western medical descriptions of madness with a simplicity that undoubtedly accounts for their success. In his study of the history of melancholy Stanley Johnson has given a résumé as succinct as the doctrine itself when he writes that these three traditional forms of madness were the basis for all nosological categories. Phrenitis meant delirium and fever, whereas melancholia and mania were differentiated from it by a lack of fever. Phrenitis was caused by yellow bile, melancholia by black bile.[6] The Middle Ages lived with an easier sense of the drama of madness than the Greeks; nor did they have a tragic knowledge of life.

Much of the rich analysis of the early Greeks is lost in these later simplifications, just as the agonistic complexity of the Greek tragedians was lost until the seventeenth century—when theater and medicine both underwent renewal. In spite of this loss, the pre-Socratic texts remained and perhaps remain the source of our basic concepts for dealing with mental illness, if "mental illness" is a concept we still wish to use. It is a Greek notion deriving in part from the a priori localization of mental illness in the brain. In the same move the pre-Socratic concept of "mental illness" redefined the rules for medical practice so that the rational doctor had to exclude divine intervention as a cause of madness. *The Sacred Disease* is quite clear on this point: epilepsy may have a divine source, but no more so than any other disease. Only charlatans would invoke the gods as a cause of illness. The gods can be a source of purification in some cases—which leaves room for going to the temple if one so desires. But all causation is natural. And all diseases have a cause, including a "mental illness" such as epilepsy. The gods play no role in bringing about these attacks.

The Development of Tragedy's Depiction of Madness

Tragedy depicts madness, structurally, in much the same manner as the Hippocratic texts. Madness is an alterity based on an opposition between a body and a self that tragedy could dramatize, if not explicitly name. Madness is a loss of equilibrium springing from an agonistic conflict. If the gods can bring about this loss of equilibrium, the later tragic hero often seems nonetheless constitutionally predisposed to hubris and delirium. In the development of tragedy the intervention of the gods lost much religious significance. A character's disposition became an implicit psychological category in the tragedies. And it should be pointed out that Greek literature never made the gods responsible for all madness, since comic heroes often seem to be insane because their bile has gone amuck. Critical theory has often seen this to be an important distinction between comedy and tragedy. Comic heroes are subject to natural causation in their deviance from reason and social norms, whereas the more noble genre of tragedy demands that the gods intervene to cause heroes to lose their reason. However, this convention should not obscure the fact that the tragic understanding of madness lost its religious basis in the development of tragedy from Aeschylus to Euripides.

Sophocles (ca. 496–406 B.C.) is the crucial tragedian in the portrayal of characters whose self is assailed by madness that takes the form of an exterior force. Critical opinion in the twentieth century has been remarkably unanimous in crediting Sophocles with the first literary portrayal of a self that defines itself in opposition to the madness that besieges it.[7] And nearly all concur that, in Sophocles' work, world and self are sorted out for the first time, especially in his tragedy *Ajax*. In Sophocles' work the Homeric hero undergoes the first case of individual alienation with such clear delineation that O'Brien-Moore asserts that Sophocles' sense of the limits of the self's autonomy is superior to Aristotle's: Sophocles can account for hallucination, whereas there is no room for hallucination in Aristotle's doctrine of the soul.

Yet, it appears that a god is involved in Ajax's fall into insanity. At the play's outset the goddess Athena speaks with Ulysses, and the spectators learn that Ulysses won out over Ajax in a dispute about who would acquire Achilles' arms. Ajax has become furious, and in his fury he has slaughtered flocks and herds of animals, believing them to be Greeks. He goes so far as to bring a ram to his tent where, believing the animal to be Ulysses, he vents his fury upon it. Thus, before the play's beginning, Ajax has already raged through a series of hallucinations that have produced a most mortifying series of absurd actions. The play's dramatic action begins then with Athena's tale that she has plunged Ajax into madness so that his fury would be directed against animals, and not the Greeks. She has directly intervened to change Ajax's consciousness. But there is something of an overdetermination to the hero's insanity. For the Greek spectator knew that Ajax's well-known hubris or raging pride—his break with logos—existed before the goddess's intervention. Ajax has a disposition, so to speak, a potential for madness, that is part of his character.

Fate is also responsible for Ajax's madness, for his insanity was inscribed in his destiny and was the object of prophecy. The intervention of the goddess Athena is the immediate cause of his going insane. In modern terms we might speak of a disposition that is actualized through some immediate determination—which should make us aware of the essentially dramatic nature of a causal schema that explains an effect as the actualization of a potentiality. Etiology is often a dramatic device that works by ordering, retrospectively, a chain of events that must be because they are. For Ajax "etiology" works retrospectively from the present, for in the present moment of the drama Ajax's self reflects back upon his mad self. The drama that his madness works is created as it is recalled, which is to say that it exists when the self seizes its own drama through narration and measures the deviance from logos that the narration tells. The limits of self are traced out, in language, in the shape of a boundary that has been transgressed. The drama begins only once the character has returned to reason and can use logos. In brief, by telling the tale in retrospective, Sophocles endows the narration with a sense of causal necessity, since the progression of simple chronology makes a series of events appear inevitable.

Ajax had earlier refused Athena's help. He insulted her, claiming that he had no need of the aid that lesser mortals might desire from her. Ajax's refusal of the divine is also a form of madness, for his refusal signifies a break with rationality. It destroys the equilibrium obtained by humanity's position between fate and the gods. In his insult Ajax spoke what the chorus, in John Moore's translation, calls words that "kept no human measure."[8] Before his hallucination then, Ajax was outside the human world of shared logos and was, moreover, guilty of desiring a break with logos. Yet his madness is involuntary, and his fate is cast such that it can be foretold by the prophet Calchas, who correctly foresaw Ajax's death at his own hand. Much like Oedipus, Ajax is guilty and innocent at the same time, guilty by the judgment of objective logos, innocent when viewed as a victim of fate.

In *Ajax* Sophocles prefigures our ambiguities about the etiology of madness and deviant behavior. We see in the play the emergence of such notions as personality defect, the role of voluntary choice, and a will to madness, as well as the belief that madness is due to an involuntary determinism due to extrapsychic forces. These determinations are all bound together in the narrative strands that interact to describe a "self," an ego, or, alternatively, a case history existing as a narrative. Central to the play's portrayal of self are the contradictions that are lived as part of madness. Reflecting upon his story, and thus upon his self as reflected in language, Ajax feels at once that some alterity has imposed madness upon him and that he is guilty of some fault. Ajax's wife Tecmessa describes his present anguish:

> Ajax, as long as his mad fit was on him,
> Himself felt joy at all his wretchedness,
> Though we, his sane companions, grieved indeed.
> But now that he's recovered and breathes clear,
> His own anguish totally masters him.
>
> (P. 20, ll. 271–75)

With the medical metaphor of clear breath she describes the hero's capacity to look upon himself, a self transparent to itself, and see the revelation of his madness. But anguish masters him as another form of alienation. This malady, the alienation of anguish, can be remedied with the sword, for, as the play twice states, the sword allows quick surgery. This medical metaphor shows that medical thought has become part of the workings of tragedy. The sword of suicide offers a remedy by excising madness like a foreign body. In suicide the resolute Ajax is his own physician who "quavers no incantations / when the malady he's treating needs the knife" (p. 32, ll. 581–82).

Nietzsche considered Sophocles' plays dealing with Oedipus to be the summit of tragic expression because in them the undifferentiated absurdity of existence comes to light. In the dissolution of all contraries, the madness of existence itself could speak. Nietzsche's interpretation underscores the commonality between Sophocles' work and the medical texts deriving from the pre-Socratics. Both use a dialectic of contraries to represent or dramatize madness. In the Hippocratic texts the dissolution of opposite forces leads to a dominance that produces madness. For the tragedian, the tension between pride and submission, hubris and reason, leads to a comparable dialectic. Tragedy enacts a madness in which there is a rupture with logos through which the hero is plunged into dementia. The direct causal agent for Ajax's madness is, to be sure, the goddess. Athena's intervention may appear to oppose the naturalism of Hippocratic medicine. Strictly speaking, this is true, and I should not wish to dismiss the conflict arising between religion and science at this early moment in our history. But it is also true that in structural terms the god or goddess is a visible emblem for some exterior agent or force that the self experiences as other than itself—what medicine named air or heat or black bile. And it is this structural determination of alterity that is fundamental for our scientific as well as the tragic experience of madness.

The Greek writers wanted to find an image of self and its seemingly autonomous self-empowerment that is commensurate with the destruction of self that madness works. The last great tragedian, Euripides (480–406 B.C.), confronted this problem after the elaboration of most of the Hippocratic texts. All of his work was probably written after *Ajax,* which is to say that Euripides came at a time when Sophocles' religious beliefs were less universally accepted. Euripides himself seems hardly to have believed in the gods' intervention in human affairs. However, he used the agency of divine intervention in the depiction of a number of cases of madness. For example, Phaedra, the scorned queen, goes insane with a semi-incestuous passion for

Hippolytus. Aphrodite is made the scapegoat for this crazed lust. Rationalistic critics are inclined to see in Euripides' evocation of the god a dramatization of what we call today the exteriorization or the projection of psychological forces or instincts. I think, however, that this modern reading is more a projection of our own psychological metaphors onto the problem Euripides was confronting: how could he depict a mad self that was consonant with the naturalism of Hippocratic medicine while respecting tragic conventions.

I would suggest Euripides thought something along the following lines. To name a god is to name something that is other than the psyche. This naming dramatizes madness as otherness; it makes intelligible the alterity of madness while respecting theatrical and religious conventions. Once an exterior agency is set over and against rational self-consciousness, the dialectic of contraries sets up a conflict in which consciousness, in opposition to some alterity, risks losing its logos or relation to the world. Now let us consider the embodiment of this dialectic in Euripides' *Heracles,* a case study of alterity. In Euripides' version of the legend, Heracles finishes his labors and returns from the underworld just in time to save his family from the murderous villain Lycus, who has just usurped the throne of Thebes by killing Creon, the father of Heracles' wife Megara. Euripides is often credited with the invention of melodrama, and it must be said that the first part of the play unfolds much like a Western movie in which the terrorized family awaits the improbable return of a John Wayne to rescue them. But he arrives at the last moment, and the villain gets his deserts: the usurper is slain.

After this justified murder of the tyrant Lycus, the goddess Hera intervenes in the action. (Zeus conceived Heracles with Amphitryon's wife Alcmene, which accounts for Hera's enmity against Heracles.) In anger Euripides' Hera sends Lyssa or Madness to strike down Heracles at the moment of his greatest triumph. Heracles suddenly goes mad: acting more like a hero of tabloid journalism than a legend, he slaughters his own family. Upon recovering his sanity, Heracles reacts likes Ajax and wants to expiate his guilt through suicide. But Theseus—whom Heracles has freed from Hades—arrives to argue that Heracles must accept his fate. In Theseus's words, as William Arrowsmith renders them, Euripides presents an argument about the gods and fate that is different from what is found in Sophocles:

No other god is implicated here,
except the wife of Zeus. Rightly you judge.

> My advice is this: be patient, suffer
> what you must, and do not yield to grief.

Theseus goes on to argue, moreover, that the gods are no different from men:

> Fate exempts no man; all men are flawed,
> and so the gods, unless the poets lie.[9]

Sophocles would not have accepted this point of view that makes men the equal of gods in their debauchery and predestined misfortune. But Heracles accepts it, for he is not even certain as to who his father Zeus is. Not only does Heracles avoid Ajax's paradoxical bind that makes him at once a innocent victim of exterior forces and guilty of insanity, he can even exonerate the gods by proposing a rationalistic justification of madness that shows that Euripides shared some of the views of the writers of *The Sacred Disease*. Heracles, in his decision to "prevail against death," offers a theodicy that lifts guilt from the gods' shoulders:

> I do not believe the gods commit
> adultery, or bind each other in chains.
> I never did believe it; I never shall;
> nor that one god is tyrant of the rest.
> If god is truly god, he is perfect,
> lacking nothing. These are poet's wretched lies.
>
> (P. 360, ll. 1340–46)

The play ends denouncing the fictions of poets, which, written by a poet, may sound like self-denunciation. These words suggest a critique of the poets' use of the gods as convenient fictions for something that should be named in other terms. Hera's intervention is thus not to be taken seriously? Is she to be taken as an image of what cannot be named? In any case, the goddess's intervention hardly seems to symbolize any modern psychological process. She enacts one part of a dialectic of contraries. And Hera points this out herself when she says that Heracles' triumphs menace the equilibrium between heaven and earth, the gods and men. According to the goddess, in the person of Heracles, a mortal came close to possessing the qualities of a god. And this is a fundamental threat to the equilibrium of contraries that sustains logos, and the world.

Euripides' view of madness is thus at least partly grounded in a pre-Socratic conceptual grid. By psychologizing Euripides' works in allegorical terms derived from our own metaphysical entities—our instincts or drives for example—we lose the sense of dialectics that characterizes the knowledge of madness that the Greeks had. This knowledge is perhaps most developed in what is probably Euripides' last extant play, *The Bacchae*. We should study this last work to see that the sense of logos as dialectical equilibrium continued to underwrite insanity on the Greek stage until its final great moment. Moreover, this tragedy brings to the forefront the social dimension of madness that will be a leitmotif in our history of discourses on madness. In *The Bacchae* madness becomes epidemic and menaces social order. The disequilibrium of the body becomes the source of a rupture with logos within the body politic.

The play consists of an action that pits mad characters against one another, characters whose fault has been to scorn the delirious wine-god Dionysus. Agave, the queen of Thebes, is turned into a furious bacchante for having denied the divine origin of Dionysus. Dionysus will brook no rejection from the women of Thebes, as he explains in his opening speech:

> This is the reason
> I goaded these women into frenzy,
> Drove them raving from their palace
> To the mount'n, their wits unhinged. . . .
> And I have stung all the women of this town
> Manic, to follow Kadmus's daughters.[10]

But women are not alone in this madness. Pentheus, Agave's son, refuses to honor the god. For this, he is accused of insanity by Tiresias, the prophet, who is quite willing to give himself over to the ecstasy that plunges all into mania—since this mania comes from a god. Tiresias and Pentheus confront each other and exchange mutual accusations of insanity. In this agon they embody the dialectic in which each side claims reason, though reason for one is madness for the other.

From one perspective, Pentheus is guilty of hubris, since in his scorn for the "girl faced" god he is guilty of the pride that leads to a break in logos. But from the opposing perspective—one that Euripides clearly suggests—there is no harmony or just measure in Pentheus's fate. Dionysus tricks Pentheus into observing the bacchantes in their revels, and, when they discover him, the women tear him into shreds. Agave kills her own son while under the delusion she is destroying a beast. There is perhaps no more powerful description of the break with logos produced by manic rage than the description of this murder:

> She fell on him.
> And he, tearing off the wig,
> So that she could recognize and spare him,
> Kept mumbling, trying to caress her cheek:
> "It's me, Mother, it's Pentheus, Mother your son
> Remember Echion, remember the palace
> Where I was born, it's me, don't kill me
> Mother, it's me your boy, I've not been good
> But don't kill me yet not your own boy."
> But she was foaming at the mouth, her eye
> Upturned, showed white, wandering wildly
> Like her wits—she was possessed by her god
> And words meant nothing.
>
> (P. 209, ll. 1115–29)

The reference to words shows that language is staked out here as the boundary of the rational self; and that shared logos is the form of equilibrium that sanity takes. Euripides gives us in this late play the most exacting image of the fall from language, from logos in all its senses, into an otherness he can only represent through a god—or an animal. Both are an emblem of non-human otherness in the classical Greek world.

This otherness is centered on a curious god, for he is split between his theatrical presence and a self that seems to be elsewhere. He addresses himself as if he were both present and absent, as when he calls up the god—himself—to drive Pentheus mad:

> Dionysus,
> —And you are not far from here—
> Now
>
> Demand your retribution.
> First, drive him
> Out of his mind into ecstatic madness.
> While he's sane he'll never accept
> To dress in women's clothes. But once
> Outside the pale of reason, he will.
>
> (P. 199, ll. 847–53)

The alienation of the sacred is offered by this image of a god who acts out on the stage the embodiment of an otherness that lies beyond what can be represented. And from the viewpoint of the Greek man of reason, Pentheus, the eruption of this otherness causes a corruption of the social order that can be compared to an illness. The comparison of social disorder, madness, and disease establishes analogies between the interruption of the harmony of logos and the destruction of equilibrium, be it of the body politic, be it of the material body that needs the harmony of humors for its health. This web of metaphors sets out the modes of representation that underpin our determinations of reason and unreason, logic and illogic, legality and exclusion. Madness in the individual body is transferred by metaphor to the social body as a whole. The body's disorder becomes the image of the social body whose existence had been taken for granted as long as the working of logos was unquestioned.

With regard to the threat to social order, the destruction of the son by the mother presents an inverted analogy with Sophocles' *Oedipus*. Killing one's son is the deviant converse of sleeping with one's mother. Both forms of deviance threaten the state or the "body politic" with disease, the latter taking the form of the plague that invests Thebes because Oedipus is in power. The threat of madness and deviance has profoundly social ramifications for the Greeks. The notion of "disease of the state" has its origin here in the Greek concept of relations among bodies that must exist in some homeostatic harmony if they are to function in accord with their logos. This medical metaphor undoubtedly has it origins in pre-Socratic thought, since the tragedians' vision that the disequilibrium of madness is an affliction of the state reflects the doctors' view that, for the body to be healthy, there must be a balancing of the mixture of qualities—or else the body falls into sickness. The analogy of body and state probably most directly derives in fact from the doctrines of the pre-Socratic physician Alcmeon. He taught that without *crasis*, or the equilibrium among the indefinite number of qualities that are in the body, sickness results through the dominance of one quality—or what Alcmeon called *monarchia*, the monomaniacal as well as the monarchal. Health is *isonomia*, or the equality of rights of bodily qualities as well as of those citizens who compose a democracy.[11] And so when Shakespeare proclaimed that something was rotten in Denmark, he was continuing a long line of medical analysis that makes the individual's insanity a source of social disorder.

Once we grasp the importance of this notion of harmony and equilibrium that is part of logos, we can also see that it works mainly as a regulative concept with which to talk about the real. But that harmony was never taken to be the real, as a neoclassical aesthetician like Winkelmann, in the eighteenth century, wanted to believe in his idealization of the Greeks. One need not be Nietzsche to see that *The Bacchae* is hardly illustrative of harmony: the play demonstrates the invasion of madness into all realms of existence and the destruction of logos. Nietzsche's criticism of Winkelmann's belief that all was harmony in Greek art needs to be completed by the insight that logos was a regulative concept describing health and sanity. The Greeks were quite aware that the contrary of harmony—madness—was always poised ready to bring about the destruction of the *isonomia* of forces that define rational equilibrium. *The Bacchae* would also suggest that, in the male-dominated culture of classical Athens, a major threat to logos came from women who might break the bonds of their relation—their logos—to the political state. From this perspective Pentheus's savage death is a representation of how the disequilibrium that destroys societal bonds also destroys the individual; in this case the male principle is destroyed by feminine forces of disorder. It does not seem hyperbolic to say that this tragedy marks the origins of a long tradition portraying the threat of feminine madness and its power to disrupt patriarchal order.

In résumé, then, the disruption of equilibrium by an exterior invader, by the god from the east, is produced by an alterity that destroys the harmony of social force; it is as much a political as a medical event. Madness was not separated out from a political threat, for any destruction of logos is a potential destruction of the foundations of the polis. Plato's *Republic* can be viewed in this respect as an utopian construct that guarantees the mutual solidarity of the city and rationality—polis and logos intertwined—by producing sanity in the souls of all its citizens. I shall deal with Plato presently, but in this context it is important to note that his views concerning the relation of the individual to the polis develop what we find in Euripides or the pre-Socratics: Platonic justice is the equilibrium of all parts existing in dialectical harmony. It is, in short, a condition of health in the soul. And to conclude this consideration of tragedy, I note that later Freudian beliefs in the superego seem to continue a tradition in which the individual self is the repository of the culture's logos. I leave it to the reader to decide if the god from the east acquires different names in our history and if the id—that Latinized alterity that lurks within—is not an avatar of the Dionysian reveler who would overthrow logos in the celebration of the dissolution of order. The repressive superego that Freud described would then be the latest incarnation of Plato's philosopher king.

Madness and the Nature of Comedy

The staging of madness in the Greek world was not limited to tragic enactment. I want to argue that madness is, if anything, more central to comedy than to tragedy. My deepest intuition, based on a fondly nourished experience of comedy ranging from Aristophanes through Harpo Marx, is that comedy is the genre that takes madness in hand and momentarily socializes it. Comedy exhibits madness within the confines of an aesthetic structure—on a stage, a screen, or within a book—and thus brings it into the purview of logos. Tragedy demands an ultimate exclusion of deviance, usually in the form of destruction. But in comedy laughter is part of our accommodation to the insane, by the curious mechanism that allows us to take pleasure in madness at a distance. This is not to say we really accept madness, since comedy demands that we observe deviance at a safe distance. But through comedy madness acquires something like a social role. In comedy the individual's madness is defined by the individual's deviance from social norms, norms that reveal the individual's idiosyncratic psychopathologies. And these norms are norms that we usually accept. Comedy's dialectic between norm and deviance shows two sides of the same coin bearing the stamp of the logos. This logos defines what should be the proper dialectical relation of the individual to the whole—a whole we must grasp and accept in order to be sensitive to the comic deviance of the nutty hero.

The dialectic of comedy has had a more continuous history than tragedy, and I should make a few remarks on this history before examining Greek comedy in detail. For my historical considerations are dependent upon the theory of comedy that I derive from this history. Comedy begins of course in Athens with the "Old Comedy," of which remain the eleven works by Aristophanes (448–380 B.C.) that survived the collapse of the Greco-Roman world. From a slightly later date we possess today one play and a number of fragments of works by Menander (342–292 B.C.), the most important Greek writer of "New Comedy." Medieval literature evolved a number of comic genres, largely independent of Greco-Roman models. However, during the Renaissance renewal of theater, writers by and large dismissed medieval models and returned to the classical models. To be sure, our Renaissance forebears largely imitated the Roman imitators of Greek comedy, Plautus and Terence. In this way the models of the comic have persisted from the Greeks until the present, right into Hollywood, all relying upon a mad deviance from logos that was originally defined by the Greeks. The continuity of the comic tradition is great, even where we often do not suspect it, because the Greek views of logos have lasted, again where we are hardly aware of it. The continuity of the Greek view of rationality means that even medieval farces are often not far from Aristophanes, and the film viewer today can recognize in the satire, farce, and romantic comedy of the movies direct antecedents in Aristophanes, Menander, and their Latin imitators. "Crazy comedy" is a staple of our culture, allowing us to accommodate ourselves to those forms of madness that place in question our social rituals and bonds. From this tradition I would conclude that our continuing need for comic laughter witnesses to our ambivalent desire for participation in and release from deviance, perversion, and madness.

Critics and theorists have interpreted the relationship of madness and comedy in various ways. The most systematic were the Renaissance writers who made the medical doctrine of humors into a theory of comedy. They found warrant for this theory in Greek, but mainly Latin, comedy written under the influence of Menander, whom the Renaissance knew only by report. The Renaissance generalized the view that the comic hero is deviant because his or, more rarely, her bile is running amuck. This is an approximate view of comedy as far as the Greeks are concerned, for no Greek writer can be cited whose work is dominated by humors theory. There are homologies between humors theory and comedy, but, unlike the Renaissance, antiquity did not see the comic hero simply as a madman "in his humor." But after the revival of Greek medicine during the Renaissance it seems almost inevitable that humors should become the basis for a theory of comedy. Or as the seventeenth-century playwright Ben Jonson put it in *Every Man in His Humor,* a humor is not a rare thing: "it is a gentleman-like monster, bred in the special gallantry of our time, by affectation, and fed by folly" (3.4). Humors cause folly, and folly feeds humors, and thus comic characters are locked into their madness by a feedback system that forever excludes their coming to reason.

Before Aristophanes, comedy apparently had its origins in ritual. During Aristophanes' life in the fifth century, comedy as theater became institutionalized in the life of the city-state. Comedies were performed at the festivals and were awarded prizes, like the tragedies. This institutionalization of comedy and tragedy takes place, then, at the moment of the birth of rationality in Greece, in the works of the pre-Socratic thinkers and the first medical writings of the Hippocratic corpus. I would propose that comedy, like tragedy, is part of the elaboration of ways of generating and codifying knowledge, in this case, the knowledge of the individual's relations to society and what the perturbation of those relations can entail—and perhaps a remedy thereof.

The institutionalization of comedy means that there was a social matrix in which Aristophanes' work was created and performed. To understand comedy one must consider the social context in which the genre was invented, since it is in that context that one can understand what was the function of the comic. What constitutes the comic is a larger question than what constitutes the literary genre called comedy, but the two questions overlap. In our context the salient fact to consider is that, in the fifth century, Athens gave birth to a literary genre that, analogous to the Hippocratic texts, focuses on the body and its imbalances and the ensuing lack of harmony between the individual and the societal body. The literary genre called comedy thus established the rules for developing the comic: the comic unfolds in a public space as the dialectical relationship between the norms for sanity and the deviant self of the comic character on stage. As a theatrical genre Greek comedy allows madness and deviance to occupy a societal space—the stage—to which the presence of spectators is essential. They *are* the societal body who embodies the norm from which the comic character deviates. (Relevantly, laughter without an audience is difficult.) The mad individual and society are mutually bound up in desiring the break in logos that the play enacts, for the break gives us pleasure even as we reprove it. Or, as Harpo Marx might have said if he were granted the use of logos, deviance is the rule of the game that comedy lets us play with impunity. The audience's laughter may be taken as a measure of pleasurable participation in, and recognition of, deviance that they could never countenance in reality. Worked out dialectically, deviance thus pays homage to the norm by destroying it. And in this dialectical play, we see, as Groucho could well have said, that the pre-Socratic dialectic of opposites is as much a guide to understanding the origins of comedy as the origins of tragedy.

A dubious reader, considering the comic to be a universal part of human culture, may well ask if I have not overestimated the importance of the Athenian context for comedy: after all, people laugh the world over. To which the reply is that all human infants are born with a capacity for laughter—hence a capacity for perceiving deviance and the comic, and for entertaining a participatory relationship with madness and insane aggression. Laughter manifests itself in the cradle, though I do not think the baby laughing at daddy's antics is performing the same act as the adult laughing at, say, Aristophanes' putting Socrates in a basket in the clouds. Neonatal laughter, like the inarticulate sounds of the same baby, shows that the human child has the innate capacity for laughter, just as the human child has the innate capacity for speech. The two capacities are interrelated. It is clear that not all adults have the same capacity for laughter, or for entering into the comic, any more than all have the same capacity for acquiring the skills necessary for playing different language games. (Try to explain why Groucho is funny if someone doesn't see it.) It seems fair to observe that the human child acquires skills in perception of the comic much like the child acquires skills in language use. Human beings must master the rules for the forms of the comic, much as they must master the rules for the multiple language games that go to make up human language. The more capacious is a learner's grasp, the more the learner will be able to enter into new realms of experience, into ever vaster areas revealed by language, including that realm of inverted logos that the comic proposes.

The rules for the comic are grounded in a societal context. I have no doubt that all cultures have produced forms of the comic, though this is an empirical question that is beyond the scope of my study. It is perhaps true that one can conceive that not all forms of the comic need be based on a perception of the deviant. But this has largely been the case in Western culture: our ideas about the comic are tied up with our notions of the rational, the conventional, the expected and with rules for their transgression. All grammars are social and historical in nature, and Western comic genres are a codification of discourses that begin for us with the Greeks. Beginning with Aristophanes, comedies are complex language games—including gestural language and visual signs—that allow us to approach and yet distance ourselves from the break with logos that comedy's madness enacts. A break with logos is a fundamental rule of the game—and by codifying the break, comedy works to make the irrational intelligible. Like a medical diagnosis, comedy proposes a reading of the irrational in the societal body.

In its dramatic specifics, then, Aristophanes' work is the inaugural work codifying comic forms for our culture. Cedric H. Whitman offers a concise résumé of the general structure of the plays when he notes, with relevant reservations, that the Aristophanic comedy always has a general shape, "to wit: an old countryman, faced with a dilemma, conceives an idea, and goes off on a quest in order to achieve it; he is opposed by the chorus (usually), and there follows the agon, in which he is successful, whereupon he sets up a whole new regime; then, after the parabasis, various 'impostors' enter, and try to share in the benefits of the new scheme, but are beaten off by the hero, who concludes the play with a celebration, usually a marriage (gamos)."[12] This description stresses the formal structural properties of old comedy, which depend on the conflict or agon between opposing forces. But, unlike the usual case of tragic conflict, in comedy the opposing forces are equally mad, for both the hero and his opponents are usually guilty of insane deviance.

A wonderful image of this double deviance from logos is presented by the example of a soaring Socrates in *The Clouds*. When the old man Strepsiades comes to Socrates' "thinkery" in order to learn the art of reasoning, he finds Socrates suspended in the clouds. Strepsiades wants to learn to think, which is to say, gain sufficient skill in the new art of sophistry so that he will be able to defraud his creditors. Several centuries of idolatry of Socrates probably make it difficult for a modern audience to consider the thinker Socrates to be as crazy as the deviant old man Strepsiades (Socrates' having been condemned to drink hemlock should remind us that not all his fellow Athenians were as convinced of Socrates' virtue as Plato was). But both Strepsiades and Socrates are mad: the double deviance is found in the way each character is characterized as breaking with the regulative concept of equilibrium and logos. In terms of polarities Socrates is drawn toward the sky, whereas the old miser is all too representative of the instincts of the netherworld. The conflict between the addle-brained thinker and the old scoundrel sets deviance in relief until their conflict leads to the elimination of one character, the levitating Socrates in this case, leaving Strepsiades victorious in his craziness.

Aristophanes does not end *The Clouds* with a resolution that suggests the triumph of reason, such as we find in the seventeenth-century comedies of Molière. In Molière's work the final marriage marks the victory of natural reason over an insane old father who has usually used his young daughter in an attempt to promote a dominant obsession. This is not to say that Molière's fathers recognize their madness, only that in the end they are defeated by the forces of reason. In contrast, Aristophanes allows insanity to pursue its course even after his victorious old dodger has recognized that he is mad. At the play's end, in Benjamin Bickley Rogers's version, Strepsiades proclaims:

> O! fool, fool, fool, how mad I must have been
> To cast away the gods, for Socrates.
> Yet Hermes, gracious Hermes, be not angry
> Nor crush me utterly, but look with mercy
> On faults to which his idle talk hath led me.
> And lend thy counsel; tell me, had I better
> Plague them with lawsuits, or how else annoy them.
> [*Affects to listen*]
> Good: your advice is good: I'll have no lawsuits
> I'll go at once and set their house on fire.[13]

This is no triumph of logos, even if for a moment madness seems to be lucid about itself. In the dialectic of opposites one force replaces another: Strepsiades gives up on Socrates' madness and sets out to pursue his own form of insanity. At the end of the play Strepsiades commits an insane act of aggression by setting fire to Socrates' house. It all ends in flames—the light of reason inverted in a final comic illumination of madness.

Aristophanes' dialectic of double deviance characterizes most of his plays. In the first extant play, *The Acharnians,* the conflict between individual and polis is enacted in the crazy old Dicaeopolis's opposition to Athens's demented warmongering. Opposition to war is not of course insane—unless your country declares it so. But Dicaeopolis is insane in pursuing the project of negotiating an individual peace treaty between himself and the enemy. Or at least the chorus judges his negotiating to be insane and tries to stone the old fellow—a practice that Bennett Simon says was reserved for the mad in ancient Greece.[14] In the convoluted dialectics here of reasonable madness and mad rationality—for Athens, like more contemporary democracies, could also rationalize an insane war—Dicaeopolis wins out over Athenian imperialism. The play's conclusion vindicates his insanity: Dicaeopolis is prospering for his troubles, and with a fine young whore to enjoy. This triumph is not a resolution that later moralizing eras could easily abide, but the play's end underscores that Aristophanes allows insane desire to enjoy victory.

The triumph of madness is rather consistent throughout Aristophanes, as one sees at the end of *The Wasps,* a slightly later play. The play's elderly father Philocleon is first locked up by his son to keep him from indulging in the insane Athenian obsession with spending all day in court at trials, a passion that paid a few obols to its citizens. The father is obsessed, but in this case his obsession coincides with, rather than opposes, a public dementia. The son seems briefly to make his father accede to reason: the father agrees to stay home, though he is allowed to stage a trial and judge his dog for a theft of cheese. But the father adjusts all too well to the rational standards his son proposes. The father becomes an aggressive party-man, drinking, cavorting about with a pretty young flutist, committing farcical assaults on all who come near, and ends with an outburst of dancing. Perhaps only the *The Birds* ends in greater triumph: logos and the gods are overthrown, not just by men, but also by the combined dancing cohorts of the entire order of *aves* in the victory of the birds over the gods. This is madness at its most celebratory.

In its most concentrated and emblematic form insanity's victory is expressed in dance. Dance is mime, which is to say, it is madness in the service of the deviant body in motion. Dance, parodistic in *The Wasps,* centers on a body that parodies the gestures of body language. In this comedy, dance seems to correspond to the role of the destruction of the body enacted at the conclusion of a tragedy—as when Ajax commits self-destruction out of shame or Oedipus puts out his eyes in penitence for the involuntary act of seeing the truth. By contrast, in comedy's triumph, dance is a controlled alterity, a madness mastered through form, though madness nonetheless.

The dancing body overthrows logos, yet remains in harmony, which is the essential paradox of comedy. Dance enacts the control over madness that we desire even as we desire the destruction of the norms that comic madness effects. For the essential revelation of comedy is a desire for madness within all of us.

Comedy after Aristophanes

Aristophanes' work frequently alludes to humors, though humors are not cited as the direct cause of the various insanities the characters manifest. The most famous writer of New Comedy, Menander, seems to have worked out the logic of madness with some reliance on the humors theory, and for his role as a largely unknown precursor, determining the history of literature largely without having been read, Menander should be considered here. His use of humors theory is evident in his earliest extant play, *The Bad-Tempered Man,* the complete text of which came to light merely a few years ago. The play's Greek title, *Dyskolos,* the peevish or discontented man, points to a monolithic determination of comic imbalance by some bodily determinant, such as black bile. Menander's work inaugurates another development of comedy, quite a major one to be sure. The obsessive father in this play wants to stymie the course of nature by thwarting the natural attraction of a young woman for a rich young man. This formula, involving a monomaniacal old man and his beautiful daughter, is so familiar that we may not see its reliance upon the original matrix of comedy: the father's singular desire opposes the dictates of universal logos. The old father embodies madness as he pursues his desire in the recurrent comic dialectic of contraries that smashes the harmony of logos and reason. Menander's comedy develops this dialectic, though by attenuating the strident conflict of Aristophanes' plays. At the end of *The Bad-Tempered Man* we find the father dancing, as marriages are arranged between the worthy young people; but this dance seems to have a different significance from the dances at the end of Aristophanes' plays. In Menander's work the father is tamed, or at least brought to reason, by exterior necessity; he is not victorious in his madness. The dance marks the victory of reason over a joyous anarchy that would overturn logos—which is to say that Menander is not very funny. In this sense New Comedy presages a development of the theatrical genre of comedy in which the comic often ends up defeated.

Menander's dialectic of contraries becomes a formula for romantic comedy. In this type of comedy what seems irrational, crazy, or destructive finally reveals itself, through an ironic reversal, to be a form of benevolent fate. Menander's *The Unkindest Cut* begins with an insane act of jealousy: the young man cuts off the young girl's hair. But this act of aggression begins a plot that leads to the discovery of who is whose father and brings about a happy marriage and general prosperity. We are close to Hollywood formulas when, at the play's conclusion, the heroine pithily gives a résumé of it all by saying to her beloved that his going crazy was the beginning of their happiness. Dialectical opposition has been reduced to an ironic twist, and madness largely reduced to a threat that hovers over the operations of reason.

Later Greco-Roman Philosophical Views of Madness and Christian Developments

In addition to the medical and theatrical discourses we have discussed, there is a third type of discourse that antiquity used to speak about madness. This is the philosophical discourse that wanted to find the origins of madness within a self that could not master itself. In the Hippocratic texts and in theater, madness is a relation, a rupture in the equilibrium that logos should encompass. But in the moralizing discourses of later antiquity madness becomes a condition lodged within the self. Our view of the centered self, of the self capable of knowing and perhaps curing itself, has its roots in these developments in antiquity. Plato is central to this tradition, for he used the pre-Socratic dialectic of contraries to describe the equilibrium of the healthy soul and, by contrast, the disequilibrium of the diseased psyche. Self-knowledge becomes in Plato the prescription for the healthy self, which for Plato means both the ethical and the sane self. For example, in *The Republic* ethics is a question of mental health—which is to say, it is an equilibrium of parts that all desire the Good if they know what it is. By way of contrast, Plato celebrates madness, or at least delirium, in *Phaedra,* provided that this delirium is sent by the gods and is not a product of bodily disease. All of this is an elaboration of the Greek views discussed thus far, for Plato's views of mental health are largely a development of the pre-Socratic medical dialectics, though with an interesting twist. In *The Republic* Plato defends the view that the soul cannot voluntarily elect evil choices. Ignorance becomes in Plato's work a determinant of mental disease.

Historically speaking, however, Plato's most influential medical doctrine is found in the *Timaeus,* the only Platonic dialogue that the European Middle Ages directly knew, though this in Latin translation. This work's medical views are largely consonant with the Hippocratic corpus. In it Plato states that folly is a disorder of the soul. There are two types: madness and stupidity (*mania* and *amathia*). These disorders can be brought on by excessive pleasures and pains. In this dialogue Plato confronts the belief that, when the soul is made sick, the person afflicted is deliberately bad. Plato again denies that intention is involved, claiming that "no one is willingly bad" (86d). This refusal of evil intentionality is consistently the central axiom of Platonic ethical thought. The Platonic interpretation of madness thus begins with the view that madness is a privative notion. This view is close to the Hippocratic doctrine that disorders of the soul are caused, involuntarily, by an exterior agency, or to quote Cornford's version of the *Timaeus* (86e),

> where pains are concerned, the soul likewise derives much badness from the body. When acid and salt, phlegm or bitter bilious humours roam about the body and, finding no outlet, are pent up within and fall into confusion by blending the vapor that rises from them with the motion of the soul, they induce all manner of disorders of the soul of greater or less intensity and extent. Making their way to the three seats of the soul, according to the region they severally invade, they beget many diverse types of ill-temper and despondency, of rashness and cowardice, of dullness and oblivion.[15]

In this summary of Platonic views of disease and madness, we find a classic statement on the involuntary nature of mental disease.

If we turn to later Roman thought, developed in the centuries after Athens ceased to be the center for the development of Western thought, we find a view of madness almost diametrically opposed to Plato. Most influential historically are Roman Stoic views, now concerned with the *anima* rather than the *psyche*. In contrast to Platonic thought, these Stoic views throw the mad back onto themselves for their responsibility for the conditions of their diseased inner self. Cicero is the central figure to this development. Today Cicero is the prototype of the Roman republican moralist, but for much of our history, at least through the eighteenth century, he also had the authority of a medical thinker, especially for the doctrine of insanity elaborated in *The Tusculan Disputations*. It is of course true that, for much of our history, it is not entirely meaningful to separate medical and philosophical discourse. For the case in point, the literary historian Ernst Robert Curtius tells us that the *Tusculanae* became part of the medical curriculum in the twelfth century.[16] This introduction of Cicero into the curriculum was part of the renewal of medical studies in the Middle Ages in the newly established universities. From the twelfth century through the Enlightenment, Cicero was as important as Plato and Hippocrates for moralistic and legislative attitudes toward madness. And Cicero is certainly the most representative thinker of the Stoic voluntarism that furnished Christianity with much of its moral attitudinizing—as well as its fear of the mad. In Cicero's work the moral subject is enjoined to take itself as the object of its own solicitude. The basic moral relationship thus consists of the subject's relation to itself. In effect the soul must seek to cure itself of its own afflictions.

To this end Cicero proposes a medicine for the soul that is different from the medicine that aims at curing the body. Few are capable of being their own physicians, and so it seems that only the elect—the Stoic elite as it were—can escape insanity. Only the sage can maintain the proper relation to *ratio* and *oratio*—reason and speech—or the logos that is the basis for social life. To escape madness, then, one is enjoined to master oneself. This imperative contains within it the circularity of all voluntarism: in order not to be insane, one must not be insane. For Cicero this means mastering all passions. Otherwise, again by definition, the mad person is not a sage; the insane person is insane, or at least suffering to some degree the insanity that entertaining a passion entails. This view of passion is an all-encompassing doctrine. When asked if any movement of the soul is a form of insanity— "Quid? tibi omnisne amini commotio videtur insania?"—Cicero answers, logically enough from his perspective, "yes" (3.4.7).[17] Before Freud, and, more importantly, before the church fathers, Cicero makes of the human species the sick-souled animal for whom it appears that there is little chance of a cure. By definition to have a passion—to be human—is to be insane.

Cicero was rewritten for the Church by Ambrose, then by countless others. Ciceronian views of madness provided rational grounds for the Christian view that we are born into sin, hence the idea that we alienated from logos at birth. Original sin means that our passions always destroy our relationship to logos, but with a difference. With help from Plato and especially Plotinus, logos was transformed by Christian theologians who identified the concept of reason emanating from the godhead with the Judaic God. From this perspective, the perspective of the Fall, to be born into sin, which is simply to be born, is to be born into madness, folly, and depravation. Alienation from logos becomes the central drama of Christianity, and madness a central metaphor for our existential plight.

There were of course reactions against this Christian Stoic view that makes us all guilty of insanity. The exemplary reaction of Christian rationalism took the form of Thomas Aquinas's rewriting Aristotle in the thirteenth century. In the *Summa Theologica* he corrected Cicero in the name of Aristotelian principles. To defend the rational soul, Aquinas proposed that the Stoics, in not discerning between sense and mind, drew no discrimination between the passions of the soul and the motions of the will. From Aquinas's rationalistic viewpoint Cicero erred in calling all passions diseases of the soul. Aquinas approved of the way that Aristotle's followers, the Peripatetics, gave the name of passion to all movements of the sensitive appetite, which they esteemed as good when controlled by reason and will. The only passions to be deprecated as evil are passions not so controlled. Hence, according to Aquinas, the most important thinker of the scholastic tradition, Cicero missed the point in criticizing the Aristotelian theory of moderation or the mean in the passions.[18]

In fine, Aquinas wanted to grant the movements of soul their own rational sphere as movements of volition and recognize their power to control the appetites. In these medieval disputes what is at stake is not merely ratiocinations of dully reasonable men, but arguments about how to articulate the nature of our inner life: is madness constitutive of most of what we find in the inner ebb and flow of consciousness, or can we chose to value some of these movements? Do we have some form of consciousness about choosing what will constitute our consciousness? To what extent is madness our ordinary state, a development of our normal passions, and to what extent is madness a pure anomaly? These are questions whose answers cannot be fixed by observation, for observation presupposes these questions and normative answers for decisions about what is the nature of what one has observed.

If philosophy can be medicine, medicine can be the grounds for philosophy, and the Western Christian tradition used the Greco-Roman doctor Galen for those purposes. Greco-Roman medicine found its fullest exposition in the works of Galen, whose death at the end of the second century of our era came centuries after the original elaboration of the Hippocratic corpus. His works fixed a medical tradition that, through Latin and Arabic translations, lasted until the Renaissance, and even later, in countless editions and translations of the original texts, into the nineteenth century. Today's textbook writers may well be envious when they note that editions of Galen's works were being used by students for some seventeen centuries or so. Galen was *the* doctor whom Christianity accepted as the touchstone of medical theorizing for some fifteen centuries. In many respects he is the most important link between the Greco-Roman world and later European civilization, and his views on insanity are central to any understanding of how the Western tradition came to construe madness.

A continuator of the Hippocratic tradition, as I indicated earlier, Galen put humoral theory at the heart of his doctrine on madness. He believed humors could exist in abnormal forms: "Acute diseases tend to be the result of the anomalies of blood or yellow bile, and chronic diseases the result of anomalies of phlegm or black bile."[19] Humors act in conjunction with the four elements, but also the seasons, periods of life, and occupations. This much is all to be found in the Hippocratic corpus. Galen, however, also developed the theory of temperaments. This theory is the first explanation of pathological character types and contains within it an explanation of comic character. The temperaments, such as the sanguine, choleric, melancholic, and phlegmatic, are not so much diseases as they are mild pathologies—pathologies that occupied two centuries of literary exploration after the Renaissance.

In other theorizing Galen developed a more varied theory of the anatomy of madness, including some notions of localization. Opposing Cicero, Galen proposed that madness can be the result of physiological changes. I paraphrase the doctor and noted literary scholar, Jean Starobinksi, from his *Histoire du traitement de la mélancholie,* to note that it may happen that the change of humor is limited to the encephalitic region of the brain, or it may be that black bile empties into the veins and circulates throughout the body. And bile can also cause an obstruction of the hypochondrium, or the area above the lumbar regions. The vapors theory of madness and melancholy apparently finds its origin in Galen's belief that, when the stomach is swollen with black bile, vapors rise to the encephalitic region of the brain, obfuscate the intelligence, and produce depression.[20] Our modern definition of *hypochondria*—the delusion of illness—thus comes from a Greek doctor for whom vapors, coming from the hypochondriac region, could produce real melancholy, hallucinations, and other forms of mental illness. The example is of more than mere philological interest, for it shows that we can obscure the origins of our ideas and beliefs when we redefine our world by giving new uses to old language games.

Galen's legacy to Western culture, after the demise of tragedy and comedy, and the rise of Christian metaphysics, was the doctrine that the body, construed as an alterity to self, is the main cause of madness. This may not seem consonant with a theology that viewed the *anima* as a part of the divine spirit; but, since Galen could be construed as showing a belief in a monotheistic God, Christian thinkers worked with enthusiasm to fit Galen's thought into the Christian worldview. In some respects this was not difficult. The Platonist in every Christian could consider the incorporation of ideas into matter to be the equivalent of the soul's fall into the material body, and hence into the realm of madness. Since the Fall, creation has shown itself to be a botched affair, and it is not surprising that the embodiment of God's logos in the material world results in a fundamental alienation. It is hardly any wonder that the mind or divine spirit called the human soul has so much trouble finding equilibrium in a material substratum—especially since it needs a delicate balance of humors to function at all. Physiology can be metaphysics, it can be theology, it can even be the grounds for political thought. Galen's medical theories about madness was the basis for all three—not to mention medicine—for the duration of the Christian consensus.

Chapter 2

Continuities and Ruptures in Medieval Folly

Modern historians often speak of a renaissance in medicine that took place after the medieval period, since during the Middle Ages after the fall of the Roman Empire, the Greco-Roman medical tradition had been nearly lost. But beginning roughly with the fall of Constantinople there was a recovery of classical medical thought. Scholars began to recover and discover Greek medical and philosophical texts. However, this does not mean there was any great renewal of medical thinking in the fifteenth or sixteenth centuries. To be sure, the Hippocratic-Galenic texts were edited in the original Greek and translated. This editing renaissance shows an advance in literacy—by and large scholars could not read Greek during the Middle Ages—but this increase in literacy did not represent a medical "advance" over medieval thought in any modern sense. On the contrary, much original Renaissance thought about insanity is an explosion of irrationality that has little to do with either Greco-Roman or modern medical and philosophical thought about madness. Some writers, such as Erasmus or Rabelais, did advance the possibility of understanding madness by redefining critical rationality in works of literature. But Renaissance medical theories of madness often seem to be as deviant as the insanity they wish to explain. The Renaissance quest for theory needs to be contextualized, first by exploring the medieval consensus about madness, and then by looking at literary discourse before turning to the Renaissance medical views of madness.

The Christian Consensus of the Middle Ages

The notion of a sixteenth-century Renaissance in medicine is misleading, since the process of the recovery of Greek medical thought had really begun several centuries before the Renaissance. For example, in his study of medical manuscripts, Marie-José-Imbault-Huart has shown that from the fall of the Roman Empire through roughly the tenth century Western medicine developed, in the monasteries, largely in the form of pharmacopoeias. After the founding of the medical school at Salerno, medical manuscripts began to circulate that offered renewed access to Greek texts, usually in the form of translations from the Arabic. The eleventh and twelfth centuries continued this recovery. With the rise of the medieval universities, editions of Aristotle mark the dominance of Greek thought, not only in medicine, but in metaphysics, physics, astronomy, and physiology. It was largely the decadence of the universities at the end of the fifteenth century that justifies the received view that a Renaissance then began as a rejection of the university and its "scholastic tradition." Manuscripts based on translations gave way to printed books as the humanists produced editions of Hippocrates and Galen that represent an advance in accuracy, if not in medical content.[1]

The printing of editions in the original of what was already largely known in translation did not effect an epistemological break with the past. Those hankering after an epistemological break would do better to look to the seventeenth century, when scientific and philosophical doctrines instituted new types of discourse about what constitute the criteria for reality and knowledge. With these new discourses, the criteria for madness were transformed—though I shall also argue that the seventeenth century's institution of new criteria for the real marks a return to Greek standards of rationality after the excesses of the Renaissance.

What is clear is that there was an explosion of interest in madness at the end of the fifteenth century and throughout the Renaissance and that madness acquired different meanings from what it had in the twelfth century. But this new interest in madness was hardly based on any new science—or at least on what we take to be science today. One must also bear in mind that, along with the explosion of new interpretations of madness in the sixteenth century, the Galenic Christian tradition remained dominant. The Christian Galenic theory of madness remained dominant and unchanged until after the Renaissance. For example, a late Renaissance writer like Robert Burton (1577–1640) continued, in his famous *Anatomy of Melancholy,* to describe madness in terms of the dichotomous point of view that was typical of the previous fifteen centuries of Christian puzzlement over madness. Is insanity a spiritual or a medical issue? To which the ingenuous melancholy stylist answers:

> It is a disease of the soul on which I am to treat, and as much appertaining to a Divine as to a Physician; and who knows not what an agreement there is betwixt these two professions? A good Divine either is or ought to be a good physician; a spiritual physician at least, as our Saviour calls himself, and was indeed. They differ but in object, the one of the body, the other of the soul, and use divers medicines to cure: one amends the soul through the body, the

other the body through the soul. One helps the vices and passions of the soul, anger, lust, desperation, presumption, etc. by applying the spiritual physick; as the other uses proper remedies in bodily diseases.[2]

The principle of complementarity neatly gives equal responsibility to the priest and the doctor, though the dualism of body and soul that Burton so neatly resolves here will soon surface to plague Western thought later, after transformations of scientific discourse have made problematic the belief in a spiritual soul and a physical body. The Ciceronian undertone in Burton's view of passion as a spiritual disease underscores the historical continuity of this discourse.

Burton's dichotomous view that divides up responsibility for madness between secular and religious authorities reflects of course the problems of assigning political and legislative authority that emerged in the Middle Ages. Actually the dichotomy was not always so neat. Earlier medieval thought makes more often a tripartite division of discourse about insanity that corresponds largely to what were adaptations of the categories of classical antiquity. For the Middle Ages the three forms of alterity that could characterize madness are described in the following ways. Madness could affect the body, or be an alteration of the body. It could also be a form of divine or, more usually, diabolical possession. And it could be the result of a diseased will. With all necessary allowances, one can say that these three forms of alterity correspond to a humoral determination of madness, to a supernatural form of possession (as in tragedy), and to the Stoic determination of passion as madness.

Christianity constantly added a superior level of interpretation to these three classical determinations of madness, since any affliction could be interpreted by a Christian as a test. The naturalism of humors theory was subordinated to a theological interpretation that construed humoral imbalance at times as directly caused by God, especially with a view to punishing the proud, damning the wicked, or testing and improving the just. With the revival of Aristotelian metaphysics, the schema could be applied in terms of Aristotle's fourfold division of causality. In Aristotelian terms everything has a final cause or telos, which meant that, for a Christian, madness had to have a purpose in God's great design. For, if madness exists, it must be part of God's plan—even if the efficient cause of madness was believed to be the usual black bile, or humor of Greek origins.

Greek thought was the basis for the naturalistic interpretation of madness, but Greek medical views were subordinated to the final arbiter for all medieval interpretations of reality: the Bible. Penelope Doob has appropriately entitled her seminal study of madness in medieval literature *Neb-uchadnezzar's Children*. It was the biblical tale of the madness of the ruler of Babylon that gave the Middle Ages its key emblem of mental pathology. According to the Bible this king was such a proud and evil ruler that God turned him into an animal—an act often cited to prove that metamorphosis was clearly in the realm of the possible. Bestiality symbolized for the Christian mind the fall from logos, and pointed to the fundamental ontological instability that menaced all taxonomies. This instability was due to humanity's fall from grace, and thus the medieval mind could also interpret humoral disequilibrium as a result of original sin. There was apparently no melancholy in the Garden of Eden. Underwriting this web of analogies was, in addition, the view that all disease can be interpreted in moralistic and teleological terms. As countless writers of theodicies, large and small, constantly stressed, madness must ultimately be an expression of some divine purpose.

The seamless nature of this web of analogies was, as far as we can tell, accepted by the insane. They, too, interpreted their madness in theological terms, as we glimpse in their depositions in later records of the trials for witchcraft and devil worship. This is undoubtedly a recurrent phenomenon: the mad live and interpret their insanity in terms of the prevailing explanatory paradigms. Perhaps the earliest literary example of this experience of madness as imposed by the medieval paradigm is found in the poetry of Thomas Hoccleve (or Occleve, ca. 1370–1450). Living his madness as a theological test, he seems to be the first European to write about his personal experience of insanity, or at least the first of whom we have record. Hoccleve is of singular value for his demonstration that a poet lives his madness in conformity with the explanatory model that his era offers him.

In his "Complaint" Hoccleve claims that he discovers in a book that Reason teaches that he must accept madness as a scourge that God uses to test him: "For god, to prove the [thee], / Scourgid the hath with sharpe adversite." And then to dramatize the process of insanity Hoccleve uses a metaphor that has found much favor with writers attempting to explain the inner experience of madness. Insanity has been a trip, a pilgrimage, or a voyage to another realm:

> Right so, though that my witte were a pilgrim
> And went fer from hom, he cam again.
> God me devoided of the grevous venim
> That had enfectid and wildid my brain.
> See hoe the curteise leche [doctor] most soverain

> Unto the seke geveth medicine
> In nede, and hym releveth of his grevous pine.[3]

Hoccleve has two explanations for his insanity. Madness is at once a product of a "venim," some physiological excess that affects the brain, but also a diseased state depending upon God's direct intervention for its coming and going. Hoccleve lives his madness as divine possession and a humoral imbalance. And at the same time his poetic rhetoric suggests that madness— the trip—has some psychological dimension that can only be expressed metaphorically by the self reflecting back upon itself in time. There is thus an allegorical dimension to this process, for the allegory of madness makes sense within the great Christian allegory in which all that happens has meaning. Hoccleve's example is instructive of the way the expression of madness is literally informed by the possibilities of discourse. Hoccleve does not live his madness as anguish generated from within the self. Rather, he views madness as a kind of normal deviance in which all must participate because all are born into sin. God is at once cause and balm, means and telos, of madness lived as a trip through sin.

Madness lost its anguishing specificity as irrational deviance in the Middle Ages. This loss is clear in Hoccleve. And the context for this loss becomes clearer if we contrast, with the insane poet, the greatest medieval poet and the supreme rationalist, Dante. It is generally recognized that the ultimate expression of the Christian consensus is the summation of the rationalist side of medieval thought found in *The Divine Comedy*. Dante is at once a Christian rationalist, drawing upon the scholastic achievement of the thirteenth century, and the most powerful poet of the human fall from divine potentiality. Aquinas's reconciliation of Aristotle with theology gave Dante a Christian standard for rationality that interprets the fall as deviance from logos. In neither Aquinas nor Dante is madness in itself a central issue, precisely because the strength of their rationalist credo has so ordered existence that irrationality is banished to the inferno's shadowy land in which alterity is hardly mentioned—though madness is constantly present as part of the self-understood universal condition of sin.

Dante's rationalism does not allow for a belief in diabolic possession. From Dante's perspective the self can lose its rational autonomy only through false love, as Marco Lombardo explains to Dante in *Purgatory* XVI:

> A maggior forza ed a miglior natura
> liberi soggiacete; e quella cria
> la mente in voi, che 'l ciel non ha in sua cura.

> (79–81)

[To a greater power and to a better nature you, free, are subject, and that creates the mind in you which the heavens have not in their charge.][4]

Mind is autonomous and free according to the divine model, and so mind is not subject to external determinants. This rationalist credo means that astrological, diabolical, and magical forces have no role in madness. One wonders if Dante would have allowed black bile a role. He would certainly have scoffed at the irrationalities of the Renaissance.

To understand the kind of medieval discourse Dante embodies means to grasp the way the rationalist current considered all texts to be a part of a great master allegory or the divine design of logos. Since language, as a part of logos, is a guarantor of right reason, any operation in language, such as in allegory, is already working on the side of logos or God's design. Madness can be understood through language, since madness must exist as part of that design, even if madness, like sin, represents a failure to live in accord with that design. (Opposed to this view stood the belief that language is fallen, a belief underlying another important medieval current.) The belief that madness, like sin, could be mediated through allegory had great consequences. For one, it appears that the Middle Ages could live with the mad.

The Breakdown of the Master Allegory

If we are all born into sin and madness, then we are all to some degree mad. How then does one differentiate between the sane and the insane? The answer is that the Middle Ages did not differentiate so sharply between the mad and the nonmad. Legal criteria for insanity existed, but the allegorical explanation of insanity promoted the relatively greater tolerance that the insane enjoyed in medieval Europe. Some were locked up, some were probably tortured, but, as a general practice, incarceration of the mad became universal only at a later date, during that late medieval seventeenth century that burned witches, tortured magicians, and locked up the straightforwardly insane. But as long as the Christian master allegory held good, as long as logos and its opposite existed as part and parcel of the same allegory of divine purpose, then madness was not a problematic issue for Western culture.

Hoccleve and Dante are emblems for the medieval interpretation of madness as a lived experience and as a global allegory. However, beginning with what we commonly take to be the Renaissance, or perhaps slightly earlier, the master allegory began to function badly, and then madness became problematic. Around the end of the fifteenth century madness became a central issue of European culture. The possibility of integrating madness into a master allegory of logos foundered on the perceived impossibility of making madness intelligible. From this perspective the term *Renaissance* then comes to mean the breakdown of medieval rationality as much as a revival in learning. And emblematic of this breakdown are the new theories of madness as well as that pandemic of irrationality known as the witch trials. With remarkable unanimity, judges and the demonstrably insane were in agreement about the devil's power to make them copulate with goats.

With the breakdown of medieval rationality it was increasingly possible to view madness as an opaque discourse having magical powers, one in alliance with various diabolic forces. Understandably concern with insanity took on new importance. First, this concern had to confront the difficulty of discerning the nonmad from the mad, and this dilemma then elicited explanations of madness that appear today as mad as the phenomena of madness that the explanations sought to explain—and this in spite of the fact that the humors theory of madness remained the mainstream medical paradigm, and in spite of the new editions of classical writers that reinforced this medical orthodoxy. It is important to understand that most advances in medicine were basically adjustments of the traditional Galenic model—say, Vesalius's correcting some of Galen's more egregious anatomical mistakes. In fact, as the Christian master allegory came apart, there was a revolt against Galen that contributed little or nothing to a renaissance in medicine. This revolt took the form of a renewal of all manner of doctrines that the Church had already condemned: alchemy, astrology, magic, mystical doctrines, correspondence theories, and the like. Of course, these condemnations bespeak the purchase that these irrationalities had on many medieval minds as well as their longevity: for nearly all these doctrines have their roots in late antiquity. In brief, the Renaissance either refurbished Galen or, in revolt, renewed the irrational paradigms of the Alexandrian parasciences. There were quite simply no new scientific or philosophical paradigms with which to explain madness, though there were new historical trends, such as those witch trials in which the irrational achieved a demonical status that it had never had before. The Renaissance was, in brief, a time of unparalleled irrationality.

The Defense of Rationality in Literary Discourse

Literary scholars, however, are inclined to think of the Renaissance as a time of unparalleled creativity, and they are right so long as they consider only literary discourse. The creativity of the Renaissance is largely a literary matter, and so we must also think dialectically and consider the great writers of the Renaissance who contributed to the birth of a modern standard of rationality founded on ironic consciousness. This was an important step toward an understanding of madness. Erasmus, Rabelais, and Ariosto are so many names that point out that the Renaissance mind engaged a dialogue with madness with an understanding that we have not seen again since. These writers imitated madness, borrowed from the irrational, and in superb self-confidence created a higher standard of rationality. Supreme dialecticians themselves, they believed that all products of the mind have a place in the creation of a literary self through a dialectical play of opposites. With the renewal of learning based on antiquity, these inheritors of Aristophanes accorded madness a value as a producer of new discourses and new possibilities. Dialectically, then, the reformer enthusiasm of an Erasmus or a Rabelais should be viewed against the backdrop of what the historian Delumeau has characterized as the "great fear," the generalized anguish that gripped their Renaissance contemporaries, to whom it appeared that the world was coming apart, if not because the Christian allegory had lost its relevance, then because the pagan Turks seemed capable of overrunning Christian Europe.[5] Or for both reasons.

What seems to be common to all Renaissance writers is their attempt to allegorize their material, and in this regard, virtually all writing, through the Counter Reformation, creates allegories that look for a center to discourse that can explain the outbreak of the irrational. The great writers do this with irony. Lesser writers—say, the German writer Brant in his *Ship of Fools*—allegorize in an attempt to explain by moralizing the challenge of the irrational that loomed on the horizon, with the "great fear" as their horizon of concern. In the case of a Brant this meant that madness was endowed with an inconceivable evil capacity for destroying rationality, including the sanity of the writer who attempts an allegory showing the manifest workings of madness. There is little irony in this fear.

The writers who concern us use irony as a rational procedure allowing one to explore madness—the dialectical opposite of the great fear of madness. In Erasmus, for example, as in Rabelais or Ariosto, we find the willingness to cohabit with and to use madness. To study this crucial side of the sixteenth century—and its invention of a new standard of critical rationality—one can turn to Erasmus's *Praise of Folly* (or *Moriae Encomium*, published in 1511). The work begins as an enthusiastic illustration of the by now familiar topos presenting the world as upside down, or a world in which all values are seemingly reversed. The praise of madness is spoken by

Dame Folly herself. In self-praise she describes her place of birth as the Fortunate Islands, a utopian space, a place for a golden age. There she was born of the god of wealth Plutus, and of Youth. Folly's claims for herself are great. She is, as she immodestly says, at the origins of life, since who, she asks, would bother to have children without the intervention of madness. And she claims that it is she who makes life bearable. Mere wisdom dries up people, like some grim philosopher, before youth has been spent.

The grim philosopher is Erasmus's beloved Cicero. The pivotal point of understanding the reversals in the first half of Erasmus's praise of madness is the ironic deprecation of Stoic thought and its notions about sanity and wisdom. In satire Erasmus reverses the terms of the Ciceronian understanding of madness. He does this by showing that the stoic Christian who equates passion with madness is quite insane. What sane person could suppress the passions, the emotions, the supposedly lower affects:

> For since according to the definition of the Stoics, wisdom is nothing else than to be governed by reason, and on the contrary Folly, to be given up to the will of our passions, that the life of man might not be altogether disconsolate and hard to away with, of how much more passion than reason has Jupiter composed us? putting in, as one would say, "scarce half an ounce to a pound." Besides, he has confined reason to a narrow corner of the brain and left all the rest of the body to our passions.[6]

Erasmus's ironic reversal of Stoic-Christian notions is a prelude to a modern critique of excess repression (to use a useful concept the revisionist Marxist Herbert Marcuse developed in *Eros and Civilization*). Erasmus's irony points up the impossible desire to control human impulses. This desire underlies Cicero's Stoic utopia from which insanity, along with passion, is banned. Christian Stoicism, deriving from Cicero, is guilty of the "double dementia" of wanting to transform human beings into gods. From this perspective madness is a counterutopia, a refuge from the destructive impulses of a Christianity that would turn its believers into rational robots.

Erasmus works with a medical understanding of madness. Folly defines madness with precision. She does not call her own every aberration of the mind, nor every hallucination or delirium. She accepts as hers only those cases where in addition to the senses, judgment goes astray, pathologically and with continuity. In other words, her insanity is medically and juridically defined—and there is nothing demonic about insanity at all. Erasmus embraces a jubilant naturalism that is not afraid of encountering the diabolical in the form of the daily madness that one meets in the streets. His is a critical acceptance of madness as a natural phenomenon; and it is based on a philosophical understanding that, continuing Greek dialectics, remains a model for rationality.

What emerges in Erasmus's "praise of madness," as *Moriae Encomium* might better be translated, is a self-reflexive irony that represents an essential step toward the relation in which the self contemplates itself in what we call sanity. This is an essential move toward the modern self, one pointing to the reason in madness that characterizes Shakespeare's interpretations of madness. Erasmus's presentation of the ironic self, created through a rhetorical relationship in linguistic play, differs fundamentally from the medieval view that sees the empirical self as a substance that is modified by accidents—a view that continued to underwrite much of the medical thinking of the Renaissance. With irony Erasmus tries to get around the medieval incapacity to view madness theoretically except as one aspect of the same allegory of sin recurring universally after the fall. For madness to emerge as difference, as a ruptured relationship, irony is the ploy that allows the sane self to differentiate itself from the world of the fall and to view its relationship to itself and the world. In Erasmus, as in the works of other literary creators, the rational self is defined as a self that can seize itself as an object of reflection in irony. This irony is largely absent from an exemplary late medieval text like Brant's *The Ship of Fools*, and totally lacking in many sixteenth-century medical texts that, for this reason, strike us today as being nearly insane in their deadpan fantasies.

The capacity of the self to maintain a relation to itself in irony becomes part of what we mean by sanity and rationality at this historical moment—and the lack thereof becomes something of what we mean by insanity. This is superimposed on the belief that madness is caused by the fall of logos into substance. Erasmus is a Christian and is willing to take on the folly of the Cross, the final ironic reversal that lies at the heart of the reformed Christianity he wanted to propagate. This folly is the rejection of reason in the name of the higher reason that the Cross represents. The defense of a renewed Christian rationality appeared essential to a Christian reformer like Erasmus, who could sense the inconceivable changes that the Reformation was about to bring about. Not only was the Church about to be torn apart by Luther, and submerged by the renewal of irrationalities like astrology and magic, but the Christian reformer had to meet the challenge of the instrumental notion of rationality that Machiavelli brought forward with *The Prince* in 1513.

Quite succinctly, logos lost all transcendence when Machiavelli defined rationality simply and perhaps irrefutably in terms of power: the rational is that which exists because it can impose its existence. Thus by self-fulfilling definition rationality is what is; or the real is the rational. To recognize the reality of power is to recognize that all standards are subject to validation by the sword that declares them to be true. For a history of madness this is of immeasurable importance. Nothing is insane if it has sufficient power to declare itself sane. In the proliferation of irrationalities that unfolded during the Renaissance, power unveiled itself as the self-demonstrating standard that nothing can deny—unless it has greater power.

New Medical Thought on Madness

My commentary to this point suggests some of the reasons why the very notion of Renaissance lends itself to much controversy. During the same few generations medieval minds were trying to keep alive the Christian master allegory and its attendant theodicy, whereas writers like Erasmus and Machiavelli were creating those works that prefigure our modern notion of self and rationality. When one turns to many of their medical contemporaries, one confronts a curious gallery of cranks, the near mad, and the obsessed. In their attempts to go beyond Hippocrates, Galen—or in Paracelsus's case—Celsus, these doctors give the impression of perpetuating the great wave of irrationality that was to eventuate in the trials for witchcraft and the legalized burning of the mad. Of course, most doctors continued to repeat Galen, but, for the purposes of our history, those who interest us here are those who proposed new theories of madness as the master allegory came apart. Little that these doctors developed appears to have much to do with the way we talk about madness today. Nonetheless, there were displacements and modifications of our understanding of madness in that their new theories of madness challenged the Galenic model. In turning to diverse representative doctors—or perhaps medical fabulators is a more precise term—such as theorists like Ficino, Agrippa, Paracelsus, or the encyclopedic monk Tommaso Garzoni, one finds that their attempts to invent new medical theories resulted in curious fantasies that mirror the madness they contemplate. However, it often seems that this mirroring takes place through the prisms of the ancient models of medical explanation. New paradigms are not easily invented: borrowing old models is more the rule than is a breakthrough to a new theory. As a general rule, it seems that, when the doctors did not refurbish Alexandrian irrationality, they usually aped the madness they wished to explain.

I propose to speak of four main currents in Renaissance theorizing. First, in the Neoplatonist Ficino's work madness is the expression of eros, and eros the driving force of bestial metamorphosis. Ficino revitalizes Plato in order to update the medieval belief in metamorphosis. But his eroticization of madness anticipates an important psychological transformation of our understanding of madness. Second, in the doctor-magus Agrippa we find a medieval reaction against the medieval understanding that the world is a book or a text; and, as a consequence, a paranoid rejection of all knowledge. Madness becomes self-praise. A third and more important current is the alchemical trend. In this regard Paracelsus represents another type of rejection of classical medicine, and this alchemically inclined doctor naturalized madness in ways that allow for a belief in the poetic power of madness. For the final Renaissance current, I want to consider taxonomic inventions. Inventing new clinical entities has been a medical pastime since the Renaissance, and I select the Italian Garzoni as one of the most fertile inventors of types of madness in the history of medicine.[7] His "theater" of types of madness is typical of Renaissance taxonomy, if unique for the individual types it proposes. Perhaps none of these scientists will figure in a history of psychiatry dealing only with the application of the Galenic paradigm to insanity, but they should be included in any consideration of the imaginary possibilities that madness has had for our culture.

If it can be argued that the Renaissance has any major thinker who shaped our way of conceiving madness, unfortunately it must be Ficino. The doctor and philosopher Marsilio Ficino did more for resurrecting Platonism than probably any thinker since his time, and most notably in his *Theologiae platonicae de immortalitate animorum* of that auspicious year, 1492. Ficino was a sometime superstitious practitioner of astrology who was, moreover, head of the Academy in Florence. Renaissance historians have made much of Ficino. Kristeller claimed Ficino invented the notion of Platonic love; and Panofsky and his collaborators want him to be the first to have seen an identity between Aristotle's association of melancholy and genius, and Plato's view of divine possession.[8] It is true that Ficino's interest in madness was singularly influential during the Renaissance; and his views of eros are crucial for a history of madness and eroticism, or more precisely, eros as potential madness.

It would not be hard to argue, with regard to eros, that Ficino is Freud's precursor in his commentary on Plato's *Symposium* called *De Amore, Commentarium in Convivium Platonis*. In this work, composed in 1469 and given in a rewritten form to Lorenzo de' Medici in 1475, Ficino wrote his own version of the *Symposium* (also called *The Banquet*). In his "banquet" Ficino distributes the roles among friends, each of whom imitates a character in the Platonic dialogue and speaks in praise of love—understood as spiritual or disembodied love. Doctor Ficino speaks as Plato's doctor Eryxi-machus in speeches that imitate the sublimated male homophilic discourse that Plato initiated for our culture (and that Freud later interpreted for our modern culture as the war between repression and the pansexual id). Throughout *De Amore* Ficino's praise of love is an apology for love among men and an attack on the body. Positive disgust with the body is one constant in the Neoplatonic doctrine of love that Ficino proposes. Since the body is given over to the agitation of desire, it is the locus for madness.

Ficino gives "proof" of this proposition in the Seventh Discourse's description of bestial love, which shows it to be a form of insanity. This also shows that man is subject to two types of eros: one bestial, the other being Plato's divine frenzy. Bestial madness is located in either the brain or the heart. Ficino concocts a medical doctrine to describe how the agitated brain reacts to an excess of burned bile, burned blood, or black bile that drives men mad—while the same excess in the heart only produces anguish and disquiet. Ficino's version of humors theory is of lesser interest than his psychologizing, for he is really torn by a vision of divine love, which is essentially mad, and the body, which is the source of a bestiality that has little to do with humors. Ficino wants to believe that divine fury might produce an ascension that would convert man into a god, leaving behind the bestial body that ties man to the carnal desires that Ficino loathes. Aspiring to divinity, the Alcibiades of the Seventh Discourse wants to put physical eros behind him for fear it might contaminate him. Drawing on sources as diverse (and as unified) as Plotinus and Cavalcanti, Ficino's final speaker clearly fears the vision of beauty in the world; he is afraid of real flesh, of the body that might persuade him to recognize himself in his fallen flesh. This obsession is also expressed as a fear of vision, a fear of the body and its "accidents" that can tear the viewer away from the vision of unity granted by eternal logos. This insanity is an atavistic part of Christianity: self-hatred becomes the primary relation of self to itself in a fear of the "false" love that inevitably turns men into a beasts.

There is probably as much of Ovid's influence as Plato's in this syncretic stew. Madness is a form of metamorphosis. The worst transformations of the human beast are produced by deviant eros. However, the desire for ascension is also dangerous, for the soul can run the risk of going mad on its own as it aspires to transcendence. Ficino's Socrates, in the Sixth Discourse, describes the danger the soul encounters in its attempt to leave its home and unite with the beautiful that lies beyond the world. Ficino's configuration of madness includes an alienation grounded in the soul's desire to leave itself: the self is split in its desire not to desire, or in its mad desire to overcome itself. Freudians might interpret Ficino's doctrine in terms of sublimation and unsuccessful repression. But this would probably be placing his Neo-platonism into too modern a mold. Ficino is trying to adjust a medieval concept of magical transformations to his encounter with Plato, an overwhelming encounter for this late medieval mind. This is one of the most characteristic traits of Renaissance medical thought about madness: we see dimly a continuity, such as the eroticizing of madness that points to Freud, but we also see, in Ficino, the attempt of a medieval mind to come to grips with a pre-Christian classical thought that it could not force into a Christian mold. The modern reader must recognize, moreover, that Ficino's thought is embedded in a matrix that does not demand coherence, that is, a principle of exclusion that rejects viewpoints that are not consonant with each other. For example, Ficino can draw upon any story ever narrated as a proof of the powers of metamorphosis, since, as the historian of science Koyré put it, the category of *non posse*—of not being possible—hardly existed in the late Middle Ages.[9] Madness is always possible at any moment, because creatures with substances subject to multiple accidents can be infinitely transformed by savage instincts.

The proliferation of concepts of the possible during the Renaissance, the credibility that could be given to any theory that had ever been printed, could lead, dialectically perhaps, to a total rejection of knowledge. This reaction against the "vanity" of the infinite stocking of knowledge characterized the doctor Agrippa von Nettesheim (1486–1535), who abolished the irrational by declaring the nullity of all rational inquiry. His stance mirrors by inversion the madness of infinite proliferation, and his position is a kind of insane negative mimicry. This position opens a space in culture, however, where the mad can gain an audience, and for this reason I turn to the magus.

Agrippa was known as a magician of extraordinary powers during his lifetime. He was, during his wanderings, at one time physician to the mother of the king of France, though he died in poverty on the streets of Lyon. His various writings, published years after they had circulated in manuscript, include everything from medical writings and gospel commentary to a treatise on mines, an essay on the excellence of women, and a work of universal history. He is reckoned, with justification, among the founders of mineralogy. Agrippa's example points up that the Renaissance economy of discourse allowed anyone to master the totality of knowledge, with no fear of contradiction, since contradiction was not necessarily a criterion for validity, a point that Agrippa's work demonstrates. For instance, Agrippa's two major works touching on medicine are totally inconsistent with each other. The first book, a work of occult philosophy, is rejected by the second, his treatise on the vanity of knowledge. The first book, *Philosophia occulta,* was apparently published in 1510, some twenty years before he wrote the second, *De incertitudine.* Adding a preface to his first work on "secret philosophy," Agrippa published both works together, in reverse order, in 1531 and 1530, respectively, with apparently no distress about contradicting himself with works that deny each other. Agrippa's treatise on occult philosophy is an astro-alchemical mishmash based on the principle that there are three worlds: the elemental, the celestial, and the intellectual. The task of medicine or natural philosophy is to discover the virtues of the elemental world by exploring the hierarchies of the various levels of being. Agrippa's peregrinations about Europe can be explained, in part, by the fact that this intertextual collage, drawing on countless sources to demonstrate the occult, did smell of heresy and might have made Agrippa fear a trip to the stake. Heresy aside, at least part of Agrippa's treatise represents one of many Renaissance attempts to bring alchemy into the realm of medicine—or vice versa.

It was a semideviant view during Agrippa's lifetime to make medicine an adjunct to magic. And equally deviant was the rejection Agrippa proposed in his attack on knowledge—occult or official—in *De incertitudine et vanitate scientiarum et artium, atque excellentia Verbi Dei declamatio.* The treatise demonstrates the "uncertainty and vanity" of knowledge by creating a typically medieval intertextual collage to demonstrate that there are conflicting opinions on any subject one wishes to name, astrology or baking, medicine or surgery. Doctors are damned for their desire to go beyond the precepts of Hippocrates and Galen; and the ancients are damned for being contradictory. Anticipating Rabelais's carnival use of verbal abuse (and Rabelais's parody of Agrippa himself), doctors are portrayed as scatophagic, avaricious piss sniffers of dubious morals—no better than poets.

In this paranoid attack on knowledge Agrippa reverses the late medieval standards for demonstration: texts can be quoted indefinitely, not to add to knowledge, but to subtract from it. And this reduction eventuates in a call for a return to the Pauline Gospels. The modern reader immediately wonders if Agrippa is sincere or if this show of Christian ignorance is an attempt to avoid an auto-da-fé. The question is misplaced. The very notion of sincerity, I think, presupposes a self that was not yet fully developed during the Renaissance, which means that one of our primary criteria for separating madness and sanity does not really apply to the paranoid system of this demonstration of vanity that rings of insanity from a modern perspective. The inference of a state of mind from this late medieval text must take place according to different rules, rules that can account for the fact Agrippa published at the same time an encyclopedia of occult science that makes claims for total knowledge, and a treatise showing a primitive Christian's hatred of learning. The self in question here is elaborating textual games in which the sanity-insanity distinction does not have a clear position. For modern readers, equipped with well-defined protocols for the genesis of meaning, Agrippa's uncentered proliferation of discourse produces the impression of madness, indeed that it is aping insanity. Perhaps this is a turning point in the history of madness, for it is possible to view Agrippa as opening a skeptical space in which the criteria for sanity and insanity are always subject to doubt. From this historical perspective, then, Agrippa would be an antecedent thinker for Montaigne and Shakespeare, and the self that defines itself as a form of interrogation about the data of consciousness. Borges noted that we create our precursors, and historians have used Agrippa to this end. Yet it is difficult to find criteria by which to grasp textual intentionality in Agrippa's case, and that, too, is a sign of madness. Signifiers floating freely, to use recent terminology, may show a decentered universe, but that can be the world of insanity.

Ficino and Agrippa represent thinkers whom we can interpret as much as markers toward the past as signposts for some future discourse. History oriented toward the future of scientific discourse usually overlooks them and is drawn toward a doctor like Paracelsus (1493–1541): he was the alchemist who systematically tried to overthrow Galen. He wanted to found medicine on the basis of natural magic, though we should not overlook that natural magic is also a doctrine of late antiquity. Proposed frequently as a model for Goethe's Faust (as is Agrippa), Paracelsus illustrates a third tendency in Renaissance medical fabulation, which is the attempt to use occult and hermetic sciences to create rather complex language games that have been interpreted as a positive attempt to found a new science. Paracelsus undertook this innovation in such a naturalistic spirit that he has been variously called the founder of chemistry, pharmacy, and medical psychology. However, except for his recognition that excessive mercury can kill a syphilitic, there is little in his vast body of work that strikes me as having any relation to modern science. Much of it—even by the standards of the Renaissance—seems again to mirror the insanity he wanted to explain and perhaps cure. To paraphrase the epistemologist Bachelard when he spoke of dead-ends in the history of science, Paracelsus's system building was more of an epistemological obstacle to the development of science, especially any science that needed quantification as its basis.

But Paracelsus's wacky free thinking does have something grandiose about it, and one cannot help but be impressed by the legend that Paracelsus burned the works of Galen—or of Avicenna in another version—at his introductory medical lectures in Basel. Moreover, Paracelsus stands squarely opposed to the Florentine humanists, the *antici,* who were editing and translating the classical medical texts. Much of his medicine derives from folk tradition, much from a deviant tradition of alchemy, and much from his own synthesis. The example is instructive. In attempting to create a new medical paradigm Paracelsus created fantasies that demonstrate the difficulty of displacing received scientific models. In recasting ancient models Paracelsus reminds me a great deal of the poet Blake and his eclectic capacity, in creating poetic myths, for deriving names and legends from all manner of bizarre and disparate sources. Paracelsus ultimately had, however, no more originality than the blind followers of Galen, even if he did proclaim the bankruptcy of classical medicine.

Paracelsus conceived medicine to be part of alchemy, which is part of astrology, and he embedded this hierarchy in a system that, refurbished with new terminology, is nonetheless a variant of the Neoplatonism that was the basis of most hermetic "research." To this Paracelsus added empirical nostrums. All this mixing of doctrines means that every reader can create his or her Paracelsus by shifting the accent. For example, Walter Pagel finds that Paracelsus's work describes a close relation between mental illness and the mad person's relation to the stars, and thus Pagel emphasizes the astrological causes of madness seen by Paracelsus:

> [Madness] . . . is due to the subjugation of man and his divine spirit by his low animal instincts, notably lust, covetousness and the passions of the soul in general. They act like drugs, notably hemlock, and are elicited by the stars. Each star corresponds to an animal with its characteristic emotional behavior and also to a single passion of man. When he falls prey to these passions, the star awakens in him the one that corresponds to its own animal nature. This action is not as acute and deadly as hemlock, but it engenders a chronic condition of mania.[10]

Hemlock aside, Paracelsus appears here as a figure who, like Ficino, combined classical thought with the revived astrological determinations of fate and character. However, Ficino revered antiquity, and Paracelsus wanted to overthrow it. In spite of this desire, Paracelsus also described the eroticization of madness in an allegorical framework that owed as much to Neoplatonism as to the gnostic tradition that saw matter as fundamentally evil.

With an innate tragic sense, Paracelsus was also a great inventor of allegories in which man and nature are in constant correspondence in a cosmic sense. Shakespeare was not insensitive to Paracelsus's dramatic sense. For the doctor was also a dramatist describing dramas based on great principles like Experience, Life, and Nature—though none of these terms means exactly what it does today, especially experience.[11] The alchemist Paracelsus claims that his medical knowledge is a direct experience of Life and Nature, not of medical texts. By *Life* and *Nature* he means allegorical actors in a drama in which madness is an omnipresent experience of nature itself. Unfortunately, Nature withholds its truths, and so we live in a world whose surfaces are illusions. The wandering doctor has discovered that the world is a labyrinth that the student must "experience," for Nature nevertheless demands that we learn from it, or forever wander in darkness and night:

> Also müssen die secreta und mysteria der Natur in uns kommen. Also werden uns die magnalia Gottes offenbart. Also kommen herfür die arcana naturae durch den, der sie in Natur geleget hat.

> [Thus must the secreta and mysteria of Nature come to us. Thus are God's magnalia revealed to us. Thus come forward the arcana naturae (secrets of nature) through the one who has placed them in Nature.][12]

Writing a wackily pretentious mixture of German and Latin, Paracelsus tells his readers that, as Christian alchemists and with God's help, they can escape the darkness—the state of madness par excellence—by standing in the revelation of nature's secrets. The word *Arcanum* entered European languages with this invention of a discourse describing how to go behind mere appearances and find secrets. Paracelsus is not Bacon: experience is to undergo an ineffable disclosure of secrets that stand in open view.

The idea that there are secrets in nature has a certain modern ring, though in the Renaissance context it can also be a paranoid version of a conspiracy. The deciphering of secrets is part of reading nature—and of the search for readable signs that can ground discourse in something certain. An old tradition stands behind this idea that, ultimately, experience is reading the book of the world. For mere written texts cannot offer certain signs, and Paracelsus appears at times to share Agrippa's rejection of the written word. This rejection is consonant with the belief that one can experience nature, and it also revives the perennial Western distrust of the printed word. The World—not any written book—is the only book speaking a living language; whereas the written words found in ancient manuscripts are merely dead letters that bring death to the already sick (a paraphrase from "Und ohn die Bucher des rechten Grunds sind's alles tote Buchstaben. Das ist: sie bringen die Kranken mehr zum Tod denn zum Leben").[13]

Paracelsus's rejection of Galen is part of a rejection of written words. Written words have destroyed a medical practice based on the living words of spoken language that enters into direct correspondence with nature. This correspondence is vouchsafed by the natural light that the Bible mentions as the source of knowledge and which allows one to "see" all knowledge directly. The astrological doctor reads Nature as if it were a living letter sent to him by the divinity. All sanity, all rationality, must ultimately be grounded in this divine light of reason that needs no books—except the Book, of course. Ultimately this kind of allegory, also borrowing from antique sources, makes us all participants in astrological dramas based on the relation of the micro- and the macrocosmos. The specificity of any illness is lost, however, when the ultimate therapy becomes the reading of nature in order to discover there the *sapientia* that will enable the alchemist to escape madness and sin.

Of greatest interest, from our perspective, is the Paracelsus who suggests that madness is an intrinsic condition of nature. For example, in *The Fourteen Books of Paragraphs* Paracelsus declares that his favored trio of salt, sulphur, and mercury are the basis for all medicine. These three substances or "principles" are in effect actors in another alchemical allegory, though one charged with the drama of a fallen humanity for whom nature is directly the source of madness. For example, "madness" such as epilepsy is caused by vapor, or wind moved by the three principles in conjunction with the four elements. In his description of mental illness, Paracelsus sees humanity thrown back onto nature—not our nature subject to laws or processes—but a nature in which sickness is an expression of natural truths. Nature is a dramatic text. And in this dramatization madness is to be read as a truth. This is conceivable because madness is part of the great fabric of a world made up of symbolizing relations:

> And this disease is like the thunder in the sky, for they have the same origin: and whoever wished to know perfectly this disease and generation, it is necessary that he consider diligently storms, thunder, lightning, and comparable things in the great world: all the more so that by the cry or song of animals, by the flight of birds, or other gestures he comes to know the signs of these things and their horrible and frightful effect, with the results that follow, to wit, he will as easily know the beginning, progress, and end [of the disease].[14]

There is a certain grandeur in this vision in which all is connected to all, though it is an irrational grandeur that would make of the witches on the heath in *Macbeth* the most accomplished healers. However, Paracelsus is no more Shakespeare than he is Bacon. In spite of a certain grandeur he is often as banal as grandiose in finding causes for illness that will replace Galen's four humors. In *The Fourteen Paragraphs,* for example, he ultimately reduces the causes of madness to a single mechanical cause: opilation, or blockage. This is really nothing more than another version of hypochondria as the prime cause for mania. Bombast and banality are two sides to this late medieval attempt to use alchemy to explain madness.

Ficino's eroticization of madness may seem more promising than the vituperation with which Paracelsus rejected the Galenic tradition. Nonetheless, Paracelsus's rejection of classical theory was probably necessary to bring about the possibility of new theories of madness in the seventeenth century. Perhaps equally useful in this regard were the changes in taxonomy such as those found in the work of the ebullient Italian Tomasso Garzoni (1549–1589), a taxonomist of madness whose displacement of Galen's thought is found in his portraits of mad types. In Garzoni's case literature and medicine are the same discourse, which perhaps points up an alliance among literature, taxonomy, and science that has always existed, and will continue to exist as long as poets and scientists want to share in naming what is.

Garzoni also follows what we have seen to be a recurrent desire to turn madness into a spectacle. In his work Garzoni described all the types of madness that were to be observed in the "theater of society's diverse and varied brains"—to translate literally the title of Garzoni's book *Il Theatro de' varii e diversi cervelli mondani*—first published in Venice in 1583, and then redone in 1589 as *Hospitale de' pazzi incurabili* (The hospital of the incurably mad). Garzoni's reputation was sufficiently widespread that there were translations of this book into French and English.[15] There was also a German translation of *La piazza universale di tutte le professione del monde* (1585) (The universal piazza of all the professions of the world), some nine hundred pages of humanist praise of the arts and sciences that can be taken as an antidote for Agrippa's attack on knowledge.

Garzoni's European fame apparently did not last beyond his lifetime, for I have found no translation of a later work, *Il serraglio degli stupori del mondo* (1619) (The seraglio of all the stupors of the world). In the *Serraglio* Garzoni discusses with encyclopedic exuberance all the things in the world that can excite stupor. This later work is a humanist collage of classical literature and contemporary legends that discusses monsters and deviants such as witches. In all these works Garzoni maintains a stance that fluctuates between rational critical awareness and the credulity demanded by the biblical and ecclesiastical tradition—though with an enthusiasm for antiquity that has rarely been matched. In all of them, Garzoni seems animated by the passion to write an encyclopedic theodicy justifying the presence of the deviant in a cosmos that a rational God supposedly made for the benefit of man.

In his works on madness Garzoni displaced the Galenic paradigm by submerging it in a taxonomy of types that breaks out of the limits of classical schema. With Rabelaisian gusto he proposes, in a theatricalization of mad types, a new typology of madness. Garzoni offers his "theater of brains" as a *fabrica*. This term calls to mind Vesalius's book *De corporis humani fabrica* of 1543, in which Vesalius published his drawings correcting, in part, Galen's anatomical errors. This probable homage to Vesalius suggests that Garzoni intended to do for medical psychology and madness what the "father" of modern anatomy had undertaken for the science of the body: to map out an original anatomy (somewhat in the sense that Burton later proposed an "anatomy of melancholy"). Was this a dead-end effort? Or was it one of the necessary attempts at forging a new conceptual system that changed the conditions of possibility for thinking about madness? Within his own historical conditions of possibility Garzoni was breaking with the medieval framework of medical conceptualization. But Garzoni's work, like many taxonomic changes since then, hardly seems to point to a future. Garzoni's example underscores the difficulty of founding a new taxonomy or conceptual system, for it shows the ease with which taxonomies can proliferate—once received models are called into question.

In rejecting scholastic thought Garzoni called upon the antiformalistic thinker Duns Scotus (1265–1308) to give him the conceptual tools to rethink medical psychology. In rejecting the past, like Paracelsus, Agrippa, and Ficino, he was obliged to call upon the past, or as he tells his book's reader-spectator: "By walking in this Hospital, you will see Foolishness as the Mother of it, buffoonery the sister, stupidity the life companion, and among them, madness finding a logical equivalency, a physical relation, and a Scotist identification."[16] The reference to Scotus indicates an effort to think through the logic of species in terms other than the logic of species developed by scholastic thought. In Scotus's case, this meant the attempt to give the individual the same type of intelligibility that Aristotelian thought had given to the species—which is to say, an identification through positive and essential characteristics, not negative and accidental traits.[17] This typology is also a literary strategy, for one can argue that allegorical literature has always sought to give the individual the intelligibility of the general. I would not argue that Garzoni was successful in his attempt to reconceptualize the logic of taxonomy and the categorization of types. In fact, if the Renaissance made little progress in biology, medicine, or the life sciences in general—as opposed to the mathematical sciences—it was because it was incapable of redoing its conceptual matrix and finding discursive models that could deal with the relations of individuals and species other than in set allegorical terms.

As Garzoni shows, he is somewhat contradictory about his method, for he wants to begin with "l'universale": "Ma perche meglio se conosce l'universale, quand si discorre sopra le specie, veniamo pian piano ai passi particolari, que cosi della passia s'havrà quella compita e perfetta cognitione che si ricerca" (*Theatro,* p. 5). Or, to paraphrase, one should go *pian piano* in bending old habits of thought, first going from the better-known universal, when speaking of species, to the particular cases of madness, in order to have that perfect and complete knowledge of madness that we are seeking. I note that knowledge of particulars hardly seems probable if one begins with allegorical abstractions.

For his taxonomy Garzoni takes us, in his work on madness, through a theater qua hospital where we can view thirty individuals who are so many types of the mad, each type itself divided into increasingly arbitrary "species" or subcategories of insanity. These types are illustrated, in good Renaissance style, by a great number of arbitrary anecdotes, taken from the ancients and the moderns, all demonstrating the nature of some absurd form of behavior. Garzoni offers an encyclopedia of anecdotes certainly designed to induce *stupore.* He recycles, for example, Galen's tale of the man who believed he was a head and thus refrained from all activity. Or the modern cases of men who change into wolves at night—lycanthropy being a late medieval obsession. Garzoni may have believed, with Duns Scotus, that the intellect can have direct knowledge of the object before it, but his evidence for the existence of the objects he categorizes is the usual collage of textual citations. He evinces little concern with any principle of relevance for the acceptance or rejection of the information he has so abundantly accumulated.

Literature is the main source of Garzoni's taxonomy, and metamorphosis is its dominant theme. The literary exploration of metamorphosis stimulates Garzoni's fertile mind and leads him in merry pursuit of types for a new taxonomy. He invokes Alcina the Fairy and finds in her palace a source of the magic that works metamorphosis. Alcina was well known to all readers in the Renaissance, for she is Ariosto's seductive fairy in *Orlando Furioso.* When properly viewed with a magic ring, this seductress shows herself to be an ugly crone. The fairy gives thus a demonstration of the way folly works seductively, as a siren song. Madness seduces, though, when properly viewed, it ultimately reveals that it is only a metamorphosis transforming the ugliness of deviance. Garzoni's theater-hospital offers an extended taxonomy whose unifying principle is the magical metamorphosis that defies the stability of rational categories.

The walk through the hospital is remarkable. In each chapter the viewer first finds a title listing one or more of the thirty types of madness that the viewer will then see through the door of a given cell. (And these ideal types of Renaissance madmen are incarcerated.) The first to be seen are the "Frenetici e Deliri," then come the "Maniconici, et Salvatici"—or the melancholic and the withdrawn. These first two cells rather much exhaust the traditional categories of insanity, but the promenade has just begun. Each chapter narrates, moreover, anecdotes, tales, and case studies that illustrate the type, ending with a prayer for help from the appropriate Greco-Roman deity for each case. In the Fourth Discourse, for example, dealing with the Dantesque neglectful or lazy, the "Pazzi Sciperati, o Trascurati," the appropriate titulary god is Apollo. For the drunk or the "Pazzi ubbriati," Garzoni invents the new "Dio Abstemio," while calling upon the traditional Mercury for the dissimulating and Mars for the furious and the bestial.

It seems as if Garzoni were seduced by the textual existence of the gods into believing in them. Existence in language suffices to confer being upon them as well as upon every oddity he can catalog. The world of literary and medical texts offers a realm of metamorphosis that illustrates the infinite possibility of transformations in the imagination of whoever beholds them. In this way Garzoni illustrates one of the common roots of literature and madness. This root is the allurement of the verbal: the ontology of language obliges one to entertain the possibility of the existence of whatever semantic combinations language can put together. In less felicitous times, such as our own, this power usually leads to paranoia, but in Renaissance Italy linguistic fantasy led to less depressing fantasies, such as the invention of new insanities and gods to cure them. Garzoni is seduced by the power of language to create types, in a language game whose principle rule is to maximize the amount of deviance or oddness involved. This rule generates descriptions of madness, by transforming the received and the ordinary, culminating in the Twentieth Discourse with its "Pazzi heterocliti, balzani stroppiati del cervello, o matti spacciati," or the heterogeneously mad, cracked brains, or incurably mad, a category that is the negation of the idea of categories. Language clearly generates these categories as semantically possible pigeonholes, which exist because they can exist in language. In the same vein the weight of language allows Garzoni, in the Twenty-third Discourse, to declare that the "Pazzi bizarri, e furiosi" are mad because the bizarre mad have within them a substance, *bizarria*, that makes them mad.

And in turn to define this new substance as a species of material that is found in the fantastic humors in the body of those who are sick with what is called bizarre and furious madness. Garzoni was hardly the first, or last, to engage in verbal circularity when trying to sort out logos and its opposite, but his example is crucial to show how the literary imagination overlaps the medical in this attempt to find a typology of the real. But the problem is precisely that the imaginary and the real are not necessarily joined by the linkings that language proposes.

Garzoni was perhaps the first writer to identify the asylum and the theatrical stage as having comparable functions in the staging of discourse. This identification was encouraged by the tendency in Italy, and elsewhere, to view the nascent natural-history museum as a theater of nature, and, conversely, nature as a form of theater. The asylum could be taken as a kind of taxonomic museum of the various species of insanity. Beyond the Renaissance tendency, however, the reading of madness as a theatrical allegory is recurrent in our culture, from the Greeks to Freud's view that psychosis is a reworking of the world to fit an Oedipal need. It is evident that Garzoni, like most late medieval minds, could not, in his taxonomy, sort out the ontology of language in terms we recognize as rational. He could not find extralinguistic criteria for the real (a caveat to literary theorists . . .). His mixing of discourses, of the deviant and the theatrical, remains part of what we today recognize as madness: madness is often considered a staging of deviance.

I conclude this discussion of Garzoni's taxonomy by noting that his creation of a special ward for women adds to the historical importance to his work. Certain specificities to women's insanity had been recognized in various and often conflicting ways since the Greeks. For example, only a woman could enjoy the special treatment employed by ancient and medieval doctors when, to cure hysteria, they used perfumed pessaries to entice a wandering uterus back to its proper position. Before Garzoni, however, I know of no other systematic separation of men and women in carceral as well as taxonomic terms. Perhaps there is an homologous relation between the belief in the evil fairy, the feminine principle of seduction and metamorphosis, and the repression of witches as practitioners of the deviant—all this promoted by the same late medieval economy of discourse that confuses the possible, the textual, and the real. Separating women from men in his theater-hospital, Garzoni groups together the "most ridiculous subjects of the feminine mad" that have ever been seen. This hyperbole is part of a fascination with the wiles of deviance, compounded by its presence in women, as well as an aesthetic of wonder based on the possibility of the impossible. The aesthetics of *stupore* underlie Garzoni's announced expectation that the viewer will leave "this inn full of great solace" and that "full of great stupor" he will go through the world preaching and glorifying the horrible madness he has seen. "Stupor" is by our standards at once an aesthetic and epistemological category, for it is an emotive reaction to what one knows the world can produce: the most mad women imaginable. The women also offer an edifying spectacle for the viewers as they go from cell to cell, reading each mad woman's name within, posted, as in an emblem book. There is also a motto above the cell's door to orient the interpretation of her insanity, so that the viewers encounter women as moral exempla. For example, in the case of the mad woman Arnolida Folscia, who in her madness is as free as a horse and is given over to libertine speech and acts, the motto reads "Nil satius." However, identified by a proper name instead of a generic name, each woman is an absolute particular that is nonetheless a universal lesson. It might appear that the desire for taxonomy has given way to the desire to moralize about the feminine particular.

Tasso and the Madness of the Counter Reformation

Theological discourse became increasingly caught up with the determinations of madness as the seventeenth century progressed. The decline of medieval rationality gave rise to belief in diabolical possession, and hence the witch trials, which in turn made a pressing theoretical and practical problem out of the necessity of distinguishing the mad from those possessed by the devil. This necessity added to the problems of medical semiology. If the devil could act in the form of a natural disease, how could the doctor distinguish between madness caused by nature alone and madness caused by the devil? Garzoni's humanistic exuberance about madness was already out of step with the late sixteenth century's anguish about etiology. The master allegory had come apart; the light of reason was defeated everywhere by night; and the diabolical reigned supreme in a world in which judges discovered that the devil seduced children into fornicating with him. Which is to say that, after the supreme ironic rationality found in Erasmus, after Rabelais's exuberant parodies of insanity, and after Ariosto's ludic lyricism about madness, there came an epic fear of madness, which found its epic in the work of Torquato Tasso. His work marks, in many ways, the close of the literary Renaissance, and we can turn to it to see how a fear of madness informs the ideology of cloture.

Tasso (1542–1595) brings to a climax the fear of madness that had grown throughout the Renaissance. By giving epic form to Tasso's own madness while expressing the hysteria of the Counter Reformation, his *Jerusalem Delivered* was probably the most influential poem of the Renaissance. His poem is another attempt to master madness through allegory—madness both personal as well as cultural. I say personal, because Tasso's own insanity was sufficiently acute that his protector, the duke Alphonso II of Este, imprisoned him for it from 1579 to 1586. In a very real sense, then, Tasso was writing from within insanity when he self-consciously created an allegory of the war of eros against reason. The eroticization of madness is dramatized as a vision of malady afflicting civilization. The belief in pandemic madness is all-embracing, and it is instructive to see that this vision of madness is even found in *Aminta,* Tasso's early pastoral drama performed in 1573. In recreating the Virgilian eclogue, with its utopian pan-eroticism, Tasso recasts the pastoral with an alienated hero. In Tasso's drama the poet Aminta is alienated from himself by being "moonstruck" and deprived of his will power. Madness is directly spoken, by a self-consciously alienated self, that speaks of itself as lost. For example, Aminta says that it would do him little good to seek a lover to replace Sylvia, the shepherdess who scorns him:

> Ohime, come poss'io
> altri troverai, se me trovar non posso?
> Se perduto ho me stesso, quale acquisto
> fero mai che mi piaccia?[18]

How, asks Aminta, can he find another if he cannot find himself, and if he has lost himself, what new acquisition could ever bring pleasure? Desire is loss; and his loss of self is concomitant with the eros that overwhelms him. It is difficult to establish a causal relationship in this alienation, for loss and eros seem mutually implicated as they drive the poet into madness.

The Tasso of alienation became a spokesman for the ideology of the Counter Reformation when he explicitly cast madness in the role of the rebellious passion that informs the narration of his *Jerusalem Delivered,* an epic poem based on the first crusade. In his "Allegory of the Poem" Tasso explains that the epic is an allegory of the warring parts of what we and the Greeks would call the psyche, though Tasso's notion of self is defined by allegory. In his view the epic is an allegory in which Godfrey, the Christian leader of the crusaders, "stands for the intellect." He "is elected captain in this enterprise, inasmuch as the intellect is by God and Nature created lord over the other faculties of the soul, and over the body, commanding the former with civil power and the latter with sovereign rule."[19] The subordinate princes stand in turn for the other faculties. Tasso uses Aristotelian terms to explain the dissidence that sets them against the Christian representative of reason: "The love that causes Tancred and the other knights to act foolishly and alienated them from Godfrey, and the wrath that diverts Rinaldo from the enterprise, signify the tension between the rational faculty and the concupiscent and the irascible faculties, and the rebellion of the two" (p. 471). But, in addition to relying upon medical orthodoxy to describe alienation, Tasso also portrays the warring elements as diabolical passions and demons, as the forces of night that Counter Reformation orthodoxy saw at work in the insanity that had swept over Europe during the sixteenth century—when the Reformation and the Turks contributed in equal measure to promote a belief in universal madness.

Jerusalem Liberated is an allegory of, and in, madness that aims at showing a way out of the dark. However, the very conflict of light and dark seems to undermine the epic's conceptual framework. Logos and authority appear inferior to the power of night: the forces of night cloud the light of reason and bring, with apparent ease, the fall into rebellion, sin, and madness. In this regard the work shares all the tensions of the baroque art in whose representations the hysterical flesh of countless sexually driven martyrs belies the allegorical drama of their salvation. In a comparable way the epic hero Rinaldo takes the center stage upon which the forces of night and madness make themselves most manifest. He allows himself to be enchanted by the erotic bliss that the pagan sorceress, Armida, can give him. As we saw in Garzoni, evil can change vision, but not substance, when the devil leads us to view metamorphosis. So Rinaldo must overcome enchanted vision, first in the illusions that eros works upon him, and then in the hallucinations that pagan sorcerers use to keep Christians from having access to wood for a war machine. Rinaldo is the irascible knight whose vision has been enchanted, though the power of eros is such that even the sorceress falls in love with her victim. She leads him to the enchanted islands where Rinaldo, a benighted warrior, passes his days in erotic alienation. These islands make, moreover, an intertextual allusion to and critique of Erasmus's work, for these enchanted islands are no longer the source of the divine benefits that madness worked, in the early Renaissance, when Folly liberated its devotees from the Stoic madness of wanting to be god. In Tasso's poem the enchanted islands are the space wherein unfolds a madness that is in league with the forces of social disorder: diabolical madness is clearly an enemy of the divine logos that founds Christian society.

The early literary Renaissance, with its ironic rationality and playful hopes, lasted scarcely a generation. Erasmus saw the Reformation unfolding before he died. Two generations later what remained of the literary Renaissance was a fearful repression, for eros was tied to madness, to hallucination, black magic, and social disorder, and the fortunate islands had become an antiutopia. To triumph over madness Tasso's Christian king, Godfrey, must repress eros and maintain his rational authority. To this end he uses a converted pagan, conversant with white magic, to empower his warriors so that they in turn can rescue Rinaldo from the maze of desire that defies reason and authority. With hysterical baroque gusto, Tasso pits the irrational against the irrational when a magus, like some follower of the magician Ficino, uses his illumination to make himself the equal of the devil and the pagans in magic arts.

Rinaldo's lascivious loss of reason is portrayed in terms that seem drawn from Ficino's vision of insanity. In his alienation Rinaldo's soul is taken from him, sucked into Armida, leaving only the shell of an emasculated animal. The animal is what Rinaldo sees when he looks at his image in a reflecting shield. The image serves as shock therapy to bring him back to reason so that this irascible successor to Achilles submits finally to order and authority. He rises to his role as the vindicating angel who can, with magical omnipotence, destroy the mad hallucinations that black magic has worked upon the paralyzed Christian army.

Tasso has written in this epic a theodicy that purports to make sense of anything placed within an allegorical framework that unites reason and madness, black and white magic, good and evil. Tasso undoubtedly lived his own madness in terms of this theodicy that makes sense of insanity in terms of God's design. In this regard Tasso has reverted to earlier medieval views. Tasso also used the late medieval belief in white and black magic to give language to his own madness. Like Hoccleve, he writes his madness in terms of the possibilities of discourse at his disposition—and perhaps works out his insanity by integrating it into the great drama of Christendom's threatened demise at the hands of the forces of darkness—pagans, magicians, protestants, witches, and all the other agents of madness. Mad Tasso enacted in his epic a symbolic triumph over madness and the magic forces that, in his own life, he could not control. But a symbolic triumph is perhaps more important for the late medieval self than for the modern, for the distinction of personal and private seems more tenuous for the self that we intuit in Tasso, a self not yet locked into the metaphysics of subjective and objective. The madness that destroys the political and social fabric could perhaps be more directly experienced as the same madness that visits voices and visions on the demented. For this self, allegory was not yet a mere rhetorical figure.

The late medieval mind, such as in Paracelsus as well as Tasso, viewed the mad as thrown back onto the elemental forces of nature, forces that are outside of logos. In this view madness has all the naturalness of a stone or a river or the fall of night. When night besieges the Christians in *Jerusalem Delivered,* madness is allied to the exterior forces of nature. The overthrow of reason is an event over which no form of reason has power, for it comes upon the world with all the inevitability of the setting of the sun. This is not yet the naturalness of a Shakespeare for whom allegory is but a figure and logos is no longer a divine guarantee of rationality: this naturalism springs from an experience of madness as a natural rhythm leading to the dissolution of being outside of logos.

Tasso's view that madness is part of the cosmic sphere corresponds perhaps to what we would call today projection, for the dissolution of the light of logos and nature can be interpreted as the poet's projection onto the world of his inner anguish and turmoil. Yet projection does not seem quite right, insofar as the late medieval self, alone in a world that was increasingly bereft of solace, if not of devils and witches, did not live clearly this distinction of self and other that is the hallmark of post-Cartesian modernity. And allegory could express that condition of self by symbolizing relations in which self and other are fused is an objective world of discourse—objective in the sense that this discourse was within the purview of all members of society. Allegory is vouchsafed its rationality since it is an expression of objective truth and logos. By writing allegory, the poet and doctor could enter an objective order that made madness manifest, and in which the individual self was in a sense not totally burdened by the weight of the sin of insanity. In allegory madness participated in the realm of ordered logos as part of God's plan. We suspect that in some existential sense Tasso's experience of madness was not totally congruent with the allegorical discourse that was supposed to make sense of it. But until the reign of allegory came to an end, there was no other form of discourse by which madness could enter the light of public experience. Literature and medicine are bound up together in this language game, in the discourse of allegory, that ordered the possibilities of experience. But this was soon to come to an end. With Shakespeare, Cervantes, and Descartes, the possibility of speaking madness was soon to be radically altered, for these three figures demonstrate reordered possibilities of discourse that allowed us to reach back to Greek rationality and to move forward, if forward has any meaning in this context, to our modernity.

Chapter 3

Madness and Early Modernity in Shakespeare, Cervantes, and Descartes

Du Laurens and the Continuing Galenic Orthodoxy

Galenic orthodoxy lived on into the seventeenth century, though it underwent a change as a form of allegory. This change in its status is essential, for the devaluation of allegory is a prelude to much that we take to be modern. Therefore, in order to give a backdrop and a context for my later analysis of innovation and changes in the seventeenth century, I want first to discuss a version of the medical orthodoxy about madness that dominated the first part of the century, one in which the change of the status of medical discourse is clear. Perhaps there is no better medical figure in this regard than the French doctor André Du Laurens (or Dulaurens), the rector of the medical school at Montpellier, a physician to Henry IV, and the author of medical treatises in both Latin and, more importantly, French. In fact, he wrote one of the first best-sellers about madness in his often published and translated *Discours de la conservation de la veue: Des maladies melancholiques: des catarrhes: & de la vieillesse* (1597). Dealing eclectically with eye problems, old age, runny noses, and insanity, this may be the first mental health manual for the nonmedical reader. Addressing himself as much to an aristocratic public as to a growing number of doctors and surgeons with little Latin, the royal physician also served an ideological function by rejecting the excesses of doctors like Paracelsus and Agrippa. This rejection took the form of a call for a return to medical and political orthodoxy. Political rebellion, religious dissent, and medical heresy, these were all interpreted as attacks on rationality—which reflected the strongly felt need for order after years of war between Protestants and Catholics (but the worst was yet to come, of course, in Germany).

In this work on madness in French as well as in his voluminous neo-Galenic medical writing in Latin, Du Laurens (dead in 1609) was not an original figure. He was, however, probably the most influential doctor of his time because of his position and his orthodoxy, especially in consolidating the position of Galen in the universities—which in effect meant the universities had largely ceased to be places where philosophical and scientific thought might develop. In theorizing about insanity Du Laurens was an eclectic who reflects the changes in the interpretation of Galen that took place after the Renaissance. The major change in orthodoxy about madness is found in Du Laurens's belief that madness is a form of bestiality. This bestiality is not to be interpreted as a theological or a Neoplatonic allegory. The mad are not allegorical animals, they *are* simply animals:

> Consider the action of a frenetic or a maniac, you'll find nothing human there; he bites, he screams, he bellows with a savage voice, rolls burning eyes, his hair stands on end, he throws himself about and often kills himself so. Look at a melancholic and how he lowers himself so that he becomes a companion of beasts and only likes solitary places.[1]

In Du Laurens's description the mad stare at us like animals, representing some incongruous rupture in the social fabric. They have fallen out of logos, and therefore they have no claim on our commiseration since they have disappeared as participants in shared social reality. In a deep sense the mad no longer have any interest for a human science like medicine.

This exclusion of the mad from medical interest corresponds to the ideology of a humanism that sought obsessively to serve the glorification of mankind. Du Laurens shares Ficino's Platonist views that eroticism is a source of madness and rivals him in looking for hyperbole describing the fall it brings about. For the humanist, man is the image of God; he is the summit and goal of creation, and in madness the spark of divine logos is extinguished as pure animal nature asserts itself. Madness is interpreted as a kind of deicide. To explain this inconceivable extension of the divine, Du Laurens draws upon Aristotelian terminology as if the Philosopher might rationalize the impossible. In madness one gives into irascibility or concupiscence, which is to say, one of the two inferior powers of the soul that can extinguish reason and its divine light. In this terminology surfaces a recurrent fear of animality, of flesh and desire, of the human body, but it also points to the insecurity of this moment when the insane hatreds of the wars of religion had made the divine a questionable category. The same fear underwrites the panegyric on the wonders of man with which Du Laurens prefaces a volume of his general medical works. In this work Du Laurens can, in an obsessive fashion, give twenty-four specific differences between animals and mankind, but he is hard pressed to find four reasons to admire the human body.

The seventeenth century begins, then, with its most influential doctor giving voice to the fear of the body that Ficino had earlier developed and to which Tasso had given epic expression. Trying to defend the rational state, in all senses of the term, Du Laurens is still writing ideology, one dramatizing Counter Reformation struggles, but this is ideology in which allegory has been demoted. Allegory still has a role, to be sure; and if the lover is more of an animal than the melancholic, it is because his lust incites him to rebel against reason. In this now banal allegory, love is insanity since it brings about sedition against the sovereign. And insanity in the individual is analogous to madness in society when rebellion tries to overthrow institutionalized reason.

I am not certain that Du Laurens would have seen that he is writing a banal allegory, or quasi allegory. In fact he believed that he could positively describe the "physiology" of love in terms of medical causality, a causality based in equal measure on Galenic physiology and troubadour notions of courtly love. The objective cause of love is first seen by the eyes. Thereupon the image is conveyed to the liver, the seat of concupiscence. The lover alone would be too weak to conspire against sovereign reason, so the liver calls upon the heart. Together these two attack reason and "all its noble powers" and take him prisoner or rather make a slave of reason (p. 162). And this process then gives rise to the well-known clinical syndrome *melancholie amoureuse*. This syndrome can also be viewed as Aristotle updated with the platitudes of medieval lyric poetry. However, Du Laurens gives it a moral emphasis that is new. His hyperbolic moral admonitions point up how problematic eros has become in a culture that could no longer accommodate dissent—or admit desire that goes beyond prescribed limits. In his desire to drive madness from the public space of cultural awareness, Du Laurens goes on, insanely one might claim, to say that no one should consider love a sweet passion, since it is the most miserable of miserable things, and not even the hellish tortures of the worst tyrants can surpass love's cruelty (or as he phrases it, "toutes les gehennes des plus ingenieux tyrans n'en surpassent jamais la cruauté" [p. 164]). Psychological distress is accompanied by physiological destruction, since love dries up the humor, and the body's temperature is thereupon corrupted.

These are hysterically well meant clichés. Platitudes are compounded here by a desire to assure a center to public discourse and to the power legitimized by that discourse. By attributing magic powers to eros, the power to transform a rational being into an animal, the physiology of insane eros also shows at the same time how it is possible that the sovereign—reason, state, Church, or monarch—can lose power to the irrational, for this allegory works micro- and macrocosmically. A complete genealogy of this dominant medical discourse would point out its Stoic antecedents with the renewal of the idea that passions are insanity. The pre-Socratic equation of state and body has also been pressed into service: in the seventeenth century the body became an intensely political allegorical figure for the state. And with this, insanity was conceived in turn as something to be driven out of the "body politick," to use the seventeenth-century metaphor. Conversely, from the confessional to the courtroom, the sinful and insane body became the object of the greatest scrutiny, a political scrutiny that looked for the insane body in hopes of eliminating it.

Late Renaissance medicine thus wanted to exclude madness from its purview by justifying its exclusion from society. Metamorphosis of the mad into animals prepared the way for some two centuries of extraordinarily harsh treatment of the insane at the hands of captors who had medical license to treat the incarcerated as if they were chattel. But I would propose that, at this moment in the early seventeenth century, medicine ceased for a number years to have any intellectual authority. Du Laurens can serve as a model as to why doctors lost their authority. This medical vacuum, I further propose, allowed other thinkers and writers to face the challenge of tracing the frontiers between reason and unreason, or the lines of demarcation setting off the rational and the irrational. These new lines of demarcation accompanied the emergence of a new sense of self: primary to this sense of self was the belief that it is located in a world that the self could affirm has a rational structure. This shift accompanied the demise of late medieval allegorical medicine. With this newly conceived self, madness became a different object of discourse. If my readers are willing to entertain the hypothesis that a new concept of self, and a new experience of the self, emerged in the early seventeenth century—and this idea has been suggested by many other thinkers—they may grant me the following proposition: it was primarily in nonmedical writers that this new sense of self allowed to emerge new concepts as to what the insane self might be. To elaborate this thesis I turn now to the work of Shakespeare, Cervantes, and Descartes, three writers in whose work madness and its relation to the world are treated in different, but innovative, ways that contributed to the developing history of the concept of madness. In brief, as allegory ceased to be the dominant mode of discourse, these three writers, perhaps more than any others, were essential for establishing modern discourses on madness.

In discussing the first important modern playwright, modern novelist, and modern philosopher, I want to demonstrate that literature and philosophy preceded medicine in the creation of the space of rationality that allows for the understanding of madness for the next three centuries. Fundamental to this process was the secularizing of madness. This secularization demanded that the world not be read as allegory and asserted that the ultimate court of truth could no longer be the great theodicy. In one sense this change is self-evident, as are the many crucial factors that brought about this transformation: the Copernican revolution, the slow demise of the Eurocentric vision of the West, the transformations of physics and mathematics, to name a few of the most obvious. My thesis about madness is perhaps less evident, though it presupposes the changing cultural matrix in which the work of Galileo and Kepler, the transformations of geographical and astronomical knowledge, and the invention of the printing press have had their effect. I propose that in Shakespeare, Cervantes, and Descartes we can read the displacements of rationality that for the first time since the Greeks allow us to make sense of madness in new ways. Shakespeare is probably the most sensitive recorder of the secularizing process that stripped madness of its allegorical and religious dimensions. In Shakespeare's work it is portrayed as a dislocation that is open to interrogation. In his plays it is subject to interpretation; and hermeneutics becomes part of the process of reading madness. In Cervantes's *Don Quixote* (1605 and 1615) this secularization is evident and in a sense completed. Madness is interpreted in a world in which truth-values have come to have universal claim. The realm of the possible and the impossible are separated out and incorporated in a worldview that, in the name of the rational, can make universal claims for its beliefs. The role of the marvelous knight of the sad countenance is to negotiate, in madness, these realms that madness cannot sort out. Finally, Descartes's philosophical works describe a world defined in terms of universal truth-values. Set against this objective world, the self is defined as a subjective enclosure that has no commonality with the world of physics. In such works as the *Discourse on Method* and *Meditations on First Philosophy,* as well as in works on psychology and physiology, Descartes inaugurated the dualism of self and world that is the starting point of medical psychology for the modern era. However, with the invention of the enclosure of subjectivity, understanding madness becomes singularly difficult.

Shakespeare and the Hermeneutics of Madness

A sense of a secular order emerges in Shakespeare's works, though in fits and starts, with remnants of late medieval thought and beliefs embedded in what sometimes appears to be a rushing torrent of secularizing beliefs. In

the plays madness is not tied to any theological allegory or belief in possession, though Shakespeare's characters may at times, reflecting their belief in
medical or religious orthodoxy, allude to the humors' determination of
character or to pathology based on humors, or they may believe any number of superstitions and fantasies about illness and madness. No medical or
religious system is proposed by Shakespeare's plays. Taken as a totality they
seem at times grounded in a belief in some order of things, though equally
often they demonstrate that, for no apparent reason, things come apart. The
gods make sport of us, and madness and dissolution are part of the elemental order of things. Against this backdrop madness is another form of disorder that all—character and spectator—must interpret as best they can.

To illustrate the omnipresence of Shakespeare's hermeneutics in his
plays, I shall deal first with a play in which madness is not an obvious problem, and then turn to those major tragedies, *Hamlet* and *Lear,* that can
focus attention on how pervasive madness is in Shakespeare's work. For
example, in *All's Well That Ends Well* the king of France is ill with some
disorder that threatens to end his life. By threatening the sovereign, this malady endangers the social order. At the play's outset the dilemma is to find a
doctor to cure a king. The play asks if there is any remedy for illness in this
era in which magical and religious cures are no longer to be trusted, or as
Lord Lafew hesitantly observes in words that are hardly joyous about the
secularization that he sees unfolding:

> They say miracles are past, and we have our philosophical persons, to make
> modern and familiar, things supernatural and causeless. Hence it is that we
> make trifles of terrors, ensconcing ourselves into seeming knowledge when
> we should submit ourselves to an unknown fear. (2.3)

The king's illness has not been explained, much less cured, for the disease
lies beyond the power of "philosophical persons" to deal with it. The
"unknown fear" remains then as the object of inquiry after orthodox medicine has lost its authority. And Shakespeare insists on the failure of both
orthodoxy and the new medicine, for the king has been "relinquish'd of all
the artists," both "of Galen and Paracelsus." With the failure of the opposing sides of Renaissance medicine the king must be given up as incurable
until Helena, a doctor's daughter, can effect a cure that saves the king and
thus the body politic.

Shakespeare grants no insight into what kind of medicine Helena practices, which I take to be another sign of the medical vacuum created by medicine's loss of credibility at this historical juncture. She cures the king, and
he in turn grants her wish to have the aristocrat Bertram for a husband. This

royal gift sets up the context for a young man's rebellion and relevant questions about his madness. For Bertram wants no part in this marriage and, rather than obey the king, flees to Italy. Through much ingenuity Helena takes the place of Bertram's intended mistress and wins him back by obliging him to fulfill his vow to have her only if she beds him and gets a ring from him. Modern viewers may find Bertram's refusal of an arranged marriage quite understandable. The king, however, finds madness in the young man's refusal to obey, as demonstrated when the king laments to Bertram's mother about the supposed death of Helena:

> We lost a jewel of her, and our esteem
> Was made much poorer by it: but your son,
> As mad in folly, lacked the sense to know
> Her estimation home.

To which the mother replies that her son's madness was a "Natural rebellion, done i' the blaze of youth" that was too strong for reason to control (5.3).

From the king's point of view Bertram's madness consists in not seeing the real, not evaluating the true, and in defying that sovereign—the king and reason—whose commands define the order of reality. This all sounds like Counter Reformation medical theory on madness, and the mother only underscores this view in interpreting her son's acts as a rebellion against reason. However, it is clear that in this context these accusations and definitions are to be taken as rhetorical: madness is defined by metaphors designating a state of blindness, or by an allegorical figure about the nature of mad action. These figures are not embedded in any larger allegory. There is no encompassing allegorical pattern to make sense of Bertram's mad rebellion or Helena's doggedness. And this is unsettling.

In *All's Well That Ends Well*, Shakespeare begins by declaring the helplessness of medical theories, which opens a vacuum, an empty epistemological space, in which doctrines are suspended. With that suspension we must seek to interpret, by our own lights, the phenomena we confront. There is no overarching allegory to tell the viewer whether Bertram is an insane rebel, an ingrate, or a normal young man. There is nothing to bring the allegory to closure and put an end to interpretation with a category that makes of him a mad rebel or perhaps the victim of a scheming young woman—or a madman for not wanting to marry the most beautiful jewel in the kingdom. The characters themselves use figural language, metaphorical and allegorical, but the rhetorical figures have meaning only in the dialectical exchange between the characters. One can argue that Bertram is a dubious case of madness, even if he is mad by Du Laurens's as well as the king's definition. The same dubiety holds for those major cases of madness that are Shakespeare's major creations: Macbeth, Hamlet, Lear. This dubiety demands that madness be interpreted: hermeneutics is a necessity in a sense that the Western world had not seen before. Shakespeare posits interpretation as a necessity in plays that propose madness as a condition inextricably linked to discourse and context. Madness is a relation that must be situated.

Is Hamlet mad? In the second scene of act 4 it would appear that Rosencrantz thinks so, for the king's servant cannot understand Hamlet when Hamlet takes him for a sponge. If taken literally, Hamlet's speech is mad:

> Ay, sir that soaks up the king's countenance, his rewards, his authorities. But such officers do the king best service in the end: he keeps them, like an ape, in the corner of his jaw: first mouthed, to be last swallowed.

If taken metaphorically in this context, however, the sponge metaphor can be interpreted to mean that Hamlet understands his situation, that there is "reason in madness" here or at least a method behind it. Rhetorical interpretation takes away from insane discourse some of its madness. The need to interpret shifts, then, the center of discourse: where do we or the characters in *Hamlet* find the criteria for reading what is rhetorical and what is madness? Moreover, Shakespeare dramatizes the danger that we and the characters create the meaning we find in mad discourse simply by imposing our hermeneutical net on it. Hamlet himself occupies no privileged place in this respect, since he is as uncertain as any other observer, at times believing he can interpret his situation, and at times doubting his sanity, for example, at the end when he apologizes to Laertes for his deeds born of madness.

By stressing Shakespeare's staging of interpretation and uncertainty, it might appear that I am arguing that Shakespeare is Kafka's contemporary. This is not entirely the case, since a late medieval worldview also surfaces throughout Shakespeare's work. Hamlet does see a ghost at the play's outset, and others see it, too. Yet Hamlet later chalks up the ghost's apparition to the possibility that it is partially produced by his madness, his weakness and his melancholy (2.2). Ghosts are subject to interpretation as much as any other phenomena. Moreover, after killing Polonius in his mother's chamber, Hamlet alone sees the ghost who chides him. This apparition seems analogous to those found in scenes like those in *Macbeth* in which Macbeth apparently sees witches, but later is visited by clear hallucinations born of near madness, first in the form of the dagger, then in Banquo's ghost. Hamlet's mother interprets Hamlet's behavior with the ghost in her chamber as a product of his ecstasy—the Elizabethan term for alienation—

much as does Lady Macbeth when the king has lost his mind. These examples point up that Shakespeare's works use medieval views of possibility and modern views of naturalistic probability by conjoining them, juxtaposing them, and letting the characters and spectators work out their interpretations.

This is essential: the guiding intelligence informing the play's action never allows certainty to characterize these phenomena. Hermeneutics are part of the experience of the phenomena themselves—of ghosts and hallucinations and mad words and deeds. Things and acts, words and apparitions themselves, demand direct interpretation, and are not to be explained by other texts, especially by the world of the transcendent text of the Christian master allegory. There is no drama of redemption. If order is to be found in Shakespeare's world, it is found in the order of phenomena themselves. Beyond itself, this world knows no allegory and no theodicy that would define and justify the relations of things in the world.

The disjuncture of phenomena and interpretation is found throughout *Hamlet,* and it underlies the way other characters interpret Hamlet and he interprets himself. Hermeneutics is staged in all the encounters among the characters. When, for example, his mother enjoins Hamlet to recognize that he "seems" to take his father's death as if it were particular to him, he rebukes her in lines that show a new sense of interpretive self-consciousness:

> Seems, madam! Nay, it is; I know not "seems."
> 'Tis not alone my inky cloak, good mother,
> Nor customary suits of solemn black,
> Nor windy suspiration of forc'd breath,
> No, nor the fruitful river in the eye,
> Nor the dejected haviour of the visage,
> Together with all forms, woes, shows of grief,
> That can denote me truly; these, indeed, seem,
> For they are actions that a man might play:
> But I have that within which passeth show;
> These but the trappings and the suits of woe.
>
> (1.2)

Exterior signs are mere "denotation." They can be aped and acted out, and thus they are incommensurate with some sincere expression of inner feelings. The self is split here, torn between its exterior expression relying upon signs that are subject to interpretation, and an inner being that should somehow be beyond interpretation—but which isn't, as Hamlet discovers to his chagrin. This demand for interpretation is a new way of defining self, and it complicates what madness and the self it afflicts might be. To use nondenotative signs, to use rhetoric to signify an inner self, is merely, as Hamlet knows, to open up more interpretive necessities. Perhaps Hamlet's madness is to be explained in part as his anguish about his incapacity to find a language expressing his innerness in ways that are beyond interpretation.

The other characters crowd in upon Hamlet with the interpretations they extract from the exterior signs of his madness. In the first act Horatio states the problem of interpretation and madness when he warns Hamlet that his interpretations of the ghost may be a snare for his reason:

> What if it tempt you toward the flood, my lord,
> Or to the dreadful summit of the cliff
> That beetles o'er his base into the sea,
> And there assume some other horrible form,
> Which might deprive your sovereignty of reason
> And draw you into madness?
>
> (1.2)

It seems that each character has a theory of madness to apply to Hamlet, and, in this context, Horatio's theory recalls a case by the Renaissance taxonomist Garzoni, one in which *stupore* cracks the brain through an excess of impressions that are too large for mere reason to encompass. The Renaissance belief that all is possible does not entail, for Horatio, that it might be possible for reason to tolerate all.

Ophelia's father, the sententious if not addled Polonius, has another theory for Hamlet's insanity, the theory of eros as madness that might well appeal to fathers with daughters as well as to Neoplatonists. Polonius finds that his daughter's rebuffing Hamlet "hath made him mad" (2.1). The cause of Hamlet's enigmatic behavior is the "ecstasy of love"—meaning quite literally the insanity brought on by eros—"whose violent property fordoes [kills] itself / And leads the will to desperate undertakings / As oft as any passion under heaven." This Stoic identification of passion and insanity, placed in the mouth of the old pontificator, says much about the status of this cliché in the early seventeenth century. Polonius is not, however, a total fool; rather, he is a compendium of received thought. In his attempts to interpret Hamlet he even senses that the rhetorical turns of Hamlet's speech convey more than mere passion or the wiles of the libido. There is method in the madness, to quote Polonius as he puzzles at the wit and double meanings Hamlet uses: "How pregnant sometimes his replies are! a happiness that often madness hits on, which reason and sanity could not so prosperously be delivered of" (2.2). Madness can display reason, and it can even suggest richer meanings than mere sanity. Or at least interpretation finds in madness new meanings, as well as a rhetoric that competes for credibility with the rhetoric of rationality.

This discovery singularly complicates the task of interpretation and of finding the line of demarcation between madness and reason. Even befuddled Guildenstern, the soon-to-be-beheaded messenger, must recognize the hermeneutic problems of dealing with what the king calls "turbulent and dangerous lunacy," but which Guildenstern suspects to be "crafty madness" (3.1). That madness has meaning obliges each character to be something of a psychiatrist, attempting to reason about Hamlet's unreason. The king has his doubts about the nature of Hamlet's affliction, for, as he puts it, there is more than mere unreason upon which Hamlet's "melancholy sits on brood" (3.1). The materialist queen thinks Hamlet's hallucination in her chamber is an "ecstasy" produced by his brain. And when Hamlet tells his beloved Ophelia to go to an nunnery, she describes his madness, in rather Neoplatonic terms, as both a form of rebellion and as a disequilibrium produced by a lack of harmony:

> O! what a noble mind is here o'erthrown. . . .
> And I, of ladies most deject and wretched . . .
> Now see that noble and most sovereign reason,
> Like sweet bells jangled, out of tune and harsh.
>
> (3.1)

In a mind "here o'erthrown," Du Laurens would have seen an image of rebellion and subversion in which the supreme part of the soul has been subjected to the dominion of its subordinates—an image of psychic disequilibrium at least as old as Plato's *Republic*. But this is hardly the final interpretation, for Hamlet himself equivocates, at once interpreting himself as deranged and then proclaiming to his mother that he is mad in craft alone. Hamlet's stance leaves open the disquieting possibility that his is the greatest madness, self-conscious, and self-denying, interpreting his own madness as feigned when he is mad.

My point is not, after several generations of psychoanalysts, to put Hamlet once again on the couch. Rather I want to stress the historical importance of the fact that in Shakespeare's work one finds the opening of a space in which contextualization demands interpretation. This demand is by and large a new way of treating madness, and this is as true of *Lear* or *Macbeth* as of *Hamlet*. Madness is not the metamorphosis of some psychic or physiological substance. It is a question of defining and then interpreting relations. It means interpreting the question as to whether, within the context of their situation, characters' acts and discourse deviate into the nonrelation of insanity—or, more interestingly, whether insanity can maintain a relation to a context of shared meanings. Hamlet's example obliged one to ask if, in this world of hermeneutic necessity, even madness can interrogate itself, with all the possible paradoxes that self-referential discourse can have. Is the statement "I am mad," spoken by an insane person, a rational statement? On the model of the classical paradox of the Cretan liar, Hamlet offers us the modern paradox of the rational madman.

Shakespeare's other great madman, King Lear, can enrich this argument. The raving king has been variously interpreted by critics as sane, as a victim of mere irascibility or, later in the play, as struck with feverish delirium. However, within the play, Kent judges Lear to be mad in the very first act (1.1). Kent sees from the outset, I think, that Lear cannot judge how language functions. Asking his daughters how much they love him, Lear cannot see that, in their answers, his daughters Goneril and Regan use hyperbole, or figural language. Lear takes this language literally. Conversely, when he hears the literal language of his honest daughter Cordelia, he takes it as figural language and disowns her for not loving him. Lear cannot interpret the literal, and I, as Kent does, would interpret this incapacity to interpret as a serious mental disturbance. Like many medieval minds, he confuses the literal with the rhetorical, the existential with the semantic. In the context of the play these confusions must be further interpreted. And all—including Regan and Goneril—pursue this deciphering.

Lear is interpreted by every character. His fool sees in him a fool, which provides an image of hermeneutic mirroring among characters who are also foils to madness. Facing this foil Lear interprets his own distress as madness and implores the gods, in an outcry that harks back to the Greek determination of tragedy, not to inflict insanity upon him. In the play of foils, then, the fool seems to be what Lear should be, which is an image of wisdom in madness. Kent himself, though he has judged Lear to be mad, attempts to defend the king's interests, and for this he is called a deranged subject and put in stocks. The disinherited son Edgar also mirrors madness in the play of foils and misleading interpretations: he chooses the role of a Bedlam beggar. He is driven to act the madman after the bastard Edmund, in villainy bordering on insanity, has falsely accused him of wanting to murder their father Gloucester.

The betrayed Gloucester has his own interpretation of madness. Blind Gloucester longs for madness as a balm that would help him through the intolerable night, and envies the madness he perceives in the king:

The king is mad. How stiff is my vile sense,
that I stand up, and have ingenious feeling
Of my huge sorrows! Better I were distract.
So should my thoughts be fenced from my griefs,
And woes by wrong imaginations lose
The knowledge of themselves.

(4.6)

Gloucester positively evaluates the comfort that "wrong imaginations" might bring. Madness is a positive experience in the world that is already invaded by night—and with this evaluation Gloucester proposes a positive experience of insanity that contrasts totally with the medical view that would make of the insane fallen animals. Shakespeare's pivotal example demonstrates that at the beginning of the seventeenth century, in spite of the sclerosis of medicine, it became possible to view madness as something other than an accident produced by humors, or diabolical possession, or animal lust, or the position of the stars—to evoke the principle fantasies that had allayed our fear of madness. Madness in *Hamlet* and *King Lear* is a position in a context, a relation that must be interpretively explored, and one that can be positively evaluated. In fine Shakespeare offers an understanding of madness unsurpassed since the Greeks.

Cervantes and the Order of the Real

The most important critique of the excesses of the Renaissance views of madness is probably Cervantes's *Don Quixote* and its portrayal of insanity and insanity's relation to the order of the real. Like Shakespeare, Cervantes often seems an ambiguous figure, at once late medieval and modern. But he is clearly modern for having written the novel that created the type of narrative embodying truth-values that make universal claims vouchsafed by rational criteria as to what truth-values are. This feat was accomplished by setting the claims of reality against the claims of madness that Don Quixote embodies. Don Quixote is the knight errant who has read all the books that once defined the ideals of Western culture. He lives in the intertextual collage of all narrations that, for the Renaissance, for Agrippa and for Garzoni, defined the real. However, the Renaissance world of interrelating texts, if taken to be the world, has become the realm of madness. Don Quixote, as all have noted, takes literature seriously; but more than that, he takes seriously the late medieval belief that all forms of textuality can enter into the realm of the possible. Don Quixote, with a mad coherence, lives out the logic of late medieval epistemology. As Foucault might have argued, Quixote's project demonstrates with comic rationality that to hold onto a worldview, once its discursive practices are no longer accepted, is to be mad. Or as Wittgenstein might have said, Don Quixote quite literally plays language games by medieval rules—but the framework of rationality, in which these rules made sense, has changed, or was rapidly changing, no doubt in part because Cervantes wrote *Don Quixote.*

Two salient facts characterize this novel: in it the modern novel is born with the demise of allegory, and its hero is a madman. His madness is literal, not figural, or allegorical. The novel states, with some self-directed irony, that Don Quixote read too many fantastic knightly romances and his brains dried up. Thereupon he decides to emulate Amadis of Gaul and becomes a knight errant. By attributing this madness to dried brains, Cervantes gives a parodistic nod to Renaissance medical theory, but the real question that this madness brings up is the relation of discourse to context, and especially to historical context. For Cervantes's comic stance marks off his distance from medical discourse, and it is somewhat misguided to believe, as have some critics, that medical theory had an influence on the way the novel represents madness.

Of course Cervantes, like all educated people at the beginning of the seventeenth century, was familiar with medical writings on madness, such as Juan Huartes's *Examen de ingenios para las ciencias,* a widely read neo-Galenic work dealing with temperaments and capacities for education. Cervantes knew that, according to Huartes, all character types and natural capacities are due to combinations of only three qualities: heat, moisture, and dryness in the brain.[2] Excessive dryness interferes with the work of reason and judgment, but not with the work of the imagination. Cervantes alludes to this theory of dried brains when referring to textually induced madness, but precisely to underscore the comic inadequacy of medical orthodoxy. No medical explanation could account for the way Don Quixote uses the rules for antiquated language games to sustain his project to live in a medieval intertextual collage. To buttress my argument, I note that Cervantes's distance from medical discourse and its capacity to explain madness is found, moreover, in the story of the *Novelas ejemplares* called "El licenciado vidriera" (The pane-glass student). In this story a student goes mad when he is given an aphrodisiac by a woman intent on seducing him. Cervantes's skepticism with regard to medical "potions" is obvious in this tale of a boy who believes he is made out of glass. A love potion is hardly an etiology, and medical discourse has nothing to add to this ironic explanation of madness.

If there is an "etiology" for Don Quixote's madness, it begins with the rules of discourse that had prevailed through the Renaissance. Like many a late medieval reader, Don Quixote is lost in a world of discourse. He is a victim of language's capacity to sustain itself with appeal to its own autonomous structure, its own rules, its own self-referential justifications. Language is reason and unreason, and Don Quixote's madness is quite literally a product of texts:

> So odd and foolish, indeed, did he grow on this subject that he sold many acres of cornland to buy these books of chivalry to read, and in this way brought home every one he could get. And of them all he considered none so good as the works of the famous Feliciano de Silva. For this brilliant style and those complicated sentences seemed to him very pearls, especially when he came upon those love-passages and challenges frequently written in the manner of: "The reason for the unreason with which you treat my reason, so weakens my reason that with reason I complain of your beauty."[3]

Don Quixote loses his "reason," for he is lost in language games for which he misapplies rules. Renaissance doctors had given ample precedent for this misapplication of rules. By the early seventeenth century it was clear to a Cervantes, as it had been to a Rabelais or an Erasmus, to what extent many readers and writers were unable to sort out the fictional, the fantastic, and the order of the real according to the rules of language use for which possible and impossible were quite separate categories. I stress process, and not rupture in this context, for if a Machiavelli announced procedures for a quick understanding of the real as objective power, it took more than a century for this understanding to dominate educated Europe. Confusion of the language of the real with literary language, with its special rules for suspending disbelief, continued into the seventeenth century—as witness the witch trials. But this confusion was also becoming a description of insanity—as witnesses Don Quixote.

This is not to say that, beyond dried brains, medical theory is not part of the novel. References to medicine are instructive. For example, Cervantes makes Sancho submit to a doctor in the second part of *Don Quixote* where, after Sancho has finally received a governorship of an island, the medical expert makes him starve. The doctor is in the employment of the duke who has arranged the deceit that makes Sancho think that he is at last a governor. But this framework only heightens the comic madness that Sancho perceives in the doctor, a follower of Galen, who uses medical jargon to exercise control over what Don Quixote's fleshy squire may eat. The doctor's Latin is the mark of abusive power, for he can deprive Sancho of food merely by uttering, "Omnis saturatio mala, perdicis autem pessima," a burlesque rephrasing of Hippocrates meaning, "All surfeit is bad, but that of partridges is worst" (p. 765). The comedy marks two forms of deviance here. First, it points up Sancho's less than ideal commitment to the earthly and the fleshly, for his first allegiance is to what the Russian critic Bakhtin called the nether regions of the body. In context this seems a mark of sanity. Second, comedy marks the deviance of medical discourse in its fraudulent claims to explain the empirical world. The critique of medicine shows that it is fraudulent, which puts medicine in alliance with the mad abuse of texts that has driven Quixote mad. Only Molière would push this point with more vehemence.

A doctor is also present when Don Quixote dies at the novel's end. His diagnosis is that the knight dies from grief and melancholy. Since Don Quixote has recovered his wits at the end, then melancholy must be taken as a condition of sanity. To this irony about diagnosis Cervantes adds Sancho's claim that it would be the greatest madness to die because one had become sane again. Erasmus's sense of the positive value of madness undoubtedly lies behind these ironic twists satirizing doctors. Don Quixote's death is due to his losing his madness, which is to say, to his being obliged to embrace the framework of empirical reality that has set off his madness in all its comic grandeur. He dies when he can finally sort out orders of discourse and levels of reality. After he has acquired that capacity, then, in simply textual terms, Don Quixote no longer exists. He could only exist in the mad language of literature—which is indeed the case.

None of this owes anything to medicine, nor to theological discourse. Don Quixote is a good and reasonable Catholic, but this is incidental to his madness. Catholicism is a common belief that makes up the backdrop of shared social reality. His madness is centered on a world of discourse allowing his belief in knight errantry, and this belief can be explained neither by humors, nor by possession theory. This is to say that medicine and theology have little to say about the ordering of truth-values that make up the empirical world of the novel, a world embodying truth-values that have a demonstrable claim to universal validity. And this demonstrability is the strength of Cervantes's exploration of madness: he shows, comically and empirically, that nothing is at work in the empirical world that is not part of the order of nature about which there is universal agreement. And universal agreement is a precondition for speaking about the empirical. Truth-values are independent of language, texts, and their (often) fictional systems. Moreover, nothing can contravene the universal order of this world. Don Quixote's belief in magic, enchantment, and the possible impossibility of contravening the world's order is by definition now a sign of madness. And since he is mad, his very belief is a proof that this contravening is impossible. Madness has become part of the criteria for truth: it is now part of untruth. With comic clarity the line of demarcation between the universal order of truth-values and the belief in the possibility of the violation of that order is clearly drawn. The very notion of boundary acquires new clarity in *Don Quixote,* and for the first time since the Greeks the line between reason and unreason exists as part of epistemology.

The line of demarcation is also embodied in Don Quixote's worldview, for he is not insane on every subject, nor is his insanity devoid of reason and consistencies that endow it with meaning. And Don Quixote can constantly use reason to adjust his insanity to the regularities of empirical reality. (Cervantes seems to prove the philosopher Quine's contention that no scientific paradigm need ever give up its core beliefs, for a believer in a theory can always adjust his theory, on the periphery, to accommodate discordant facts.) Reason acquires in this context an instrumental meaning as Cervantes complicates in various ways the dichotomy of reason and unreason. Consider how, for example, in probably the most famous episode in the novel Don Quixote sees windmills and proclaims them, to Sancho's chagrin and to the reader's delight, to be giants. He rushes to charge them. The order of nature is not long in establishing its primacy with an empirical demonstration: Don Quixote finds himself on the ground, battered, and needful of adjusting his belief to his current state, not to mention justifying this defeat to a reproachful Sancho. Sancho "saw" that they were windmills, to which the knight replies:

> Silence, friend Sancho. . . . Matters of war are more subject than most to continual change. What is more, I think—and that is the truth—that the same sage Friston who robbed me of my room and my books has turned those giants into windmills, to cheat me of the glory of conquering them. Such is the enmity he bears me; but in the very end his black arts shall avail him little against the goodness of my sword. (P. 69)

Don Quixote is rational when he evokes the truth as the standard by which to measure his statements, though truth here means the standards of the world of texts in which enchantment is a category of the possible and a principle of explanation. Yet Don Quixote also understands that truth means adequation to the empirical world that Sancho sees. He can see when the world of texts has lost its purchase on the empirical world. Don Quixote's adjustment of the world of texts to the world of empirical reality is at once rational and insane, rational as a necessary operation, and crazy in its results.

The presence of reason in madness, in Cervantes as in Shakespeare, demands a sorting out of signs, although the reader is never in doubt as to Don Quixote's madness. Rather, Cervantes complicates the interpretation of his madness by ironically embedding forms of *sapentia* and reason into Don Quixote's speech and his interpretations of reality. At an inn, for example, Don Quixote takes an ordinary girl for a princess and thinks that he has fought a giant when he chops up wineskins with his sword. But at the evening meal he can meditate upon the familiar topos of uncertain knowledge and apply his conclusions to the present guests:

> For who is there of all men living upon earth who would judge us and know us for what we really are, if he were to come in now through the gate of this castle and see us as we appear at present? Who would be able to guess that this lady at my side is the great queen we all know her to be, and that I am that Knight of the Sad Countenance, so trumpeted by the mouth of Fame? (P. 343)

Don Quixote sees his dowdy companions as they empirically appear, or sees them as they might appear objectively to others—which does not stop him from also seeing them as they appear when transformed by the necessities imposed by living in romance. Reason is present in his use of conventional wisdom, though it is in the service of madness. The pertinent nature of his question remains: what allows one to interpret exterior signs, how does one recognize enchantment or madness?

Don Quixote's most sustained demonstration of reason in madness in the same context occurs when he begins to reflect on that favored Renaissance topic, the superiority of arms or letters, or whether the exercise of the sword or the pen is the superior activity. That Don Quixote's insanity makes of him a man of arms produced by literature establishes the ironic backdrop against which the knight errant gives a quite rational argument in favor of arms. Arms are necessary to guarantee peace. With Don Quixote's display of eloquence, all forget he is mad, and this would apply as much to readers as to characters, for "no one listening to him took him for mad": "ninguno de los que escuchándole le tuviese por loco."[4] But the insanity exists here as a dialectic of reason and madness in which one pole generates the other, and Don Quixote, waxing on about the hardships of war, finally passes from reason to unreason when he begins cursing the invention of artillery. This diabolical invention can take the life of a valiant knight with cowardly anonymity. A knight errant judges the deviance of the modern world, again with some logic, for it is indeed difficult to be a knight in a world in which a cannon can pulverize him in one shot. However, this demonstration uses this logic in the service of madness.

No reader doubts that Don Quixote's world of giants, sorcerers, and enchanted princesses is a product of insanity. This certainty is essential, for the comic view depends on establishing a worldview about which there are no doubts. In *Don Quixote* Cervantes achieves this construction in part through self-reflexive procedures. The novel uses self-reference to call attention to itself as a novel, which is to say, a verbal construct that demands from the reader a relation of critical distance. With *Don Quixote* critical distance comes to be defined as part of the stance of sanity. With this critical distance the novel brings about a focus on a framework of rational certainty that is universally shared. There are many such self-reflexive procedures in the novel: Cervantes's constant allusion to the novel's fictional author, the supposed translator's comments on the text, the fact that characters in the second part of the novel have read the first part. These devices establish the critical distance that is essential for the rational evaluation of the world and allow the ironic complications that promote that evaluation.

It does not seem hyperbolic to claim that the establishment of this critical distance, as a way of reading or viewing the world, was as important for the creation of a modern worldview as were the revolutions in astronomy or geography. Critical distance is concomitant with the emergence of the belief in the uniformity of nature. For nature is uniform only when scrutinized with the same distance that also allows ironic understanding. This critical distance is part of the *Don Quixote*'s demonstration of its own relation to reason. This is all the more necessary in a book about a hero who has gone insane after reading too many books. The self-referential problem in this respect is to use a fiction to show the nature of fictions, to create a credible text that rebuts the authority of texts, or to make writing show that writing cannot have a truth-value simply by being a text. The novel must self-consciously deal with its own truth-value and ponder on its relation to the empirically real. Perhaps all of this was necessary in a world in which there were no fixed criteria for differentiating levels and types of discourse; and hence no clear criteria for sanity and insanity, or the real and the hallucinatory. *Don Quixote*'s self-reflexivity is the first step in a bootstrap creation of a typology of discourse that opens directly onto a modern grasp of the real.

This formulation is another way of saying that *Don Quixote* appeared at that moment in history when myth and fantasy were being separated out from other discourses, and when allegory began to lose its dominance. It is revealing with regard to the belief in fantasy to compare Tasso—mad Tasso—with Cervantes. The historical distance between Cervantes and Tasso is small—Tasso died in 1595, some twenty years before Cervantes—but the difference between the two is extraordinary. Even if one reckons that much in Cervantes was anticipated by Ariosto and Rabelais, the shift from Tasso to Cervantes might tempt the historian to speak of a rupture. Tasso was still attempting to maintain a worldview in which fantasy is not perceived as such and in which madness invests the world as a nocturnal force of evil. By contrast Cervantes gives us a novel to which, for the first time perhaps, Wittgenstein's famous aphorism applies: the world is all that is the case.

Of course Cervantes was aware of the enchantment of texts, and if through self-referentiality and irony he completed the creation of a standard of rationality for literature, he did so by depicting the madness that is at the heart of literature. Cervantes offers the insight that literature may originate in the same sources as some forms of madness. Literature's suspension of disbelief depends on the slippage by which one loses a grip on empirical reality and begins to entertain a belief in a worldview that may be different from the one that defines the empirically real. Much of the power of any worldview is generated by language's seeming capacity to define the real by simply decreeing what is the real. Fiction derives its power from the same source. *Don Quixote* shows that the power of madness is that it can replace rationality, or our worldview based on interpretive constraints and critical distance, with a circle of self-sustaining fictions that can be as powerfully self-justifying as any linguistic construct. The slippage from one worldview to another is Don Quixote's story: he moves from a belief in a worldview of which knight errantry is a constitutive part, then embraces the vocation of knight errant, and finally comes to *see* embodiments of this worldview in our everyday world—while continuing to see this same world as it is viewed by everyone else. Belief can impose vision, and it might appear that for the late medieval mind belief often preceded vision: people could, in generalized madness, see what texts said they should see.

Descartes's Double Legacy for Understanding Madness

A generation after *Don Quixote* the French philosopher René Descartes (1596–1650) joined Cervantes in demoting immediate vision, for Descartes's rationalism suspected that immediate perception could give rise to monsters. Descartes's refusal to grant truth-value to immediate vision would in itself be enough to make him a major figure in a transformation of our understanding of sanity and insanity. But Descartes also wrote a body of philosophical and scientific work that is especially important, in a history of madness and medical psychology, for his reordering of the mind-body question. Descartes's separation of mind and body—known as Cartesian dualism—set the terms for much of medical thought about madness through the Enlightenment, and beyond. In a sense his meditations and philosophical writings theorize the axioms of the worldview that made *Don Quixote* possible. Like Cervantes, Descartes defined the self as a place where madness can occur without the structure of the world ever being involved. However, in Descartes's view, reason can dominate the world, a world defined through mathematical rationality, without madness being able to touch that rationality.

Cartesian thought provided the grounds for new thought about madness. Conjoined with the new science—physics along with hydraulics and mechanics—Cartesian metaphysics offered the basis for a new "philosophy of madness," as it was put in the eighteenth century. In defining the world as a place in which the laws of nature hold unquestioned sway, Descartes developed what Galileo and Cervantes had begun. But he went beyond them when he established an ontological dualism between the realm of extended matter, subject to the laws of mechanics, and the realm of the soul wherein freedom rules. Mind and body are defined as belonging to two separate realms of being. Cartesian thought marked out the epistemological space in which medicine came to conceive of the physiological body in terms borrowed from mechanics. In addition, Cartesian views of the soul and the functioning of the passions challenged Christian-Stoic notions of insanity, for if passions are to be understood causally in mechanical terms, the soul is subject only to its own absolute freedom. Finally, the Cartesian revolution, if that is the right term, meant that madness was henceforth a relationship to be interpreted in terms of the objective and the subjective relations constituting an immaterial soul's relation to a physical world.

Having made this outline of Cartesian thought, I need to add nuance to my argument about Descartes's importance for a history of discourses on madness. For, in arguing that Cartesian thought allows reason to function even when invested with madness, I do not intend to imply that the effect of Cartesian dualism was to humanize the relations between the insane and their doctors. This was a possible effect, but the Cartesian legacy is double. In formalizing the philosophical dualism that separated thinking and extended substances, Descartes set up the conditions of possibility for considering human beings to be machines as well as for recognizing that the soul can never be truly touched by madness. Descartes allows the argument that a rational being is always to be found somewhere behind the wall of insanity that encapsulates it. But his physiology also suggests that the mad are merely dysfunctional machines. Descartes's legacy is a double inheritance that both promotes the humane views of Shakespeare and Cervantes, and conveys a fear of the deviant machine that can be seen in a mad person. Descartes's legacy at once affirms and denies what we have seen in Shakespeare and Cervantes.

Let us pursue this in some detail, since Cartesian dualism poses all the problems of the relation of mental illness and medical physiology. As a Cartesian, a doctor could relegate madness to the body and make of it a problem of mechanics or physiology. Or the doctor could make of madness a problem of the soul. This solution necessitates reconciling the presence of reason in a free soul with the demonstrable presence of unreason. Descartes's own argumentation about the presence of reason in unreason is still the classic demonstration. Wanting to show that there is within the self a source of certain knowledge that lies beyond mere visual or sensual perception, Descartes tried to prove that the rationality of the soul cannot be affected by deceptions that might come from dream, madness, and hallucination. He hypothesized that all that one perceives could be a product of dementia just as much as the result of empirical observation—and with this, Descartes discovered that there are no criteria for distinguishing valid perception from rampant hallucination.

In his *Meditationes de prima philosophia,* written before but published after his *Discours de la méthode* (published respectively in 1641 and 1637), Descartes developed his method for finding rational certainty by subjecting to radical doubt any knowledge the self might garner through sensation. This moment of doubt entails entertaining the hypothesis that the self is plunged into hallucination, into madness and dream. This moment of doubt has been interpreted in several ways. In his *Histoire de la folie* Michel Foucault sees this thought experiment as the moment in Western thought when madness is excluded from discourse.[5] Foucault made Descartes a villain insofar as this exclusion "silenced" madness. But the *Meditations* are sufficiently ambiguous to impose the doubly legacy I refer to. This legacy is clear from the moment Descartes, in the First Discourse of the *Meditations,* looks for a first principle upon which to base certain reasoning. He decides to doubt everything, since nothing seems certain. Unlike Agrippa or Montaigne, however, Descartes had a different epistemological order in mind when he rejected textual authorities and tradition as well as immediate experience. His doubt represents a radical break with the Renaissance, and one must return to Greece (or to Augustine) to find any comparable attempt to base certain knowledge on the forms of reasoning alone. And in rejecting the testimony of the senses, Descartes's reasonable doubt aims first at the testimony of vision. Any reader of *Don Quixote,* not to mention Galileo, would have found this doubt about vision quite convincing.

In his need for certainty, Descartes decides in his *Meditations* to undertake unreasonable doubt, which is to doubt the veracity of even the most immediate sensations; for example, to doubt that he is present to himself as a body:

> For example, there is the fact that I am here, seated by the fire, attired in a dressing gown, having this paper in my hands and other similar matters. And how could I deny that these hands and this body are mine, were it not perhaps that I compare myself to certain persons, devoid of sense, whose cerebella are so troubled and clouded by the violent vapors of black bile, that they constantly assure us they think they are kings when they are really quite poor. . . . But they are mad [amentes], and I should not be any the less insane [demens] were I to follow examples so extravagant.[6]

In this passage Descartes says he does not wish to take the mad as a model for uncertainty. Using this same passage Foucault appears basically correct in his romantic interpretation charging the rationalists with the exclusion of the mad from the privileges of discourse. Descartes does not wish to base his doubts on a dysfunctional body—and his image of the mad here appears to call upon the humors physiology that makes of them victims of their own body with its "violent vapors of black bile."

However, the necessity of radicalizing his doubt brings Descartes back to the idea that our sensations might be hallucinations, such as in sleep and dreams. After all, dream is an ordinary state, a state in which even a healthy philosopher might find himself at any given moment, and perhaps even at the moment of writing his treatise. To his astonishment Descartes finds that there are "no certain indications by which we may clearly distinguish wakefulness from sleep" (p. 146). At this moment, providentially, Descartes slips in his proviso that all composite things are capable of being produced as illusions, whereas simple things, such as the objects of mathematics, are indubitable whether one is dreaming or not. In other words, hallucinations, dreams, and madness cannot affect the products of pure reason. With this proviso not even a mad deity could contrive to make two plus two equal five.

However, given the dream hypothesis, might we not be constantly living in madness? In making a critique of Foucault, the contemporary philosopher Jacques Derrida answers this question affirmatively, since Descartes's dream hypothesis constitutes an extension of the hypothesis that we might always be mad. Descartes continues his thought experiment so as to justify the most radical of doubts about truth, which permits him to define and defend reason as it might exist even within madness. Descartes frames the hypothesis that an evil genius is using all his powers to deceive him. Nothing apparent is true, for, as Descartes writes, "the heavens, the earth, colours, figures, sound, and all other external things are nought but the illusions and dreams of which this genius has availed himself" (p. 148). Descartes's doubt is possession theory pushed to its extreme limit: all that one perceives is produced by an insane deity. But even if all we perceive is caused by delirium—produced by humors, dreams, or possession—Descartes's first principle retains its validity. The proposition that "I think, therefore, I am," remains true even in madness, dream, and hallucination. The first principle of a knowing subjectivity, the cogito, is established as the first principle of certain knowledge, whatever be the vision that madness and dream foist upon a subject who cannot trust perception.

Descartes thought that in the cogito—I think, therefore, I am—he had found a transcendental demonstration of certainty, beyond place and history. Turning to the world, Descartes introduces a second principle, his idea of a perfect God whose perfection would not, by definition, allow him to deceive. We need give little attention to this revival of the ontological argument to prove God's existence, nor the extra "proof" that it brings to Descartes's now certain principle. Descartes had already found the extra certainty he needs by quietly granting language the role of guarantor of truth. In his Second Meditation, having arrived at his first principle, or the cogito, Descartes ponders on what he believes to be the "I" that thinks:

> Undoubtedly I believed myself to be a man. But what is a man? Shall I say a reasonable animal? Certainly not; for then I should have to inquire what an animal is, and what is reasonable; and thus from a single question I should insensibly fall into an infinitude of others more difficult; and I should not like to waste the little time and leisure remaining to me in trying to unravel subtleties like these. (P. 150)

In effect Descartes pushes aside the question of how the interrelations of semantic networks determine the fabric of reasoning. Perhaps with Don Quixote in mind, Descartes does not want to face the question of how language might foster beliefs and impose visions upon the mind. By avoiding the question of language, Descartes implicitly affirms that reasonable thought is coterminous and coincident with language and its nonproblematic functioning. This view of language is all-important for the history of rationalism, in the narrow sense of the term, and its determinations of madness for the next two centuries. Logos is not subject to doubt.

Madness may invest the world, but, from the Cartesian perspective, language will continue to function unperturbed. Language functions much like God and mathematics in Descartes's system, since none of them can apparently deceive. The identification of God and logos, of divine certainty and the operations of reason through language, is a recurrent theme in our culture, and it is hardly surprising that this rationalist belief survives implicitly in Cartesian thought. It is the foundation of Christian rationalism: God is the nondeceiver who underwrites the certainties of logos, the same logos that defines the nature of God. This circular axiom guarantees, mathematically as it were, the primacy of reason. And like the biblical belief that finds man to be the image of the deity, this rationalist credo makes of the divine soul in man—but rarely woman—the repository of logos in all conditions. This side of the Cartesian legacy joins Cervantes and Shakespeare in humanizing the mad, for it encourages the attempt to find reason in every form of insanity.

The other side of the Cartesian legacy does not recognize reason in madness. This legacy is found in the physiological doctrines of Descartes, which make of the body the center of the imagination. In asking who he is, Descartes purports to discover, in the moment of hyperbolic doubt, that nothing brought to him by the imagination belongs to his essence as a thinking subject. In the Sixth Meditation as well as in his physiological writings all imagining belongs to the realm of extended substance, for example, the body:

> [T]his power of the imagination which is one, inasmuch as it differs from the power of understanding, is in no wise a necessary element in my nature, or in [my essence, that is to say, in] the essence of my mind; for although I did not possess it I should doubtless ever remain the same as I now am, from which it appears that we might conclude that it depends on something which differs from me. (P. 186)

This separation—perhaps better named a schizoid severing—of mind and body, of pure understanding and imagination, is the other side of the Cartesian legacy. Through this separation, understanding is made impervious to madness, and madness is transformed, in its imaginings, into a question of physiological dysfunctions. Imagination becomes the most dubious of faculties, for, like an evil genius, it can dazzle the understanding with an array of illusions. Descartes banishes magic from the understanding, but the possibility for deception, through the imagination, is unlimited.

This dualism is stressed in Descartes's later writings such as the *Traité des passions* and the *Traité de l'homme,* expository treatises respectively on the passions and on the nature of man in which Descartes set forth what was implicit earlier: human beings are essentially machines with a soul in the pilot's seat; or, in a different version, the humanoid machine is a hydraulic apparatus with the soul acting as the *fontainier* or engineer directing the moving stream of animal spirits. In these writings Descartes is recasting Renaissance thought, for which hydraulics and mechanics represented innovations with regard to Greco-Roman antiquity. Descartes's model of physiology based on mechanics hardly seems consonant with his metaphysics, for how can a spiritual, thinking substance be influenced or afflicted by a material, extended substance? The interaction of mind and body was the thorniest dilemma that Cartesian ontology gave succeeding generations of thinkers—and even today one can hardly find a philosophical or neurological treatise on mind that does not begin by attacking Descartes. Cartesian ontology obliges one to ask how can madness even be possible. How can the machine affect the pilot, or how can there be madness in reason?

With or without a soul, man is a machine. Mechanical physiology is incorporated into the metaphysics of the Sixth Meditation: "[T]he mind does not receive the impression from all parts of the body immediately, but only from the brain, or perhaps even from one of its smallest parts, to wit, from that in which the common sense is said to reside." Having hesitantly made of the pineal gland the point of contact of mind and body, Descartes develops this a priori physiology by using a mechanical model to imagine the workings of mind:

> [I]n the same way, when I feel pain in my foot, my knowledge of physics teaches that this sensation is communicated by means of nerves dispersed through the foot, which, being extended like cords from there to the brain, when they are contracted in the foot, at the same time contract the inmost portions of the brain which is their extremity and place of origin, and then excite a certain movement which nature has established in order to cause the mind to be affected by a sensation of pain represented as existing in the foot. (Pp. 196–97)

Analogies taken from physics simplify the relations of mind and body. With the Cartesian revolution, Platonic or Aristotelian divisions of mind or soul into multiple faculties go by the board. The soul is intellect. The rest of a human being is a machine subject to mechanics. The two are separated into hermetically tight ontological realms.

Human understanding is in contact with the world thanks to those mythical beings that flow in the nerves and reach the brain: animal spirits. Harvey's model of the circulation of the blood provided one impetus for this a priori belief in animal spirits, just as measurements accomplished in mechanics provided a justification for attempting to explain the body as a machine. Motivations for Descartes's thought are clear, but there is also a great deal of imagination at work in anatomical descriptions like the following one that attempts to explain how the immaterial soul has an effect on a material body:

> [W]hat is here most worthy of remark is that all the most animated and subtle portions of the blood which the heat has rarefied in the heart, enter ceaselessly in large quantities into the cavities of the brain. . . . For what I here name spirits are nothing but material bodies and their one peculiarity is that they are bodies of extreme minuteness and that they move very quickly like the particles of the flame which issues from a torch. Thus it is that they never remain at rest in any spot, and just as some of them enter into the cavities of the brain, others issue forth by the pores which are in its substance, which pores conduct them into the nerves, and from there into the muscles, by means of which they move the body in all the different ways it can be moved. (*Passions of the Soul,* p. 336)

In various versions this metaphysical fantasy presides over the next two centuries of mechanistic medicine that displaced, but never replaced, the Hippocratic-Galenic tradition. And this is as often true of Lockean empiricists as of pure Cartesian rationalists. In effect, most effort at elaborating medical theory henceforth would be essentially reconciling Hippocrates and Descartes.

To conclude these considerations, I stress that Cartesian imaginations are the work of the body. They are perceptions mechanically or hydraulically caused by the nerves. They can be independent of the will, for will belongs to the soul alone. Imaginations are products of agitated animal spirits, such as in dreams, reveries, or wandering thoughts. Descartes did not specifically mention madness in his later physiological writings. Perhaps the rationalist in Descartes felt the question had been settled with the relegation of madness to the realm of sensation, perception, and imaginings. And certainly it was easier not to face the fact that madness does not have any easy explanation if the soul is a substance that is totally different from matter. Can merely material imaginings so easily cloud the thinking substance's capacity for rational thought? Moreover, Descartes further complicated the interpretation of madness by introducing, in his later writings, a view of the passions according to which they are not insanity. Passions are, to be sure, products of the body and the realm of mechanically functioning matter, but in his treatise on the passions Descartes concludes with an anti-Stoic position. He maintained that, when the passions are under the control of prudence, they may be a source of joy. This anti-Stoic position lies behind seventeenth-century debates about madness, and concomitant debates about freedom of will and determinism, or beliefs about the causes of madness. The Cartesian position is clear in its radical affirmation that the soul's freedom is absolute. The rational soul is totally free, and any errors in judgment spring from the realm of the senses. Any malady that interferes with freedom can only come from a dysfunction in the human machine's extended substance. Logically—or illogically—the will should be able to master the passions.

This voluntarism, if taken seriously, would also seem to make it very difficult to go insane—insofar as insanity is understood to involve aberrant judgments or pathological passions. Descartes's attitude anticipates in a sense the repugnance with which the neoclassical thinkers in Europe, and above all the Augustans in England, envisaged madness. Theoretically madness should not exist in a rational being, or at least a rational being should be able to will that insanity not exist, that it cease to be a blemish tarnishing the rationalist image of the perfection of man. The Augustans despised Descartes, but they probably would have agreed that the infinite power of will that Descartes granted the soul means that the mad are mad because they will to be mad.

As the seventeenth century unfolded Shakespeare, Cervantes, and Descartes became received names, even if Shakespeare's reception on the continent had a checkered history of resistance, and Descartes's influence in England was often to spur doctors and scientists to refute him. Nonetheless, the mad, if not their doctors, became sensitive to the need to interpret their discourse, and by the end of the Enlightenment this demand becomes a leitmotif of literary history. Medical Cartesians and anti-Cartesians also set up a debate based on Cartesian axioms that dominated the seventeenth and eighteenth centuries. The influence of Cervantes as well as Descartes can be felt in the belief henceforth that one must interpret madness within an empirical space that is characterized by the uniformity of nature and the sway of natural law. And that truth-values are universal and do not depend upon language and textuality. This "rationalist" era, an era that soon found in Newton's work the greatest demonstration of the rationality of the universe, continued to confront the question that Shakespeare, Cervantes, and Descartes had brought to the fore: is there reason in madness? Or, conversely, how can madness come to inhabit the reason that should be out of the reach of madness? Uncomforted by Descartes, many of our great rationalists were obsessed with thoughts of madness, for one power of reason is, as we have seen in Shakespeare and Cervantes, its capacity to demonstrate its own fragility.

Chapter 4

The Iatro-Mechanical Era and the Madness of Machines

The problems associated with the application of mechanical physiology to an understanding of madness occupied doctors and philosophers from Descartes well into the Enlightenment. Groups and tendencies as diverse as the iatro-chemical and iatro-mechanical doctors, the Augustans, and the Enlightenment writers associated with the philosophe movement attacked each other in the acceptance and rejection of mechanical medicine and its views of insanity. In dealing with the central paradigm of mechanical philosophy and physiology, I want to map out here the developments of medical and literary thought about madness beginning roughly in the wake of the literary quarrel of the ancients and moderns, in the seventeenth century, which came a century after medicine had experienced the same quarrel. The issues for medicine and literature in this quarrel were much the same: were the European moderns superior to the Greco-Romans upon whose achievements the moderns built? The quarrel had by no means been settled in medicine by Descartes's time, nor was it quickly resolved in literature. In medicine, after a seeming defeat, the ancients made a return when medical neoclassicism came to fruition in the revival of Hippocratic thought at the end of the eighteenth century. This is, however, a reprise that will concern us in the following chapter in which, in analyzing another side of the Enlightenment, I want to investigate the preromantic literature of Goethe and Rousseau and the medical thought of Philippe Pinel at the end of the eighteenth century.

Before the Hippocratic revival, moderns were generally dominant in medicine, especially after Descartes provided a metaphysical framework for a psychology and physiology that seemed consonant with Galileo's physics and Harvey's physiology. The problem that the moderns faced was that Cartesian metaphysics did not explain how the rational soul could go mad if it were not part of extended matter. For most medical purposes, it mattered little if the soul were considered to be separate from the realm of extended matter, and thus not subject to the mechanical causality that physics describes mathematically. Disease afflicted matter alone, which is to say, the body, leaving the soul (and theology) intact. Insanity seemed, nonetheless, to be a disease that affected the soul. So the problem remained: was insanity an affliction of extended matter or of thinking substance? Doctors motivated by Christian ideology, often partisans of the ancients, were obliged to consider the soul separate from the body. Theology dictated that the eternal soul must be free from any blemish such as insanity. So the medical task for these doctors was to describe insanity in such a way as to leave the soul intact and free from any permanent damage. Nonreligious and materialist moderns did not face this problem. Since the materialist accepted only Descartes's concern with extended matter, for all practical purposes the materialist need not be concerned with a soul, but simply with mechanical causality working itself out in the body. Hence there is no problem with madness that is not a medical problem. Madness afflicts the body, the body is a machine, and that is a problem of medical mechanics.

There were of course many variants on these responses, but the polarities of ancient and modern, and of Christian and materialist, set out the dichotomous range of descriptions of madness that characterize the first part of the Enlightenment. There were many critiques of Cartesian metaphysics. But Cartesian dualism remained the starting point for much medical and philosophical thought about the relation of mind and body. Even English empiricism had to work out its nominalism in terms of this dualism as it tried to imagine how mind could be something other than a soul, untouched by the material world. These dichotomies allow one to make sense both of the dominant modern medical paradigms dealing with madness as well as the Augustan lampooning of these moderns. The Augustans Swift and Pope represent the ancients undertaking their most contradictory attempts to exorcise madness, and especially the madness of the science of madness. These polarities also establish the context for reading continental writers, a generation or so later. From these writers, the paradigm of "machine man" elicited entirely different responses. These mainly French moderns pushed the mechanical paradigm to its illogical logical consequences. Machine man gives rise to an insane deviant in the works of the most brilliant of the philosophes, Diderot, whereas in fictions by the Marquis de Sade machine man is only rational if he or she is insane. The oppositions within the neoclassical attempts to understand madness—oppositions that eventuate in the founding of psychiatry and in permitting the dreams of madmen to enter literature—set forth the essential tensions of the Enlightenment.

An Exemplary Iatro-Chemical Understanding of Madness

The Christian medical response to the problems Descartes developed began during his lifetime, and at times developed independent of any direct response to Descartes. Given the importance of the Christian response to the challenges of mechanistic physiology, I turn to a Christian scientist who, in trying to circumvent the materialism of mechanistic thought, also founded a major medical school. Descartes's contemporary Van Helmont (1577–1644), a physician known for his work in chemistry, is exemplary in this regard. Using chemistry—and alchemy—he tried to elaborate a model of medicine that offered an alternative to the mechanical view of physiology that became dominant only a generation later. Van Helmont is usually considered in medical history to be a founder of the "iatro-chemical" school that competed with the "iatro-mechanical" movement in medicine. Van Helmont proposed that human physiology is as much explained by chemistry as by mechanics. The two schools are actually not very far apart, partly because iatro-chemical views were taken over by the later developers of the mechanical paradigm. This eclecticism is evident in the work of the doctor who dominates the eighteenth century, Boerhaave, for whom man is a machine composed of both fibers and liquids.

Van Helmont was a modern, and his views of madness were grounded in personal experience. As a Christian modern, he also found it repugnant to believe that mere pagan doctors might have discovered some significant truths. With Paracelsus as a precursor, Van Helmont elaborated a psychiatric doctrine that is as inventive as any we have considered thus far. According to this doctrine a living being is presided over by a "generative spirit," or what Van Helmont called the *Archeus faber,* the producing principle that directs the development of every naturally born creature—as opposed to those born of spontaneous generation. The notion has logical necessity: everything that is must be what it is, or it would not be. Thus there must be a "principle" from which it emanates. The *archeus,* or principle, is part of a strategy to save the biblical version of creation and to find an explanation of madness that preserves the soul as God's creation, eternally exempt from any physically caused blight such as insanity. In the human *archeus* is found the soul made in the image of God, and this cannot be touched by insanity. Emile Guyénot has described Van Helmont's "model" for disease in terms that show that the iatro-chemist fused together mechanical images with Neoplatonic harmonics:

He supposed that the living body is tied to a sensitive soul, which is dominated by the immortal soul. This *Archeus* would have its quarters in the pylorus of the stomach. Dominated by this authority, a secondary archeus, called *blas* or *vulcan,* would reside in each organ and would act as an intelligent mechanic in controlling their functions. Every organ, thus equipped with its archeus or "local president," would constitute an individual endowed with a kind of autonomous life. So long as all the archeus obey the principal archeus, the organism will function in harmony. Disease will result, on the contrary, from the revolt of a local archeus.[1]

Guyénot's description properly stresses the way a mechanical metaphor is replacing a political metaphor as the dominant metaphor for talking about psychic and physiological functions—though they coexist here. Van Helmont's example points up that, even in iatro-chemical discourse, the engineer is about to replace the king as the organizing metaphor for understanding dysfunctions in the body and in the mind. Harmony is still the key metaphor, one describing logos and reason, but the supporting cast of metaphors is changing. The machine is about to replace the kingdom.

Van Helmont also illustrates the permutations that arise with the classical concepts for the analysis of madness. For example, he places reason on the side of the senses by saying that contact with the world is made through the sensitive soul wherein are found reason, imagination, and perception. Reason is joined with the senses, and the intellectual soul is left alone and pure. Reason can be corrupted by madness, for excessive passions such as assiduous contemplation or great fear can besiege the sensitive soul and drive it insane. But even during madness the divine spark of the intellectual soul remains unmoved. From a theological point of view this is a satisfactory way of avoiding the Cartesian dilemma, but Van Helmont's essentially materialist view of madness is also a prelude to the Enlightenment view that it needs no soul at all to explain madness. A materialist reading of Van Helmont would find the soul physically situated in the upper orifice of the stomach.

Van Helmont did believe in the truth-value of empirical data and used it, as did Descartes, to localize the soul. He claimed empirical proof for this localization, since one day, while he was busy with chemical research, he did some drug experimentation. He was preparing some aconite (or monkshood), a plant reputed to be deadly, so deadly that Furetière's dictionary claims a famous beauty once chewed it and then killed people by breathing on them. (The plant in question is *Aconite napellus.*) Van Helmont tasted this plant, whose relationship to mental illness was already established in the seventeenth century, since Avicenna had declared it a cause of epilepsy.

After tasting the plant, Van Helmont felt pressure on his cranium; then, after some activity, he suddenly noted a lack of feeling in his head: a total lack of conceiving, feeling, or imagination.[2] He felt that all these functions were taking place in the precordium and that they extended from there toward the upper orifice of his stomach. This revelation was proof for Van Helmont that the intellectual soul is found in the epigastric region.

I cite this jumble to show that "experience" often confirms ancient views, for Van Helmont's epiphany recalls the ancient doctrine that finds in the hypochondrium or lower abdominal area the seat of the vapors that rise into the brain to cause melancholy and insanity in general. In the Enlightenment context this proof could also confirm the mechanical doctrine, since it relies affirmatively upon the hydraulic model of physio-psychological functions in which spirits are pushed by the heart, seat of the will, to the brain. However, to get around this materialism, Van Helmont invented for the intellectual soul a spiritual means of passage since a spiritual substance would not use a mechanical canal. He allowed the soul's "light" to travel freely, as in sleep, meditation, ecstasy, syncopes, mania, delirium, rage, et cetera. This list underscores that Van Helmont, like most Christian doctors after him, could not figure out how to reconcile his belief in a spiritual soul with the empirical reality of a state of madness. He is contradictorily obliged to attribute physical characteristics to the soul for its localization and spiritual characters to it, even in madness, to explain its functions. Van Helmont was a major scientific mind, and I do not wish to denigrate him. But one sees in Van Helmont's medical work a defense of an ideology in contradiction with the basic impulses of the new science. Van Helmont had to defend theology and at the same time respect the axiom of medicine that made no separation between mental and organic illnesses. This resulted in the elaboration of a mystical materialism that located the soul with a literalism that seems incredible (though I would not contest the interest of the same charge made against some of today's simpleminded doctrines of mental localization, making use of one-variable causation).

Van Helmont's attempts at localizations point up the fact that, in the seventeenth century, iatro-chemists were trying to make progress in anatomical knowledge and to use this knowledge for medical psychology. Drawing on Harvey, for example, one of the founders of clinical medicine, Sylvius (1614–1672) attempted to reshape Van Helmont's medical doctrines by getting rid of the *archeus* and founding a medical psychology using mechanical conduits to explain the flows in the body. Harvey's demonstration of the circulation of the blood also contributed significantly to the rise of the mechanistic paradigm by offering a hydraulic analogy to explain the nervous system and correlated mental functions. The most famous English contributor to iatro-chemistry, Willis (1622–1675), made positive contributions to the description of brain anatomy; and he, too, proposed to explain madness as a condition of the blood. Medical history likes to make much of the differences of these doctors and the iatro-mechanical thinkers, but, as I suggested, one is struck as much by the commonalities as their differences, especially as the century developed. Significantly, the "English Hippocrates," as Sydenham (1624–1689) was called, took his distance from humors theory and was willing to endorse the generalized view that a disturbance in the flow of animal spirits can cause madness by producing vapors—or hysteria in women and hypochondria in men. Syndenham's eclecticism parallels the way most of the iatro-chemists also offered a mechanical view of humanity driven mad by a perturbation of the inner flow of spirits and other juices. But, in defending the nearly gnostic ideology of a Van Helmont, they often tried to protect a principle of divine light in the machine by putting the soul in an organic box that ultimately might not be contaminated by those juices and vapors emanating from the principle of darkness—or matter itself.

The Iatro-Mechanical Consensus on Machine Man's Madness

The iatro-chemical models finally merged with the main paradigm of medical psychology that dominated the eighteenth century: the model of "mechanical man." This model was bound up with a physiology based on fibers, though it frequently had recourse to hydraulic metaphors, calling on modern engineering terminology describing how machines function. The work of the mathematician Borelli (1608–1679) was fundamental for his comparison of bones to levers moved by muscles. After Descartes and Borelli, two names dominate mechanical medicine: Hoffmann (1660–1742) and Boerhaave (1668–1738). Boerhaave was perhaps the most famous doctor of the time, a grand eclectic, combining mechanical and chemical models in order to concoct the potpourri that most of the educated public accepted as medical truth during the Enlightenment. Hoffmann, however, was a more rigorous thinker. Facing the dilemma of reconciling theology with materialist science, he declared that the Christian doctor's first obligation was to know mechanics, to which end he recommended Leibniz, Borelli, and Descartes.[3] Hoffmann saw in the human body a machine endowed with "active forces" that, in their reciprocal interaction, produce movement. These active forces are translated and controlled by those ever vigilant engineers, the animal spirits. Even for a Christian, in the early eighteenth century medicine demanded the study of mechanical principles dealing with matter, and theology relied upon the laws of motion. After Descartes, Newton's natural philosophy swept the field and made mechanists of even those most recalcitrant to Cartesian thought.

Medicine then worked with a new unity to produce an image, a kind of phantasmagorical fiction, that we can call machine man—to translate the title of a book, *L'Homme machine,* that made Boerhaave's pupil La Mettrie famous in philosophe circles. Boerhaave's mechanical explanation of madness in his *Aphorisms* had already given wide circulation to an image of the human machine whose soul is situated outside the realm of material causality. Insanity was reduced to an affliction of the physical machine. Delirium, for example, can be explained as a lack of conformity between inner and outer ideas and occurs when there is an obstruction that stops the blood's movement to the brain and its transmission beyond.[4] A coma is due to the same cause or to anything that stops the spirits from separating out of the blood in the nerves (p. 207). Boerhaave could also freely use iatro-chemical explanations, as when he declared "idiopathic phrenesy" to be due to an inflammation of the pia mater and dura mater, the membranes covering the spinal cord and the brain (p. 232); whereas "sympathetic phrenesy" is due to the presence, in the meninges, of phlogiston—the material substance, recently invented by the vitalist doctor-chemist Stahl, that explained burning (p. 236).

These examples are instructive for a history of reasoning about disease and madness. Boerhaave combined some empirical insight—the presence of inflammation seen in some cases of delirium—with a priori constructs that could answer the question "what if?" What if the body were a hydraulic machine transporting animal spirits, or subtle fluids, or phlogistic matter, or other perhaps unknown substances through real blood vessels and logically necessary small tubes? Given this image of the material body, what constructs then make sense of disease? The modern epistemologist Bachelard thought that Boerhaave's use of essentially verbal constructs make of him a primary example of a prescientific mind.[5] However, Bachelard's impatient judgment does not take into account that nearly all scientific constructs, once superseded, fall into a strange domain in which they are always prescientific in the banal sense that they have lost the validity of what replaced them, and, in an ontologically interesting sense, that they often resemble some fictive fantasy. These models have a role in the development of science. Boerhaave's medical science consists in his borrowing metaphors from what are positive sciences and adjusting them to classical medicine. What the ancients took to be black bile, for example, Boerhaave could explain in terms of residue left by the blood; or classical hypochondria, in the sense of a mental illness, could be explained as essentially a question of clogged-up pipes.

Some of the ideological consequences of the medical vision of machine man were worked out in the work of an atheistic disciple like the doctor-philosopher La Mettrie (1709–1751). La Mettrie's *L'Homme machine* of 1748 is a culminating point in the development of materialist physiology. Using basically Cartesian arguments, La Mettrie rebutted Descartes. With comparative anatomy as a guide, La Mettrie notes that men and animals share the same structures, whence he concludes that they are basically the same: both are machines endowed with sentience. This conclusion also follows from the basic materialist axiom for explaining life, according to which, as fellow philosopher Diderot put it, sensibility is a general and essential quality of matter. Even a stone feels—which must logically be the case if inert matter organized as a human being has sentience.[6] From today's perspective materialistic medical mechanics proposes as fantastic a view of humanity as iatro-chemistry. This is evidenced in the assurance with which La Mettrie explains the "mechanism" of passions in his *Histoire naturelle de l'âme*. In this *Natural History of the Soul* he notes that contemporary mechanics has, with regard to nerves and passions, shown that "as soon as one knows, for instance, that chagrin squeezes the diameter of the tubes—even if one does not know the first cause that makes the nerves contract around them, as if to strangle them—then all the effects that follow, such as melancholy, black humour, and mania, are easy to conceive."[7] The mechanical nature of emotion is spelled out. From some first cause, an emotion causes a mechanical reaction, such as the constriction of the spirit-carrying nerve tubes, which in turn brings about a change in a mental state—such as madness. With grand assurance La Mettrie describes how mental states determine mechanical reactions, which in turn are the causes of mental states.

This same materialist assurance led La Mettrie, like many of his contemporaries, to have a dismissive attitude toward the mad, to a flippant devaluation of their dysfunctional nervous systems that reduced them to defective animals. A few grams of gray matter are all that separate man from the lowest of beasts. The hyperevaluation of human characteristics is the converse of his scorn for the mad animal. This contempt for animality leads La Mettrie, in his *L'Homme machine*, to a celebration of the superiority of the anatomically determined features that allow humanity to have language: "Nothing is so simple, as one sees, than the mechanics of our education: everything can be reduced to a question of sounds, or words, that from the mouth of one person pass through the ear of another into the brain, which receives at the same time through the eyes the shape of the body of which these words are the arbitrary sign."[8] Language is the glory of mankind, even for the atheist who does not seem aware that, in this materialist semiotics, he is repeating the praise of logos. The scope, if not the certainty, of language is limited by the materialist, for logos is given only through a mechanically determined education that empowers one to use arbitrary signs. Without education, humanity, as in the case of wolf men or those with blocked hypochondria, is only apparently human, for logos is what separates humans from those beasts with a human face—the mad or "bêtes à figures humaines" (*Oeuvres philosophiques,* p. 316). More sharply than the Greeks, the Enlightenment philosopher conceives logos as a realm separate from a nature of which he is deathly afraid.

Moreover, La Mettrie observes that mad humanoid beasts have no place in a rational taxonomy. They merit no special class in scientific attempts to categorize reality. This observation shows wherein lies the materialist's hatred or fear of the mad. It is not merely that they are animals who are not capable of speech as he conceives it. In addition, madness and the mad threatened to topple over the rational construction of the world to which the philosophes were dedicated. To what rational taxonomy do the deviant belong? In what rational arrangement of existence do the mad find a logical place? For the Christian doctor madness threatens divine logos lodged in an eternal soul, but for the materialist the threat is perhaps more dangerous. For insanity makes a mockery of the principle of rationality that led one to become a materialist rationalist in the first place. The perfect order of mechanics and the rational harmony of being in which this order is embedded could not really account for deviance. And thus reason had to distance itself from madness and avoid a challenge it could hardly meet. Madness is an epistemological threat. La Mettrie counters it finally by refusing to deal with the mechanical determination of the madness of all those who think they are werewolves, roosters, vampires, or who, believing they are made of glass, sleep on straw for protection (p. 291). Invoking by his examples a tableau of obsessions that haunt the imagination of the iatro-mechanical doctor, La Mettrie concedes that the "medullary canvas" of the brain is quite capable of imagining all those things that he does not wish to discuss. For this would mean discussing the "soul," a mere concoction of the imagination and its workings.

The Development of a Science of Insanity

La Mettrie represents the dominant rationalist attitude that is not so much concerned with "silencing" madness, as Foucault argued, as with refusing to face the taxonomical implications that irrationality forced upon the Enlightenment. However, there were trends within medicine leading to a different encounter with madness. This encounter resulted in the institution of a special science of madness. One can call this discourse "psychiatry," though the word is a coinage of the German romantics, and much of what we mean by psychiatry came into being after the French Revolution. Let us say that contained within iatro-mechanics and its rationalism are the beginnings of psychiatry, though in ways that have little to do with the modern medicine that came into existence in the nineteenth century with the work of Bichat, Magendie, and Virchow. The formation of a science that took madness as its object occurred before the creation of experimental medicine and attendant disciplines such as histology, pathology, or microbiology. By special science I mean a discourse that established the diagnosis and treatment of the mad as a discipline separate from the general nosology or taxonomy that treated madness as one or several diseases among all other diseases. There were a number of doctors who contributed to the establishment of a medical discipline concerned with madness as its primary focus. Among the earliest was the rather obscure Antoine Le Camus who published in 1753 the first edition of his *Le Médecin de l'esprit*—or *The Mind Doctor*. His goals were clear. In his work, he declared, he wished to find the mechanisms of the body that have an effect on the functions of the soul; Le Camus's clarity shows that psychiatry was born as a branch of mechanical medicine.

In terms of influence, however, my candidate for the first protopsychiatrist would be the English doctor William Battie who published a *Treatise on Madness* in 1758. I nominate this book for the designation as the first psychiatric manual, written by a distant disciple of Locke whose name has obviously outlasted his fame. Battie's book is a general work on madness that entertains no other nosological considerations. Unlike Hoffmann or Boerhaave, Battie does not consider madness—meaning, basically, melancholy, phrensy, and mania—as one disease among others, to be considered somewhere between colic and cholera.

Battie's removal of madness from the general taxonomy of disease is also part of the development of iatro-mechanical thought. Battie's insane are humanoid machines. His machine is run by small fibers connected to larger fascicules that in turn make up larger bundles. These are, or rather must be, in turn connected to the "medullary substance"—that canvas on which La

Mettrie saw images projected. One understands why Battie's contemporary, the skeptical philosopher Hume, made his acerbic critique of the metaphysics of causality when one examines the abuse of causality that underlies most iatro-mechanical doctrines, including Battie's. The principle of necessary causality is constantly invoked by doctors to explain what is because it must be. Battie declares that all that "occurs" in the brain must be explained in terms of cause and effect. All perceptions must take place in the inner world of the medullary substance, though their causes must be found in an outer world. Relying upon the a priori assumption that there are inner and outer worlds, the doctor may then logically assume that there must be something that connects them in causal terms. (And Locke provides ample precedent for this move.) From this configuration the doctor can deduce the necessity of connecting fibers. There is a veneer of empirical justification for these deductions. After Willis a fair amount of positive description of the anatomy of nervous system was available to doctors, and Battie makes appeal to anatomical descriptions by Vesalius and Willis to give plausibility to his logically necessary physiology. But he finally decrees that fibers as communicating vessels explain how the machine *must* function. Madness is explained by this a priori system when Battie simply defines it as false perception. With this definition Battie can then look, in all good logic, for causes of madness in either the outer world or the inner world—and engage in the search for what are called proximate and remote causes of madness.

Some medical historians have saluted in this separation a distinction between organic and functional disturbances of the psyche. This is, I think, a projection of modern concepts, though it may well correspond to a possible genealogy of the concepts of organic and functional—concepts that today denote either a discernible physical cause of insanity, such as a lesion, or the lack of a physical cause in the etiology of madness. Battie's distinction of inner and outer is metaphysical. Not surprisingly, much like Descartes, he has no criteria by which he can say if perceptions are caused in the inner or outer world. Battie declares nonetheless that once one can decide wherein the cause of a perception lies, one can decide whether madness is curable or not. False perceptions arising from causes within the nerve fibers cannot be corrected, since the rationalist's a priori knowledge that nerve fibers exist does not extend so far as to discern what actually occurs within the fibers and their subtle fluids. Therefore, the doctor can only know that something is amiss, but not what is amiss and is causing false perceptions. This view leads to the conclusion that in most cases of madness the doctor cannot intervene except through what Battie calls management of the insane. With this he endorses the Hippocratic hope that, in a beneficent milieu, nature may offer some remedy.

Battie's position is at once humane and disquieting, and in this ambiguity his work seems to embody the double aspect of the Cartesian legacy. His position is humane in its recognition of a specificity to madness within the economy of human disorders. Moreover, madness does not transform the insane into animals, nor is it a result of sin or error. In the history of dealing with the mad this is a major achievement. And one need only contrast Battie's philanthropic attitude with the extravagant medical practices of the time, when rationalism had led to the bloodlettings and the beatings in use regularly at Bedlam and elsewhere. But Battie's position is also disquieting, for, in reducing madness to a question of dysfunctional fibers, Battie has effectively corroborated the view that the mad are machines, and thus, in spite of Battie's humane criticism of such practices, he has corroborated the views of his contemporaries who saw in madness a comic bestiality to be placed on exposition for a few pence.

The Augustans' Derision of Madness and Theories Thereof

By the early eighteen century the mad had become, for much of Europe, the mirror image of machine man's comic derisiveness, the degraded image of what the modern philosopher Bergson later, in defining the comic, called the mechanical grafted onto the human. Even after they rejected the medical philosophy behind this vision, the English Augustans could revile the mad and, at the same time, go to Bedlam to dodge their excrement and laugh at them. Fibers physiology made of every humanoid a potentially comic puppet, and Bedlam was the emblematic theater in which these puppets could present their farcical spectacles. The linkage of theater and madness seems intrinsic to our need to transform the disaster of madness into spectacle. But, of course, it is one thing to see, like the Greeks, the comic as based on madness, quite another to view the insane as comic. Many Augustans had, in reversing these terms, lost the Greek understanding of the relation of madness and comedy.

None of the medical models that transformed the mad into defective machines silenced them—on the contrary, slack or shortened fibers seemed to release creativity. During the eighteenth century the mad began to speak, to write, and at times to publish. Madness acquired all the appeal of a mode with the new bourgeois reading public. And with writers such as Swift, Pope, and Johnson in England, or Diderot and Sade in France, to name only the best known, madness entered the literary arena. Ancients and moderns confronted in literature madness and the image of the dysfunctional machine humanoid with varying reactions, but it is generally true that the "ancients" gave little credence to the claims of medicine to explain madness, whereas the "moderns" were likely to adapt those claims to their own agendas.

To offer the example of a partisan of the ancients who preceded the Augustans, one can turn to Molière. A hostile stance toward doctors and philosophers can be found, with interesting complications, in Molière's version of Don Juan. Molière was on the side of the ancients, but his Don Juan seems to be a modern. This libertine atheist is scientifically literate, yet he shows a dismissive attitude toward doctors' incapacities when he addresses Sganarelle, his servant, who, upon dressing in a doctor's robe, finds himself solicited for medical advice. Don Juan scornfully comments:

> And why not? For what reason shouldn't you have the same privileges as other doctors? When the sick get well they have no more part in it than you do, for their entire art consists in mere grimaces. They do no more than take credit for fortunate successes, and you can take advantage, as much as they, of the patient's good fortune, and thus see attributed to your remedies what may come from the good grace of chance and the forces of nature. (*Don Juan*, 3.1)

Doctors have, from the point of view of rationalist skepticism, nothing to say about the sick, even if this modern rationalism is voiced by a character created by Molière, a believer in the superiority of the ancients. Both ancients and moderns could embrace skepticism, for the possibility of scientific rationalism had created—in the wake of Cervantes and Descartes—the conditions of possibility for a skepticism that was larger than one's position about the relative inferiority or superiority of the classics.

The widespread skeptical dismissal of much of medical theory did not resolve, moreover, any questions about what the mad represented. The mad were very visible, even when locked up, and they often demanded a voice. Indeed many neoclassical writers found in themselves the voice of the melancholy they attempted to consign to Bedlam. Depression, hallucination, and manic guilt were ready to invade the neoclassical writer's well-ordered world, and at times these forms of madness seem far more prevalent than the celebration of the best of all possible worlds that rationalists like Leibniz, the young Voltaire, or Pope described.

My argument is, then, that the neoclassical world is the world in which madness begins to gain a nonironic literary voice, even if it speaks as a combatant in a dialectical arena in which reason tries to gain mastery. And, later, with the writing of Cowper, Smart, Sade, and Hölderlin, one can argue that madness came into its own during the Enlightenment. For the first time certifiably insane writers explore their madness in texts. To sharpen this argument, in the rest of this chapter let us first give consideration to the work of the two major Augustan writers who dealt with madness, Swift and Pope; and then deal with their continental opposition, the materialists like Diderot and Sade, the first sane, the second demonstrably mad. And in the following chapter we can then see how madness gained a voice in the exploration of singular voices created by Goethe and Rousseau as well as the new insane asylum.

The insane ironies of the saturnine antimodernist Swift (1667–1745) highlight crucial ambiguities showing how fluctuating were the lines of demarcation between what neoclassical reason could stake out as its domain and what it wanted to relegate to madness. In his *Discourse Concerning the Mechanical Operation of the Spirit,* published in 1704 along with *A Tale of a Tub* and *The Battle of the Books,* Swift set out to conjure the powers of madness through satire and irony directed against the partisans of machine man—partisans, in his view, of madness itself. But the reader can hardly be sure what to make of *The Mechanical Operation of the Spirit,* in which Swift promises to explain the operation of mind, but offers the explanation as an omitted paragraph that is neither safe nor convenient to print, and then concludes with a parody of religious enthusiasts. His satire aims certainly at the *virtuosi,* or the iatro-chemical and mechanical thinkers, of whom the chemist Boyle is a primary example:

> It is the Opinion of Choice *Virtuosi,* that the Brain is only a Crowd of little Animals, but with Teeth and Claws extremely sharp, and therefore, cling together in the Contexture we behold, like the Picture of *Hobbe's Leviathan,* or like Bees in perpendicular swarm upon a Tree, or like a Carrion corrupted into Vermin, still preserving the Shape and Figure of the Mother Animal.[9]

With vitriolic satire, Swift takes on the scientific moderns, using an irony that aims at the text that produces the irony—his own—as well as the world of the moderns that the text, in nearly insane rage, would destroy. The writing mind is supposedly a product of heat-driven animal spirits—a condition for madness—and so are the minds of those who produce such insane theories about the origins of madness. Madness produces theories of madness, which in turn demonstrates what Swift calls the usefulness of madness.

Don Quixote stands as one rhetorical model for writing that in reflecting upon itself reflects, ironically, upon madness. Unlike Cervantes, however, Swift offers no access to a referential world of universal truth-values. And his writing often seems maniacally on the edge of coming apart under the weight of its ironies and satire, at once directed against the insane, and against those who would explain insanity, and finally against his own insane attempt to conjure all this away. In the midst of the imitation of delirium that Swift proposes in *A Tale of a Tub* the reader must wonder if this dialectic really is an attempt to bring reason into mad discourse, or if, in Swift's attempt to test reason itself as a principle of discourse and narration, he has not passed over into delirium, real delirium. In writing this madness, he seems to have wanted to see if the rationality afforded by narrative structures can bear up under the brunt of insanity's assault upon it.

From another perspective *A Tale of a Tub* can be viewed as one of the first experimental works of fiction in English history. It is experimental in the sense that it is a testing of reason and the categories and constraints that reason imposes on discourse, especially on narrative discourse. And all this experimentation is undertaken in a spirit of nearly demented hostility against the physiology of the new science. *A Tale of a Tub* is usually considered part of the battle of the ancients against the moderns. This quarrel itself is part of an epistemological argument about what are the criteria for reference, truth, and rational operating procedures for certifying what is to count as knowledge. Though overtly a partisan of the ancients, Swift's recourse to experimental literature is a singularly modern procedure. For, in his rage about the way the sciences of physiology and medicine have become the measure of what can be said about reason and unreason, Swift is at once a reactionary critic of science and the inventor of a modern discourse in madness. By this latter term I mean that he has, or so I am tempted to argue, created the first narration of mad discourse without irony—probably despite his intentions.

A Tale of a Tub is a discourse in madness, thus one ostensibly narrated by a modern, which means that he has studied at the academy of Bedlam. In this narration composed of digressions and digressions about digressions, the reader confronts a demonstration of the modern's madness, especially in "A Digression Concerning the Original [*sic*], the Use and Improvement of Madness in a Commonwealth." The use of a mad narrator, in this tale and in *Gulliver's Travels,* to test the limits of reason seems to me to be Swift's signal invention. The digression concerning the improvement of madness begins with notice that Jack, one of the three representatives of religion in the tale, is mad, for Jack is the religious dissenter who is deviant by the rational standards of official Christianity. The mad narrator then offers an explanation of this madness, for, as he would have it, all new schemes in philosophy and all the inventions of new religions are the product of vapors rising to fertilize the brain, much as all fruits of the earth arise from rain. All history can be analyzed through a prism focusing on vapors-induced madness. The narrator has easy work showing that all thought is the product of dementia, from Epicurus through Paracelsus and "Des Cartes." Conquerors and religious fanatics, doctors and philosophers are all interchangeable madmen. The narration revels in its metamadness, or dementia about dementia, showing the alchemist Paracelsus making perfumes from excrement and Descartes wrapped up in the vortices with which Cartesian physics filled cosmic space. Rejecting the theory of machine man as the product of a diseased mind, the satire then uses the image of machine man to explain how that diseased mind was produced in the first place.

This savage circularity mimics rationality that is grounded in a series of self-evident truths. The satire produces a negative version thereof, a self-evident madness that proves itself. Madness is the obvious motor force of history. It produces schools of thought, for example, when the vapors strike upon a "peculiar *String* in the Harmony of Human Understanding, which in several individuals is exactly of the same tuning" (p. 339). The vibrating chord induces sympathy in those with the same fibers, producing those groups of individuals who are fools in one group, but philosophers in another; which is to say, groups who share the same worldview, the same set of beliefs that are wisdom or folly according to the social context. Swift seems to endorse, in this mockery, a relativistic view of truth. Relativism is another rather modern development that occurs when, in the eighteenth century, the foundation of cultural anthropology forced Europeans to look at the relativity of the criteria for reason and madness. Cultural relativism demands a justification of one culture's claim that its beliefs are superior to those of another culture. Swift's solution is to proclaim all worldviews deviant, even as he accepts the rectitude of the official Anglican worldview—which undoubtedly explains some of Swift's personal difficulties. Madness makes all points of view equal, but the curate Swift could hardly proclaim this view from his pulpit.

A sense of relativity underlies much of the satire. Religions, military conquests and empires, science and philosophy in this view are all produced by graduates of Bedlam who have not found an acceptable social context for their talents. To improve madness, then, one must find a better way of fitting Bedlam's inmates into the world. After all, the difference between a lunatic and a military hero is only the context in which he waves his sword. Or the difference between a doctor's examination and an act of insane scatophagy is one of circumstance: after reading Willis's treatise on urines, those so disposed can taste urine without being accused of coprophilia. Central to Swift's satire is his constant attack on Warwick Lane—the Royal College of Physicians—where medicine has garnered the power of practical reason. And by now this power is the power to differentiate the relatively mad and the relatively sane in view of incarcerating the former in Bedlam. But neither sane nor mad come off unscathed in Swift's world of pandementia, for the modern urine-sniffing doctor and the ordure-eating lunatic look at each other in an act of mirroring that Swift holds up in jubilation as the image of universal madness.

In pursuing the dialectic of madness and reason that levels all rational distinctions, Swift shows an understanding of the double deviance characterizing the work of Aristophanes. Swift is perhaps unique during the Enlightenment in this regard, an era better known for its wit and irony than for comic savagery deriving from madness. This understanding of deviance is lacking in most Enlightenment writers, such as Alexander Pope (1688–1744), who interests us precisely for his understanding of the task of reason. Pope, the most important Augustan poet, wanted to conjure madness while creating the most rational form for poetic expression. The fascination that madness worked on the rationalist poet brings to light the fragility of the reason that the ancients believed was embodied in tradition. A friend of Swift, Pope is the embodiment of neoclassicism: he was the aggressive proponent of an aesthetic doctrine declaring that there are forms that embody what reason dictates to be the rational forms for poetry. I formulate the doctrine so as to stress the rational circularity of wanting to use reason to reveal reason so as to justify its use. This aspect of neoclassicism, first in Boileau, then in Pope, makes of art a form of logos. His commitment to logos suggests that Pope's fear of the irrational was born of an insecurity that is the other side of Enlightenment confidence. In fact, Pope is quite clearheaded about his rejection of the horrors the inner world might reveal if pressed. Finding the revelation of poetic logos in Horace and Boileau, believing that reason is a matter of properly using transparent signs, Pope shared with Swift the axiom that the writer should not look for interior worlds, in the depths of the self or in hidden meanings beyond the luminous surfaces illuminated by reason itself. In *A Tale of a Tub* Swift's narrator observes that a certain woman, when flayed, did not look at all improved. We can take this observation as emblematic of what the neoclassical thought about revealing the inner self, or what lies beneath the surface.

This refusal of what cannot be clearly formulated by reason has many implications. For example, in attacking fibers physiology, Pope refuses to grant modern medicine any role in knowledge, or as he says in the prologue to his poem *An Essay on Man:*

> The science of Human Nature is, like all other sciences, reduced to a *few clear points:* There are not *many certain truths* in this world. It is therefore in the Anatomy of the mind as in that of the Body; more good will accrue to mankind by attending to the large, open, and perceptible parts, than by studying too much finer nerves and vessels, the conformation and uses of which will for ever escape our observation.[10]

Pope has more than a distaste for depths; he rejects in loathing any search for the hidden and the nonevident. This viewpoint might be called the neo-classical axiom of antiprofundity. Pope is hardly an anti-intellectual. Though an ancient, he celebrated Newton's achievement in bringing a new order to the world with his celestial mechanics and laws of motion. It is not the outer, but the inner world that Pope declared to be a realm of necessary ignorance. Pope was in agreement with Battie's later formulations that one must be forever ignorant of what transpires in the nerve vessels—to which Pope would have added a scornful rejection of Battie's rationalist assurance about describing the human machine in a priori terms.

In spite of his refusal of profundity, Pope was fearfully fascinated by the delirium that lies in the inner depths of humanity. His concern with madness is matched only by the revulsion he felt for the medical science that claimed to explain this delirium. This revulsion underlies *The Dunciad*, first written in 1728, and then done in another version in 1743. In this comic work Pope tried to exorcise the madness that threatened his neoclassical confidence. Appropriately dedicated to Swift, this poem is an ironic celebration of the goddess Dulness, a deity who propagates imbecility, stupidity, dementia, and madness. She incarnates the barbarous principle of unreason. But, in an ironic dialectic, unreason is to be understood as the boundless claims of reason to order the world. And the goddess condemns those who would limit their quest for knowledge to the surface of things and scorns those who are "By common sense to common knowledge bred, / And last, to Nature's Cause thro' Nature led" (4.467–68). Rather, Dulness exhorts her followers, such as Descartes and Hobbes, to flights into vision, into the invisible reality of the world of inner imagination:

> We nobly take the high Priori Road,
> And reason downward, till we doubt of God:
> Make Nature still encroach upon his plan:
> And shove him off as far as e'er we can:
> Thrust some Mechanic Cause into his place;

> Or bind in matter, or diffuse in Space.
> Or, at one bound o'er-leaping all his laws,
> Make God Man's Image, Man the final Cause.
>
> (4.469–78)

Reason follows its course, revealing its capacity to invert itself in the dialectic in which madness reveals itself in reason. In *The Dunciad* Pope's inversion of reason gives rise to what is another experimental text, one really at odds with Pope's neoclassicism that initially motivated the burlesque of the foolishness produced by the moderns' hubris.

Reason gives rise to madness, to a world gone awry, and finally to an apocalyptic finale in the fourth book. This total destruction is the mad outcome of the dementia of those who seek knowledge beyond reason. Much like *A Tale of a Tub* in this regard, the final version of *The Dunciad* loses itself in ironies about ironies, with its prefaces, footnotes, and other procedures that turn the destructive parody constantly against itself in an explosion of self-incrimination. This self-destructive irony goes out of control, and not simply because Pope wanted to write a satire of a few writers whom he found boring or trite. The poem is far more ambitious: it wants to conjure the demise of reason, the *Umnachtung* when night emerges and darkness asserts its superiority over the light of day. Poetry's task is universal exorcism, but poetry is written by the "dull poet" who, a footnote says, lives in a miserable hall in the neighborhood of the Magnific College of Bedlam, for which the poet's father did the statues that adorn the entrance into the asylum. The poet is led on in his task by insanity itself, by the mad Sibyl who preceded Dulness, "in lofty madness meditating song," on to a vision of the triumphs of Barbarism over Science (3.16). Barbarism is the triumph of poetry, by which the poem denounces itself, along with most of science, as a form of madness spun out by the deficiencies of reason.

The self-contradictory rage, with its decentering of any firm interpretive standpoint, and its final vision of the victory of madness, probably corresponds little to what a biographer might say about Pope's intention in writing the poem. He probably intended to decry the stupid, the mad, and the poor, all of whom he loathed.[11] Beyond intent, however, these paradoxes, born of an attempt to denounce the madness of reason, are generated in a cultural matrix over which a writer can have little control—as both the examples of Swift and Pope demonstrate. In denouncing the fraudulent excesses of the doctrine of machine man, they were obliged to use the image of machine man, which led to rhetorical procedures that produced the unreason they abhorred. This led to the paradoxes of ironies about ironies, irony that abolishes itself, and the contradictions of self-referential incrimination in which poetry demonstrates logically the madness of poetry.

Pope seemed obliged to embrace the image of machine man as the subject of poetry, for no other theory was available to explain how, in the sway of Dulness, the poet comes to repose, curtained "with Vapours blue." Vapors cause "raptures" to overflow "the high seat of sense," which in turn causes the poet to hear oracles and talk with gods. And then, like the benighted maid's romantic wish and the mad chemist's flame, the poet's "vision of eternal Fame" comes upon him (3.5–12). The poet's inner world is a space in which monsters find their likeness as joy surges up (3.249–51). The world of interiority reveals itself in the eruption of madness. Carried in upon the wings of madness, the Cartesian metaphysics of subjective and objective worlds forces itself upon Pope in these lines. The rationalist psychology Pope expounded in *An Essay on Man* is inadequate to explain the madness of the world, for how can a psychology based on the principles of self-love and reason explain the turbulence of inner desire? Finally, Pope seems to accept the metaphysics of machine man while berating the barbarism of the science that leads to such a view: only something as insanely comic as machine man could in any case come up with the materialist physiology that invents machine man in the first place. So Pope attacks the mechanical humanoid as a comic character in hopes of making of interiority a matter of public purview. True reason should be able to cast light on the madness of the soul, and all the more so if dysfunctional fibers are responsible for the madness that leads to the belief that fibers are responsible for the inner world.

The finale of *The Dunciad* is apocalyptic. Machine man is comic, but he truly menaces reason with the apocalyptic reign of night. Once the mechanical dunce triumphs in his madness, no light is left to illuminate the world. This affirmation of logos as light, reviving the belief in the heliocentric nature of reason, also renews the biblical vision of final judgment as the loss of logos in the world:

> Nor *public* Flame, nor *private*, dare to shine;
> Nor *human* Spark is left, nor Glimpse *divine!*
> Lo! the dread Empire, CHAOS! is restor'd;
> Light dies before the uncreating word:
> The hand, great Anarch! lets the curtain fall;
> And Universal Darkness buries All.

(4.651–56)

In this Augustan fear of madness can be read the end of the English form of neoclassicism, a doctrine that came to an end earlier in England than else-

where. The end is marked by an apocalypse that must recur each time reason gives rise to its own demise by overstepping the bounds of reason. The
rupture in logos is total, and reason is incapable of explaining the presence
of its contrary in a world for which evil and insanity are incommensurable
with anything the rational mind can entertain. The Enlightenment did not
like the dialectic of reason and unreason that it could never master. We find
this dilemma in Pope, and will presently find it in Diderot, though developed
conversely from a materialist viewpoint.

Literary Materialists and Machine Man's Madness

Swift and Pope illustrate the paradoxical difficulty of rejecting the dominant
medical paradigm for madness. Writers on the other side of the English
channel offer the equally interesting dialectical paradoxes of modern materialists who positively embraced the model of machine man, such as
Diderot and Sade, respectively the most brilliant and the most demented of
the philosophes. Thus I propose that we turn to these two more than exemplary figures to complete our understanding of how the image of machine
man figured the Enlightenment understanding of insanity, and first the
ardent materialist rationalist Diderot (1713–1784). He is the prototype of
the intellectual for whom all discourses offer models for experimenting with
discursive games in order to see their logical implications. In this regard
Diderot brings to literature the type of experimentation that was beginning
to characterize science. First a materialist, and then an atheist, Diderot was
conversant with virtually all Enlightenment fields of knowledge. He was the
ideal editor for the *Encyclopédie,* that compendium of rational organization
designed to bring the "lights" of the Enlightenment to the world. Diderot
had warmed up earlier for that task by translating the medical encyclopedia
of Robert James, giving the continent in 1742 a six-volume *Dictionnaire
universel de Medecine* dealing with medicine, surgery, chemistry, botany,
anatomy, pharmacy, natural history, and medical history, all this with
plates illustrating medical practices. In Diderot's version James work was a
major source for the neo-Hippocratic revival at the end of the century. Not
only does this medical encyclopedia present an intelligent and sympathetic
appraisal of the Hippocratic corpus, it severely criticizes Boerhaave's medical mechanics, noting skeptically that nobody had ever demonstrated that
fibers are conduits in which animal spirits flow. In the *Encyclopédie*
(1751–1765) Diderot drew upon many contributors, and it is noteworthy

that the articles on medicine generally reflect the iatro-mechanical viewpoint. For example, the article on dementia defines it as a state resulting when impressions no longer properly follow fibers to the brain and thus are no longer transformed there into intellectual notions. Machine man is unquestioned in the *Encyclopédie*.

Of greater interest for an understanding of the revels of madness are Diderot's fictional writing and philosophical dialogues. They enact thought experiments testing the theories about machine man and madness. Diderot's skepticism is especially fueled by a sense of the contingency of propositions: rationality is a question of varying contexts. For example, Diderot's narrator in the *Lettre sur les aveugles* (Letter on the blind), pursues the idea that if all ideas are dependent on sensations, then all ideas are contingent on the context and the means of production of those ideas. Imagine a people composed of only the blind. Then let one of them have vision for a brief period of time: "If a man who was possessed of vision for only a day or two found himself mixed with a society of blind people, he would either be obliged to remain silent or to pass for a madman."[12] Materialist Diderot reverses the position of Christians like Swift and Pope, for this image of madness characterizes those who, in the centuries of darkness preceding the Enlightenment, might have encountered the light of rational truth. For the philosophe, persecution of reason by darkness has been the history of reason.

The sanity of propositions depends on a social context that approves the propositions, on a relation between the origin of those propositions and their context, and finally a worldview that embraces the total context. The mad can be visionaries, then, who encounter a worldview that will not countenance them. For Diderot, there is nothing intrinsic in what people say that marks it as mad, only its relation to a context can determine that. But relativizing is only one way of describing madness, and Diderot's playful mind also wanted positive knowledge of the machine. He wanted to know how fibers produce in humans such varying interpretations of reality. How do they produce madness? One thought experiment about fibers occurs in the posthumously published *Paradoxe sur le comédien* (Paradox about the actor), in which Diderot plays dialectically with the question as to whether the actor dominates his role intellectually or if he really feels the role. Diderot draws upon Haller's physiology and Bordeu's vitalism to hypothesize that sensibility is an intrinsic characteristic of living matter. Considerations of physiology must lead to the conclusion that madness is an intrinsic part of the human constitution:

Sensibility, according to the only definition yet given to the term, is, it seems to me, this disposition, this companion of our organs' weakness, this result of the mobility of the diaphragm, of the vivacity of the imagination, of the nerves' delicacy, which inclines us to feel sympathy, to resonate, to admire, to fear, to be disturbed, to cry, to faint, to help others, to flee, to cry out, to lose one's reason, to exaggerate, to scorn, to disdain, to have no precise idea of the true, the good, and the beautiful, to be unjust, to be a madman. (P. 182)

Madness lurks within sensibility, that intrinsic property of animate matter, and hence at the heart of the sensible matter making up machine man. This conclusion is not far from what we have seen in Pope and Swift: reason, in pursuit of understanding, finds madness at the heart of itself. The important question for Diderot is what this means.

With much good humor Diderot pursues these thought experiments in works like *Rêve de d'Alembert* (D'Alembert's dream) and *Suite de l'entretien* (The continuation of the conversation with D'Alembert). Diderot here proposes that dream is a form of madness produced by loosened fibers that allow the mind to roam. He introduces the contemporary doctor Bordeu as a character so that, like a vitalist precursor of Freud, the doctor can listen to D'Alembert while the mathematician sleeps and dreams. As D'Alembert speaks in his sleep Bordeu comments on the production of madness in dream by the work of the fibers. In dream D'Alembert's soaring mind shows the effects of madness at work, for the mathematician's mind pursues hypotheses about the production of his own ideas. These works are a whir of theories, as D'Alembert dreams them and Diderot and Bordeu explain them: fibers theories, vitalist variations thereupon, Ciceronian moralizing, allegories of reason and passion, and others. However, in these dialogues Diderot is drawn most strongly to the materialist hypothesis that sensibility and madness are somehow two sides of the same coin. The irrational endowment of fibers with sensibility is a rational explanation of vital phenomena—even if this means that reason is grounded in the ultimate irrationality of vital processes. In the face of this irrationalism Bordeu attempts to defend the Stoic view that the "great man" can render himself master of his diaphragm and dominate his bundles of fibers (p. 314), which means that the less than great are simply sensitive beings, which is to say, Ciceronian madmen—"les êtres sensibles ou les fous."

Diderot's most ambitious thought experiment about madness takes the form of *Rameau's Nephew,* a work that explores how madness might logically be a superior way of life if machine man really exists. This satire is an extraordinary challenge to Enlightenment confidence, or at least a challenge to Diderot's confidence, since this satire, written as a dialogue, was never published. Written over a period from 1762 to 1776, the work first saw print when Goethe published a translation on the basis of a manuscript he had acquired. The work was thus first known in the nineteenth century to German romantics like Hoffmann. In fact, the original manuscript was not discovered until the end of the nineteenth century.

In this dialogue the philosopher Diderot confronts a madman who, reversing Ciceronian platitudes, defends his right to be deviant. It is up to Diderot to defend reason against madness. This is not an easy task. The madman, the nephew of the famous musician Rameau, is a depraved parasite who, while conversing with Diderot, makes fun of Diderot's bourgeois morality and goes so far as to recommend that Diderot prostitute his daughter. Armed with iatro-mechanical theories of madness, Diderot, the reasonable philosopher, faces a deviant who takes pride in his capacity to provide his rich, debauched patrons with all the entertainment they might find at "les petites Maisons," or the Paris equivalent of Bedlam. Diderot recognizes that insanity is entertaining, it is comic, a form of divertissement that challenges the philosopher to assert his mastery over it. Drawing upon scientific theories of deviance, Diderot also tries to justify the superiority of what he sees as the rational life. Defending deviance, however, the nephew's cynicism makes short work of the dull world that the philosopher holds up as the ideal. He points out that the philosopher's ideal is a product of his vanity. And borrowing from the rationalist philosophers, the nephew can declare that in this best of all possible worlds, whatever is, is right—which provides a witty inversion of Pope. Therefore, the parasite, a part of that world, is fully justified.

With this cynical inversion of rationalism the nephew willfully indulges in whatever deviance or perversion his sensibility moves him to. In his descriptions of the nephew Diderot borrows from medical theory by dramatizing the play of sensitive fibers when he depicts the nephew's eruption into paroxysms of pantomime. This theatricalization transforms the nephew into a gesticulating player imitating madly some reality of which he is the delirious double. The nephew's body is a pure machine for reproducing sensations. His self is lost in the play of fibers by which the body is frenetically moved in the acts of representation. Diderot is aghast before these outbreaks of insanity in which artistic forms—music, poetry, dance—are reproduced by a parasitical machine. His only defense of his own sanity is to explain in rational terms how this degeneracy can occur.

Diderot's attempts at mastery have little pragmatic value, for the nephew can readily agree that his fibers are amiss or that his hereditary background is deficient; and with that he can exult in his talent for depravity. Upon asking the nephew how, with such sensitivity to artistic beauty, he can be so insensitive to the charms of virtue, Diderot receives an iatro-mechanical justification of deviance. The theatricalization of madness is just a question of fibers, and so the nephew turns the tables on Diderot in his defense of his madness:

> Apparently others have a sense, a fiber that I don't have, a fiber that wasn't given to me, a loose fiber that one can pinch all one wants and which won't vibrate; or maybe it's that I've always lived with good musicians and with bad people; so it happened that I have a sharp ear and a dull heart. And of course there's the matter of race. My father's and my uncle's blood are the same. Mine is the same as my father's; the paternal molecule was hard and obtuse, and that cursed molecule assimilated everything else.

The nephew hardly omits a current scientific paradigm in this self-justification. Using this science, the nephew can move quickly from a de facto description of himself to an inverted moral exhortation in favor of depravity and corruption as models for the superior life.

Diderot's dialogue is a key moment in the history of mad discourse, for in this thought experiment, the mad person is allowed to assent to the power of reason and then appropriate it to justify his madness. The nephew uses the strategies of reason to assert the power of deviance. Machine man recognizes the madness intrinsic to the machine and proclaims that he wants to be entertained by his own dancing fibers. This is the logical outgrowth of a materialism developed to its deviant consequences.

A comparison with Pope and Swift's rejection of machine man is revealing. In their satires involving a mad narrator, experimental form delimits the space of folly and attempts to set reason somehow on the other side of a space informed by madness. They do not succeed, or at least that is my interpretation of their self-abolishing ironies. But one believes that Augustan reason should be victorious, even if it isn't. In Diderot's *Nephew*—a work also paying homage to neoclassicism by its very desire to master the irrational through satire—the comic dialogue entails a competition in which reason appears overtly bested by the willingness of madness to accept itself as a state caused by perturbed fibers or vapors—and then to declare that this justifies being mad. Only the nephew's sadness, momentarily a sadness close to despair, suggests that there is something amiss in deviance; and this is perhaps merely because the nephew is not nearly as successful in depravity as he feels he should be. This satire does not involve any paradoxical praise of folly, as with Erasmus. Madness is affirming its demented rights in the face of the claims of reason. It is only a step, a seemingly logical step, by the logic of machine man, to affirm the claims of madness to be the claims of reason. This is the step undertaken by the Marquis de Sade, of whom the parasitical nephew is a precursor in the inverted sublimity that makes of insane depravity the ideal, or to quote the nephew:

> If it is important to be sublime in some genre, it is above all in evil. People spit on the petty thief, but nobody can refuse a kind of consideration for the great criminal. His courage astonishes you. His atrocities make you shiver. His unity of character in everything is greatly esteemed. (Pp. 94–95)

With the idea that deviance can be sublime, the nephew inaugurates the belief that madness can set aesthetic and moral standards.

Evil as art, madness as virtue, these are questions entertained by vibrating fibers. They are not questions that Erasmus or Cervantes, nor most of Diderot's rationalist contemporaries, would have sensibly entertained, even if the nephew is developing the implications of his contemporaries' physiology of machine man. Animal spirits convey impressions that mechanically become perceptions and judgments. And physiology has no way of saying why deviance and folly should not spring from these mechanical transactions.

All the currents we have discussed so far—mechanical physiology and the dialectical triumph of madness over reason—seem to culminate in the work of the Marquis de Sade, the writer who was willing to pursue madness as an ideal in his own life. In life, as in literature, deviance was the inverted rational ideal for Sadean machine man. It was with a rare chronological irony that Sade was born in 1740, the year in which Diderot's favored novelist, Samuel Richardson, gave the world *Pamela,* a work of "sensibility" that publicized virginity as a synonym for virtue. This symmetry offers in résumé the dialectics characterizing the Enlightenment, for sensibility can designate both the source of virgin virtue and the source of the pleasure that the nerves find in flagellation. Or consider dialectically the fact that we began this chapter with the pious Van Helmont, attempting to free the soul from the ensnarements of the body, and end it with the "divine Marquis," dreaming of converting the body into the source of endless perversions that reason commands as the ideal. Sade is the dialectical end product of the thought about machine man, of iatro-mechanical medicine, and a materialism that believed it could exhaustively and reductively describe the world.

There have been many interpretations of Sade, with laudatory ones given by surrealists and, more recently, by radical feminists who want to make Sade into a precursor. From this perspective Sade's black humor is the sign of a liberated mind that reveals forbidden realms of discourse in which desire acquires new meanings, freed from the constraints of bourgeois or paternalistic rationality. The projection of the surrealist or a feminist agenda onto Sade is not very convincing. From a historical perspective there is no doubt that the Enlightenment considered Sade to be mad, both for miserable criminal acts he perpetrated—criminal by today's standards—and above all for the insane manuscripts in which Sade inverts all standards of rationality and ethics.

Sade's revels in madness thus present an exemplary case study in which literature seems to be in the service of an existential commitment to deviance. To illustrate this point, let us turn to a typical example of sadism, say, *Juliette ou les Prospérités du Vice* (Juliette or the prosperity of vice). Published in 1797 in Holland, this novel was probably as much responsible for Sade's imprisonment as was his delight in flagellation or in poisoning prostitutes. *Juliette* is a first-person narrative by one of the most liberated heroines of world literature—an anti-Pamela. First debauched in her convent, Juliette then learns the joys of prostitution in a "maison de tolérance" where she makes a series of encounters that leads her to enter into an alliance with the homicidal libertine Saint-Fond. Their cruel orgies encompass every form of sexual perversion as well as such crimes as cannibalism. During a moment of weakness Juliette hesitates to approve Saint-Fond's ambitious plan to starve to death most of the population of France. Therefore she must flee, and the rest of her tale relates her skillful manipulation of her charms in treachery to become rich again: she arranges rape, incest, murder, and even helps the pope satisfy a taste for blasphemy. The novel ends with an inverted apotheosis in crime in which she murders her own daughter. And, for the benefit of less than subtle readers, Juliette can finally cry out, "je l'avoue, j'aime le crime avec fureur, lui seul irrite mes sens" [I admit it, I love crime with furor, it alone excites my senses].[13]

The search for excited senses or for "irritated nerves" is physiology applied in the service of hedonistic delirium. The novel's plot is merely the framework that allows long disquisitions proving that physiology is essentially the science of pleasure. Juliette and a multitude of libertines indulge in interminable ramblings on the nature of nature and man, to conclude that the pursuit of the joys of deviance is the only logical deduction that follows from the premises about the machine nature of man and, in this case, woman. Juliette's teacher, Madame Delbine, is for instance an exponent of La Mettrie's materialism and demonstrates to her student that conscience is merely a question of "nervous principles" that the enlightened mind can reduce and eliminate as a question of mere physical effects:

> All moral effects . . . depend on physical causes to which they are irresistibly bound; it's like the sound that results when one strikes a drum with a drumstick. If there is no physical cause, then there is no vibration, and then necessarily there is no moral effect, that is, a sound. Are we masters of these secondary effects when the first causes make them a necessary result?
>
> Can a drum be struck without giving out a sound? And can we oppose this shock when it is the result of so many things that are foreign to us and so dependent upon our physical makeup? Therefore it is really insane, really quite extravagant, for us not to do whatever we feel like doing or to repent of whatever we've done. (P. 35)

Insanity is not to be insane. The reasoning may not be impeccable, but that matters little. What is clear is that the reversal of reason and unreason informs the argument here: insanity would consist in adhering to the norms of sanity in the world of machine man precisely because those norms have arbitrarily mechanical causes. Ergo the rational physiologist should take out the whip and pluck, if not beat, those fibers that increase the mechanical causes that give pleasure.

There is an egalitarian side in Sade's work, for men and women are companions in these orgies during which heroes and heroines never hesitate to philosophize. At the drop of a whip both are willing to reason that, since victims are necessary in the scheme of natural equilibrium, it is proper to create more victims. More than Pope or Leibniz ever dreamed, all is justified by nature's grand indifference. Whatever is, is right, and this truly all-inclusive "all" justifies that one do whatever one feels like, knowing that, as Sade puts it in *Justine,* one day science will show that all laws, all ethics, all religions, and all gallows and gods are the product of the flow of a few fluids, the arrangement of a few fibers, the composition of blood and animal spirits.[14]

With insane repetition Sade narrates the demented dream of machines coupling with other machines, enjoying the pleasures brought about when the machine recognizes that it is beyond good and evil. In his madness Sade is, however, hypocritical, for his work depends on the existence of taboos, interdictions, and rational norms—the full moral and rational culture of the Enlightenment—for the existence of the transgressions that offer the full spectrum of delight. There can be no "crimes of love," to quote a Sadean title, if there are no laws. There can be no rationally justified transgression if reason also decrees there are no norms to be transgressed. As Georges

Bataille knew, the fundamental narcissism of the Sadean text demands the existence of rationality and norms so that the transgressor can feel the shiver of delight at being beyond the norm, at daring to go beyond the law whose existence the Sadean philosopher denies in the same breath. Sade's exaltation of vice as the only stimulant capable of bringing full vibration to one's fibers entails the recognition of virtue, for in dialectical terms the notion of vice is meaningless without it. Pamela must precede Juliette. Machine woman receives her vibrations from nature—from the givens of physiology—but then Sade demands that she enjoy them because of their criminal nature. This step means that in his arguments Sade is constantly moving from culture to nature and back again to culture. He denies the existence of culture even as he affirms the necessity of the opposition of nature and culture for the existence of pleasure. This ongoing contradiction is at the heart of the mad ratiocinations of Sadean characters, machines capable of endless deviance, and even more of endless discourse about deviance. They are insanely incapable of finding a closure for this discourse, other than in death. The inverted discourse of insane repetition ends a certain easy Enlightenment acceptance of the universality of reason; though this was perhaps not apparent at the time. Sade could not really be read for some decades after his life. For better or worse Sade is our Enlightenment contemporary. The late eighteenth century still believed in reason—it enshrined it as a god during the French Revolution—and had the good sense to keep the insane marquis locked up most of the time.

Chapter 5

Neoclassicism, the Rise of Singularity, and Moral Treatment

The Marquis de Sade is a contemporary of the doctor who is often credited with being the founder of modern psychiatry, Philippe Pinel (1745–1826). Pinel gave the modern psychiatric clinic a symbolic image when in 1793—the year of the Terror—he removed the chains from the mad incarcerated in the asylum of Bicêtre. Pinel's reforms at the asylum of Bicêtre were really a culminating moment in the ongoing philanthropic movement that was changing the treatment of the insane throughout Europe. And his *Traité médico-philosophique sur l'aliénation mentale ou la manie* of 1800 also marks the high point in the neoclassical revival of Hippocratic medicine. To understand this transformation of Enlightenment views of madness, we can gain much if we study this double orientation of Pinel's thought and practice. First, however, in order to understand the context in which Pinel's work unfolded, it is necessary to examine some of the discourses on madness that precede Pinel's work. Especially important in this regard are certain literary texts from the second half of the eighteenth century. In granting the mad a voice, if even a fictive voice, these texts precede the medical reform that took place during the final decades of neoclassical thought. Increasingly in the second half of the eighteenth century, literary voices emerge that are not afraid to speak madness and demand recognition of its human singularity. The changes in medical treatment of madness were accompanied by a reevaluation of madness that was prompted by literature and its demands that madness be heard. This reevaluation took place largely in opposition to the medical doctrine of machine man. Rejecting madness as a condition of dysfunctional fibers, writers began to shape a myth of madness conceived as a form of revelation of the singular self. This myth, emerging at the end of the neoclassical period, was destined to become a defense of madness: it is conceived as a privileged state of epiphanic vision.

The same historical categories can be used to describe the major trend in medicine and literature at the end of the eighteenth century. There was in both fields a renewed interest in Greco-Roman models of thought that, during the French Revolution, culminated almost in caricature. Courageous Cicero, defender of the Roman republic, and eternal Hippocrates, inventor of clinical rationality, were public heroes. In medicine and literature this inflection of neoclassicism also renewed a rationalist view of the self. Neoclassicism promoted a vision of an imperial self that claimed capacities for itself well beyond those vouchsafed by the mechanical physiology of machine man. The development of this concept of the imperial self continued beyond neoclassicism, well into the nineteenth century. But it is at this moment in the history of consciousness, in the latter part of the eighteenth century, that the artist began to entertain the belief that the self could be a locus for revelation, of transcendence, and that madness could be a means of access to that realm of revelation. The late eighteenth century saw the development of a cultural matrix, blending antiquity and modernity, that was unique in its accent; and with regard to the mad, unique in that for the first time it gave the mad a voice and encouraged them to speak, as poets and as patients.

The Demise of Machine Man

Machine man died a rather slow death. His demise was brought about by the rise of competing medical and physiological models, as well as literary and philosophical reactions against him. A number of theories contributed to these attacks, especially interpretations of the vitalist work of Stahl (1660–1734) and of the physiology of Haller (1708–1777). Though neither broke clearly with the mechanical model of physiology, both were important for giving impetus to later nonmechanical theorizing. Stahl was a vitalist chemist who proclaimed that a "vital force" distinguished man from a machine. Haller gave a new twist to the notion of sensibility by making irritability an intrinsic property of muscles and sensibility a property of nerves. Competing with physics and mechanics as models of rationality, the protochemistry and physiology of these scientists underwrote the vision of "sensible man" that dominated the end of the Enlightenment. Moreover, the vitalism that underwrote the then nascent science of biology was the precondition for conceiving of insanity as an illness caused by something other than organic dysfunctions: vitalist forces are not reducible to mechanically caused motions. And "life" could thus be a category unto itself. In this regard Stahl's phlogistic chemistry and vitalist physiology opened onto the future, even if these sciences, especially his chemistry, disappeared, leaving little trace in the organization of contemporary scientific discourses after Lavoisier and Magendie.

Stahl's vitalist doctrine can also be interpreted historically as a rewriting of Aristotle and Hippocrates within the neoclassical matrix. His doctrine of the emission of phlogiston to explain burning is a way of restating the Aristotelian doctrine concerning the existence of a negative substance in matter. Stahl's neoclassicism refurbished an ancient language game with repercussions for medicine. Matter is a negative notion. Movement is, by distinction, spiritual and immaterial. This viewpoint means that living matter is not subject to the laws of chemistry that rule over inorganic matter. Rather, the laws of the sensitive soul hold sway in living matter—which is largely a way of restating Aristotle's doctrine of the psyche. Some version of Stahl's doctrine of the *anima* came to be accepted by nearly every continental doctor by the end of the eighteenth century, by Pinel in France, or by Reil, the German romantic who invented the word *psychiatry,* or by an innovative scientist like Bichat who refused to use a mechanistic tool like the microscope in setting forth the basic concepts of histology.

Haller's work, on the other hand, had stronger affinities with the doctrine of machine man; but his theory of the irritability of muscles and the sensibility of the nerves was also used to buttress the vitalist model. The notion of sensibility could be interpreted in vitalist terms to show that sensibility depended upon consciousness for the observer to note its existence. Therefore, sensibility was taken to be a unique mental phenomenon showing that mind could exert influence on matter. The doctrine of irritability and sensibility seemed to grant autonomy to the nerve fibers as bearers of some vital force that could not be explained in mechanical terms. Moreover, as the historian of science Canguilhem has argued, after Haller function could no longer be derived from form. After Haller, the image of the mechanic's workshop no longer seemed the appropriate image to explain physiological functions.[1]

The vitalist consensus was probably necessary for the invention of something like "mental disease." But literary voices at the end of the Enlightenment were equally as important in the change in attitudes toward madness. A number of literary texts propose that within the mad there is a principle, a self, or a form of consciousness, that can listen to its own madness. Whatever be the state of the mad body, there is within the mad an inner distance between madness and some vital center that allows the mad to speak reflexively about their madness. This view parallels the notion that the function of mind is separate from any organ to which it might be attributed, for the vitalist principle also makes functions larger than any single determining form (which might appear to be an early model of the now fashionable complexity theory). The rejection of the mechanistic model of mind meant that mind could function even in the presence of "lesions" of the understanding—lesion being a medical metaphor that seemed alternately to have a physical or a metaphysical meaning. Literary and medical vitalism meant that the mechanical image of mind could no longer be invoked to explain madness as the garbled production of ideas by a dysfunctional machine. Or as Pinel decided, neither Locke nor Condillac could explain madness.

Singular Literary Voices Speak Their Madness

Accompanying the change in medical thought was a willingness to hear the mad, to allow them to speak, and, in literature, to grant them occasionally the right to publish. The mad hero gained a central voice in literature, as one sees in the English poets of sensibility and among German writers, especially those associated with Sturm und Drang, an early revolt against neoclassicism. Moreover, in every European country the faddish affectation of melancholy became the mark of an enlightened stance toward the world. Melancholy offered the properly disenchanted note of world-weariness in which the joys of active madness gave way to despair, or to quote the neoclassical poet Delille (1738–1813):

> Ils sont passés, mes jours d'ivresse et de folie:
> Viens, je me live à toi, tendre Mélancholie.[2]

> [My days of intoxication and madness are gone:
> Come, I shall give myself over to you, sweet Melancholy.]

Is this pure period style? Undoubtedly, and yet this cliché bespeaks the common desire to explore mental illness, a desire in part motivated by the revival of the Aristotelian canon, and especially the *Thirtieth Problem* that associates genius with madness, and poets with melancholy.

It is difficult to evaluate the authenticity of claims to madness that recur with platitudinous insistence during the latter part of the eighteenth century. The poetic stance expressed, in part, the historical discovery of the possibilities of madness that we can all find within ourselves once we conceive of our self as a vulnerable singular self immersed in time. It is important to correlate the literary discovery of the singular self with the rejection of the universal rationality that underwrote machine man. Machine man was a fantasy derived from a vision of the universal machine, as transparently explainable as the mathematics that can describe the roll of a ball down an inclined plane. With the slow demise of this belief in total explanation, the necessity of defining the truth of the singular became crucial in literature and in psychological medicine. (In classical mechanics an analogous, if rather theoretical, crisis was to occur when it was discovered that it is not possible to find the equations capable of solving the three-body problem of celestial mechanics.) In poetry this quest for truth took the form of a debate with rationalistic science about the truth-value of what the singular self could know. In medicine, it meant the corresponding advent of a philanthropic psychiatry that was willing to listen to the unique mad voice expressing its singular experience.

For an understanding of the notion of singularity in literature, the work of Johann Wolfgang von Goethe (1749–1832) is historically of the greatest importance. His work allows us direct access to the singular mad voice that the mad came to recognize as their own. If Goethe dominated for several decades world literature—a notion he invented—it is in part because he endowed the pathological with a philosophical dimension. This is much what Jean-Jacques Rousseau did when he depicted his own deviance in his autobiographical writings, and so, after dealing with Goethe, we shall turn to Rousseau for an understanding of how literary confession also contributed to the rise of the belief in singularity. In Goethe's work the pathological is the center of a conflict between the universal and the singular that was increasingly at the heart of the late eighteenth century's understanding of madness. And all of Europe became interested in singularity when in 1774 Goethe wrote one the first best-selling novels, *The Sorrows of Young Werther*. In its portrayal of despair and suicide this novel elevated the pathological to a category of popular understanding. Later in his play *Tasso* Goethe also gave to Europe the first serious work of literature in which the poet or the writer is a hero—and in which he is, as Aristotle might have predicted, quite mad. (At least I have found no earlier example of a poet dramatized as a tragic hero in a work of European literature.) Insane lover and mad poet: both are seemingly platitudinous figures who appear for the first time in Goethe's work as nonmythological examples of deviance as such. Moreover, in *Tasso* the poet enters for the first time upon the historical stage as if to dramatize the madness that produces literature itself. It would appear that the poet only enters literature as a subject once his madness can reflect back upon itself and meditate the singular work to which it gives rise.

Werther, our first prototype of the antirationalist hero, is the protagonist of a simple tale. He suffers intolerably from the limits of existence and kills

himself to escape them. The clearest manifestation of these limits is his failure in love. He falls in love with a woman who is betrothed to another man.
He loves her intensely until, to escape this melancholy dilemma, he borrows
her fiancé's pistols to kill himself. One reading of the symbolic purport of
this narrative would stress that the seeker of the infinite, Werther, founders
on the presence of reality—the fiancé Albert—until he borrows the pistols.
Werther has to borrow from the representative of reality the means with
which to end his flight from reality, which is to say, his life and his insanity.

Why did all of Europe harken to this fictional outcry of madness directed
against the limits of existence? The answer lies in the way Werther's defense
of his vital singularity found a resonance among those who refused to be
defined in terms of Enlightenment rationalism and its universal categories.
Werther claims the right to singularity, the right to a deviance that Enlightenment rationalism could not recognize because this demand is not
grounded in a rational universal. Rameau's nephew would have understood
this demand, but not Condillac's statue becoming endowed with reason, nor
Kant's ethical man, nor, for that matter, the Marquis de Sade whose defense
of depravity is grounded in the universal reason of machine man.

This defense of singularity endows a pathological discourse with a voice
that dramatizes its attempt to find a language suitable to its impasse.
Werther has a voice that can express both sides of a split self, a self that is
capable of self-observation and then of speaking across the distance
between a mad self and an observing self. The observing self espouses the
viewpoint of those characters in Goethe's texts who represent the reality
principle, the fiancé Albert or, in *Tasso,* the aristocratic man of action Antonio. The inner observing self is obliged to consent to the point of view of the
man who commands reason, and hence the power of the universal and
objectivity. Werther, the split hero who is deviant and yet clairvoyant, has
within himself a self that understands the position of universal reason, but
his singular self prefers what is other than reason. He understands with
lucidity the meaning of objective demonstration, but prefers the realm of
singular interiority.

Werther's defense of his singularity takes the form of a bitterly ironic
praise of folly. This praise is ironically underscored when Werther encounters a madman in the road. Recently released from an asylum, this madman
considers the time he spent in the *Tollhaus* to have been his happiest years.
The madman is a Shakespearean foil to Werther. His praise of insanity is
reflected in Werther's relations with others. When the fiancé, the rationalist
Albert, depreciates the passions as the equivalent of madness or drunken-

ness, Werther responds with a challenge to the voice of reason that resonates like a manifesto for the right to be mad:

> "Oh you sensible people!" [vernünftigen Leute] I exclaimed with a smile. "Passion! Drunkenness! Madness! You stand there so calm, so unsympathetic, you moral men. You condemn the drunkard, abhor the insane man, pass by like the priest and thank God like the Pharisee that He did not make you as one of these. I have been drunk more than once, my passions have never been far from insanity, and I regret neither; for on my own scale I have come to appreciate how it is that all extraordinary people who have achieved something great, something apparently impossible, have been decried as drunkards or madmen.[3]

Werther's positive evaluation of madness is a defense of his own pathologies, a defensive outcry from someone incapable of ordering his life, but also a defense of what Werther takes to be superior values. He trenchantly refuses, at the cost of going mad, the mechanical rationality of a world that thinks only in instrumental terms. Goethe disowned Werther later in life, but Werther's outcry remains the starting point for understanding the outrage the mad could feel during the Enlightenment when judged by a rationality that refuses their singularity.

This praise of folly in the face of uncomprehending reason, with its universal categories and maxims, contributed to creating a dialogue in which madness speaks about itself. The structure of dialogue was essential for the foundation of a new psychiatric practice in which the medical listener might hear a self that has lost its relation to reason. The philanthropic doctor had to be capable of listening to a self lost in singularity. The medical listener had to be capable of negotiating the inner distance between the singular self and a rational self for whom the self is lost in its own eyes; and to understand that the measure of madness is the distance between a self lost in singularity and a self capable of judging itself. This view of madness encourages the belief that communication with the mad is possible. But Goethe's work also shows that this communication is most difficult. Werther's madness takes the form of a lamentation by a self that believes there is no mediation possible through discourse. Werther describes this fallen state with clarity:

> I am in the state of mind of those unfortunate creatures of whom it was believed that they were possessed of an evil spirit. Sometimes I have a seizure; it is not anxiety, not desire—it is an unfamiliar, inner raging which threatens to tear my heart asunder and constricts my throat. Woe! Woe! And then I roam about in the terrible nights of this inhuman season. (Pp. 219, 221)

Werther has an acute sense of the history of madness, comparing himself to a medieval case of possession, when he tries to describe a state beyond language, beyond logos and its mediations, in which he is isolated in his singularity. But there is no explanation, theological or other, for his deranged state that rages beyond the capacity of reason to order it in a well-regulated taxonomy.

There is a historical dimension to both Werther's and Tasso's cases. Each finds himself excluded from a historical world whose dominant worldview is defined by reason in functional terms as the power to manipulate the real. Reason is an instrumental power whose main function is to adjust means to pragmatic ends. This concern with the historical determinations of madness undoubtedly accounts for why Goethe dramatized Tasso's plight, the poet whose madness occurs at that moment when rationality, as defined by Machiavelli for the prince, was defined as power and its effective use. The historical Tasso went insane at that moment when art lost its relation to the sacred. With this alienation art was also alienated from power. Instrumental reason relegated art to the realm of mere ornamentation, produced for the satisfaction of the imagination—which is to say that art was relegated to the same sphere shared by the productions of the insane: fantasy. From this perspective art can justify itself only when it is in the service of power. This is made clear in Goethe's *Tasso,* when the play's man of action, Antonio, describes the function of art according to the pope, who is also the most powerful prince: "He values art insofar as it is decorative, and enhances his Rome, and makes his palaces and temples into marvels of the earth. He allows nothing near him that is not useful!" (1.4.667–70). If artists are not useful to a rationality defined as power, by power that decides what is real, then they must live in a shadow realm that borders on madness. Without power, artists are by definition excluded from the real and hence from rationality. Goethe's play suggests that, after the Renaissance, insanity and art are two expressions of the same historical powerlessness.

Goethe's Tasso, like an artistic Hamlet, has no power and consequently finds nothing upon which to exercise his will. Paralyzed in inactivity he is conscious of his dysfunctional nature. His self-judgment causes him, in revolt, to praise the madness that is the ultimate category for his singularity. This consciousness of singularity in the eighteenth century underlies a new aesthetics that rivaled with, and then replaced, the neoclassical belief in aesthetic forms fixed by reason. The new aesthetics is often called an expressive theory of art: it justifies art as the outpouring of the singular self, of the genius, who can somehow attain the universal by expressing his or her singularity. The artist had to accomplish in effect what the mad needed to do if they were to communicate with their doctors. The singular self was conceived as the place in which revelation could spring forth. This was a paradox, if not a form of madness, when judged by the traditional standards of neoclassical aesthetics. From the standpoint of neoclassicism the immediate expression of the contents of the singular psyche could only give access to dream, to subjectivity, to madness—a view the nascent romantic movement hardly assented to. But, for neoclassicism, it was contradictory to say that the expression of immediate subjectivity could result in propositions having universal truth-value. Neoclassicism viewed the expressive theory of art as a desire to ally art even more closely with madness—a view the neoclassical Goethe endorsed when, late in life, he said that romanticism was an illness.

As a poet Tasso must live in the sphere of dreams. This is a contradictory state, since he must also be a vessel that expresses—in the etymological sense of pouring out—truths of an objective and universal nature. The contemporary theorist of schizophrenia, Gregory Bateson, would have spoken of a double bind in Tasso's case, since the poet receives contradictory injunctions from his milieu. His prince, a father figure embodying reason and power, orders the poet to be true to his dreams at the same time the prince wants to cure the child-poet of his fantasies. Rejected by the men who embody power and hence reason, Tasso can hardly be blamed for believing that the demands of reason and the necessities of art cannot be reconciled. The contradiction is too great, or so Tasso tells the Princess, herself half-mad, when he says he cannot finish his epic poem, since it will destroy him. By pursuing art he will lose himself in imagination, or alternatively, madness—which is what reason bids him to do while censuring him for the same activity, for abandoning the real for the phantasmagorical world of his dreams.

Both *Werther* and *Tasso* propose theories of madness and, in so doing, make discourses on madness into a self-conscious staple of Western literature. First, Werther is a theorist of his own madness, capable of a self-reflexive discourse that dramatizes the distance between the sane and the deviant part of the self, all found in one breast. Refusing a separation of body and mind insofar as pain is concerned, Werther tells the play's man of reason, Albert, that there are limits to the amount of passion or pain a person can endure before being destroyed. Therefore, as Werther says, blaming a person who commits suicide is the same as chastising the sick when they die of fever. Albert finds this all rather paradoxical. He cannot see how one can be driven to the necessity of suicide. It is beyond his ken that the irrationality of suicide can be a rational response to anguish. In his singularity Werther knows that he cannot find a common measure of understanding with the man of reason. Holding fast to his worldview, Albert lives on this side of the line delimiting reason, and so Werther knows that he cannot be known:

> It is useless to hope that a calm, rational person could grasp the condition of the unhappy man, useless to counsel him. Just as a healthy man at the bedside of a sick person cannot impart to him even the slightest quantity of his strength. (P. 115)

And so Werther tries to draw an analogy between his own desperate feeling and that of a young girl he once knew. Jilted by her only lover, the girl committed suicide. To Albert's remonstrances that the girl lacked the intelligence to bear her fate, Werther replies that the little understanding a human being may have is of little avail when passion rages and "the limits of one's humanity press in upon one" (p. 18). Communication between reason and unreason demands that Werther employ, seemingly in vain, all the strategies rhetoric can suggest.

In attempting to express knowledge of madness, Werther is struggling to go beyond the limits of comprehension, using figural language and stretched comparisons to bring the reader, if not Albert, to an understanding of his singularity, which is to say, his pathology. To this end he brings to the foreground a theory of limits, a theory about the lines of demarcation that separate the realms of the norm and the deviant. These realms are associated, in rhetorical terms, with figural and literal language. The man of reason inhabits the realm of literal language, whereas the singular hero is obliged to inhabit the realm of the figural, for it is only through tropes and analogies that he can try to explain his condition. So that one sees that it is a rhetorical move that brings Werther to compare his mental state with the involuntary weakness of a person having a physical illness. And it is with this kind of rhetorical move that the metaphor of mental illness is born.

The confusion of literal and figural language in *King Lear* was central to the hermeneutics of madness. With Werther and Tasso the refusal of figural language is now part of the domain of reason, and it is the mad hero who must attempt to point out the confusion that rational men may make when they judge figural language to be mere imaginings, which is to say, insanity. In *Tasso* the representatives of reason and reality are concerned with curing the insane poet of his imaginings. Their humane concern for the poet parallels the type of moral treatment for the insane that was gaining currency at the end of the eighteenth century. Alphonse, the prince, rejects recourse to a "harsh doctor" for Tasso. He describes a cure for insanity that would respect Tasso's humanity:

I do what I can in order to fill his breast with security and confidence. I often give him, in the presence of others, clear signs of my favor. If he complains of something here, I have the matter examined as I did, when he recently thought that his room had been broken into. And if nothing turns up, then I calmly show him how I consider the matter. (1.3.335–48)

Sounding like a precursor to Pinel, Goethe's prince uses the tone of reasonable patience to create the atmosphere in which one can make moral claims upon the mad and demand that they heed reason.

Tasso takes the moral claim seriously and even tells the prince that he is healthy. But this is a pose. One part of Tasso hears the moral appeal of reason. But Tasso turns to himself and recognizes his own dissemblance. His insane self comes to the fore and encourages Tasso to hold fast to his mask. Dissimulating is hard, as he puts it, only the first time (5.4.3100). This is the crux of the moral dilemma: Tasso can recognize the moral claims of the prince, hence of reason, but he also feels that by obeying the universal he is betraying himself and a duty to his mad singularity.

In Tasso Goethe confronts us with madness's counterclaim to its authenticity, or, if that is too modern, with the desire that madness has to retain its own singularity. To this end madness must define itself in the face of reason and its power to define the real. The role of power is placed in the foreground in Goethe's work with rare clarity. The real and the rational are defined in circular terms as the power to decide what is the real. For, by definition, power can proclaim what is the real and impose that decision. The mad may have always felt the intrinsic powerlessness of their situation, but, with Goethe's work, the capacity of power to define madness is defined as an intrinsic part of the nature of power. Werther and Tasso live their madness as alienation from the defining spheres of power—or from the real.

I now turn to Rousseau, for, from my perspective here, he is the other great source for the definition of the self to emerge in the latter part of the eighteenth century. To turn from Goethe to Rousseau is to turn to a revolt against the Enlightenment understanding of the real. And in this revolt is developed another important version of the modern self as one that defines itself through its deviant singularity. I refer primarily to the self found in Rousseau's autobiographical and confessional writings that came to crown his career as the most influential writer of the late eighteenth century. All published after Rousseau's death in 1778, his *Confessions, Rêveries,* and *Dialogues* span the Enlightenment in their narration and paranoid defense of Rousseau's life. The first complete edition of the *Confessions* was published in 1789, the year that saw the outbreak of the French Revolution, that historical rupture that Rousseau's political thought had seemingly called into existence. However, Rousseau first made his mark against the Enlightenment in 1749 when, in his thoughts out of season known as the *First Discourse,* he attacked the instrumental notion of reason that the Enlightenment held up as the primary instrument for its moral and material progress. The progress made in the arts and sciences was, for Rousseau, only progress in deviation from the origins of humanity, a time when men were transparent to each other, when a purer reason held sway, and when humanity was not a slave to a form of reason demanding increasing progress—or what Rousseau saw as increasing alienation from humanity's natural origins. Rousseau began his career with an attack on Enlightenment rationality for its deviance from truth and ended it with his writing defending the truth revealed in his own deviance. Rousseau's imperial self encapsulated all of world history, for nothing less could explain his singularity. And for this vision of self, there has been a consensus that Rousseau was in some sense mad.

Since the end of the eighteenth century there has been no lack of doctors to analyze the origins and development of Rousseau's madness and, by implication, to reduce Rousseau's grand irrationality to a question of a contemporary mental illness. Jean Starobinski has shown that Rousseau has been a litmus test for successive generations of psychiatrists, each of whom has projected on Rousseau's madness and somatic problems one of the syndromes most in favor at the time the doctor was working. Starting with Pinel's diagnosis of Rousseau's melancholy and going through Morel's theory of his degeneracy and Janet's analysis of his psychasthenia, the clinical description becomes more modern with Demole's discovery of Rousseau's schizophrenia or Laforgue's diagnosis of latent homosexuality and hysteriform obsessions and reactions—and one could go on at length.[4] In refusing instrumental reason's power to define the real, Rousseau is clearly the mad writer who has challenged every nosological system of the past two centuries to use him as a test case for the system's power of explanation, and perhaps thereby refute Rousseau's view of rationality as deviance.

For our thesis about the importance of literary discourses in the understanding of madness, Rousseau's importance is that in his writing he made autobiographical singularity the center of the quest for the revelation of truth. And this quest served to validate the romantic belief in the power of madness to effect disclosure and bring about vision. To demonstrate this proposition I turn first, not to Rousseau himself, but to the greatest mad poet of all time, Hölderlin (1770–1843) and his way of reading Rousseau, which can set the stage for our reading Rousseau. No one has better interpreted the powerful effect of Rousseau on European thought than did Hölderlin in his "Rousseau," written ten years after the beginning of the French Revolution:

> Und mancher siehet über die eigne Zeit
> Ihm zeigt ein Gott ins Freie, doch sehnend stehst
> Am Ufer du, ein Ärgernis den
> Deinen, ein Schatten, und liebst sie
> nimmer.

Or, in Michael Hamburger's prose translation:

> And more than one there is who can see beyond his own time. A god shows him the way into the open, but yearning you stand on the shore, an offence to your own time, a shadow, and do not love them.[5]

Hölderlin presents a Rousseau who is oracular. In his madness Rousseau points the way to a space—the Open or the Free—beyond logos in which the singular hero's word receive divine inflection. Rousseau was not understood by his contemporaries—and in this sense he was mad—but, according to mad Hölderlin, Rousseau's madness carries him beyond the collectivity to an unmediated relation with the Word. This is necessary since the collectivity has declared its own deviance to be reason; but Rousseau shows that the historical process is a deviance from reason that has come to be called progress. History is really a fall from the gods and origins. Hölderlin's Rousseau, the divine prophet, returns to a relation to language in which singularity is empowered to understand the higher reason that the gods reveal with a hint, for "hints have always been the language of the gods" (p. 76). In short, Rousseau's madness is relative to this moment of decadence, and Hölderlin, himself sliding into insanity, finds in Rousseau's hatred of his contemporaries the prophecy of a time when passion will be restored to purity and deviance will come to an end.

Rousseau's historicizing of madness was seized upon by the romantics. Rousseau's view of history may seem to parallel the Judeo-Christian view of the Fall, but it also naturalizes the fall from grace as a philosophy of history. The Enlightenment had secularized the myth of the Fall in a number of forms. Rousseau is hardly alone in this mythologizing, which derives from many sources. For example, before Rousseau, medical thought had already taken over this myth and had made deviance and history synonymous. In George Cheyne's *Natural Method of Curing the Diseases of the Body and the Disorders of the Mind depending on the Body*, published in London in 1742, or in his earlier work on melancholy called *The English Malady*, from

1733, the doctor anticipated Rousseau with the idea that there is more disease in a state of society than in pure nature, as exemplified by societies of savages or animals. Cheyne proposed that in a state of nature, where personal interests need take no account of others, there are few madmen, whereas in civilized societies mental derangement is among the most common of maladies. It remained for Rousseau to emphasize the historical process that underlies this fall from nature leading to the madness of society. This Rousseau did in his *Second Discourse* of 1755, dealing with the historical process that has resulted in the inequality characterizing European societies. In his essay he adumbrated a theory of history that is implicitly a theory of societal madness. Only madness could account for our loss of natural origins. Or, in other words, in his philosophy of history Rousseau brilliantly rationalized what was becoming a medical cliché: madness is increasing because of civilization. Disease is increased by progress, hence by history.

This historical judgment also informs Rousseau's view of madness and his presentation of self in his autobiographical writings. He conceives that his good intentions could have been misconstrued only during an era in which passions have become corrupt. This is especially evident in the last writings, the *Dialogues,* in which Rousseau ruminates obsessively on the persecutions of which he believed, rightly or wrongly, that he was victim. Kafkaesque in their repetitive delirium, these dialogues dramatize the inner distance of madness I evoked in speaking about Goethe's characters. A character named "Rousseau" can speak of his folly in a direct conversation with a third party, a Frenchman, as they together judge "Jean-Jacques"—hence the curious title that the citizen of Geneva gave the work, *Rousseau Juge de Jean-Jacques, Dialogues.* The dialogue form imposes a distance by obliging the speaker to distance himself from his interlocutor, as he speaks of the madness—and persecutions—that the other, who is also himself, has known.

At the outset of the *Dialogues* Rousseau evokes a hypothetical primitive world in which "primitive passions all would tend toward our happiness."[6] In his singularity Rousseau believes that he has remained in contact with the felicitous world of nature that has disappeared for the rest of humanity. The phylogenetic description of humanity's deviance from happiness implies that, in ontogenetic terms, every individual must repeat the Fall of the species. And, in fact, in his *Confessions* as well as in *Emile,* Rousseau spells out that every development, from child to adult, recapitulates the Fall from paradise. Rousseau deduces from the drama of his singularity the most extreme conclusions, finally finding that he alone, in this time of fall and deviance, has undergone the unique development that differentiates him from all others. His unique development allows him at once to understand history and to be persecuted for it.

It is in this light that the famous opening lines of the *Confessions* take on their full potential for giving access to madness:

> I am commencing an undertaking, hitherto without precedent, and which will never find an imitator. I desire to set before my fellows the likeness of a man in all the truth of nature, and that man is myself.
>
> Myself alone! I know the feelings of my heart, and I know men. I am not made like any of those I have seen; I venture to believe that I am not made like any of those who are in existence. If I am not better, at least I am different.[7]

A devotee of Linnaeus, this singular man proclaims his place in a natural taxonomy in which he is the only exemplar of his species. However, Rousseau's defense of singularity is really a refusal of the entire movement of natural science in the eighteenth century. For if the mad person is a singular species, if each case of insanity is individual, one must wonder how one can frame a general taxonomy that allows analysis of mental illness and makes it amenable to rational discussion.

Rousseau theorizes the etiology of his singular state. Or rather he theorizes the normalcy of his singularity when compared with the historical development that has led to the present state of generalized depravity. Rousseau uses a familiar Shakespearian tactic: the voice of deviance defends itself, in a dramatic reversal of polarities, by proclaiming that the voice of reason is really the voice of madness (cf. *Oeuvres*, 686–87). Doctors and philosophers bear the brunt of Rousseau's defensive attack that, in denouncing materialist physiology and philosophy, privileges the voice of sensibility, the inner moral voice of singular man. In physiological terms, the singular man represents the highest form of the vitalist life force that escapes the operations of mechanical reason. But the voice of sensibility has been nearly extinguished by a historical development that has eventuated in those philosophers who spend their energy stifling this inner voice that a "nondepraved soul" could not resist (p. 687). In Rousseau's view philosophers are obviously depraved, and their reason is a form of pathology that refuses to recognize the truth of the heart. Or, to paraphrase Pascal, Rousseau seems to say that deviance has reasons that reason does not know. Rousseau defends the inner voice, the singular voice of sensibility, that slumbers under the crushing weight of historical development.

The reform movement in the medicine of the late eighteenth century cannot be separated from the literary defense of madness such as we find in Rousseau. Not only did Rousseau's attack on materialist physiology contribute to the rise of vitalist doctrines, but, in making a distinction between two sensibilities, the physical sensibility and the active moral sensibility, Rousseau promoted a doctrine that argued for the separation of mental and physical illness. The physical sphere is the area of passive responses whose goal is the conservation of the body through pleasure and plain. By contrast, the moral sensibility is "nothing other than the faculty of attaching our affections to beings who are strangers to us" (p. 805). And the study of nerves cannot make one acquainted with this empathetic sensibility. Rousseau's rejection of mechanistic models did not, however, entail a total rejection of science. The influence of the Newtonian paradigm was so powerful that neither Rousseau nor Goethe could resist the temptation to compare empathetic sensibility to the attraction exerted by material bodies on each other. One might speak in this context of the development of scientific eclecticism. For example, the rise in vitalism also coincided with the development theories about animal magnetism and mesmerism and other such "paradigms" that came, briefly, to fill the gap left by the demise of the doctrine of machine man. And with this, the dominant medical paradigm is found, in the last decades of the eighteenth century, in the neoclassical "Hippocratic revival."

Pinel and Philanthropic Views of Madness

This revival coincided with a reform in the treatment of the mad. Doctors such as Tuke, Chiarugi, and Reil are among the best-known reform leaders. For a discussion of psychiatric reform and its homologies with literary developments, however, Philippe Pinel offers an especially relevant example: in this doctor we find at once a philosophical nosologist and the doctor that many would consider the first psychiatrist. Educated at Montpellier, Pinel was a vitalist and, in the monumental nosography he published in 1798, initially a follower of the Scottish doctor Cullen. In his written work and in his practice Pinel brought together all the currents characteristic of late neoclassicism: a vitalist rejection of the necessity of lesions to explain the etiology of madness, a revival of the Hippocratic practice of clinical study, a Ciceronian concern with moral cures, and a literary sense that madness can express itself in narrative and drama. Or as he wrote enthusiastically in 1798 in the second volume of the *Nosographie philosophique*:

What a close union, what reciprocal dependency, between moral philosophy and medicine, as Plutarch noted. How important it is, in order to prevent mania or melancholic or hypochondriac affections, to follow the immutable laws of ethics *[la morale]* to maintain dominion over oneself, to master one's passions, in a word to make oneself as familiar with the works of Epictetus, Plato, Seneca, and Plutarch, as with the luminous results of the observations that have transmitted to us by Hippocrates, Aretaeus, Sydenham, Stahl or other famous observers. Does not Cicero, in the third and forth book of the *Tusculanae,* consider the passions as maladies and does he not give fundamental rules for treating and curing them? (1798 ed., 2:12)

Some modern interpreters of Pinel have wanted to see in his work a belief in a talking cure; that there is in madness a voice that speaks across the inner distance and that, in the act of speaking, finds a therapeutic balm. There is undoubtedly something of this in Pinel's idea of "moral treatment," but, as this ebullient passage shows, there is also in Pinel a desire to return to Stoic thought. Pinel's thought recycles classical ethical notions in what is largely a reprise of the dominant themes of the history of madness. Moral treatment means that an appeal to reason should be sufficient to motivate a desire to return to reason. This was also the Kantian moral position, and it points up the central dilemma of the late Enlightenment: how can revolutionary republics or insane asylums make appeals to those who deviate from reason so that they will pursue their own enlightened self-interest? Pinel was notably more humane in this regard than the *Comité de salut publique* in 1793.

It is important not to take the above-cited nosological work of 1798 for Pinel's later *Traité* or the treatise on madness published in 1800. Pinel published two separate works, the first a general nosography dealing with hundreds of diseases, the second a treatise dealing exclusively with madness. He kept both in print and felt apparently no inconsistency about being a proponent of two different medical systems. In the first work, the *Nosographie* of Year VI (1798), madness is classified along with hundreds of other maladies. In the book there are six classes of disease that we would call mental disorders. The fourth class, *névroses,* is broken down into four orders: vesanies, spasms, local nervous anomalies, and comatose affections. These orders give rise to no less than some eighty-five genres. Under the order of vesanies are included such things as hypochondria, melancholy, mental alienation, and hysteria. This was all recast in a new edition in 1818, but that is of little interest here: what is important is that, in borrowing from Cullen, Pinel tried to set up an all-inclusive system of classification that might rival the taxonomy of the naturalists. Historians Charles Singer and

E. Ashworth Underwood contend that Pinel's classification of over twenty-five hundred diseases was in no way possible in Pinel's time, "when there was little anatomical background on which to base it."[8] But anatomy is not the issue with regard to these classifications: his system was an a priori language game based on the combinatory properties of semantic models. It had little to do with the specificity of disease.

Totally independent of his nosography is Pinel's *Traité médico-philosophique sur l'aliénation mentale ou la manie*. This book was first published during the ninth revolutionary year (or 1800), and then again, without reference to mania in the title, in 1809 in a longer and revised version. This *Medical-Philosophical Treatise on Mental Alienation, or Mania* has been one of the most successful classics in the field of medicine. The first edition is an important part of the Hippocratic revival. Showing a clear sense of historical continuity in the treatment of madness, the *Traité* can be said to initiate historical consciousness in the practice of medical psychology. Especially in the introduction, Pinel displays a sense of the historical development of medical concepts, which undoubtedly explained Hegel's enthusiasm for Pinel's treatise. Pinel recognizes that the return to Hippocrates is also a form of historical inquiry into the foundations of medical discourse:

> Hippocrates appears, and an eternal barrier arises between the merely empirical use of medicines and true medical science. I mean the study in depth of the character and the process of diseases. The immense scope that was opened to his research did not allow him to give special attention to mania, but he gave the general example of his severe descriptive method. And those capable of appreciating it took it as the model of their first attempts to sketch out the history and treatment of mental alienation.[9]

This historical sense is rooted in the desire to return to the origins of medicine, there to find the history—in both senses of story and natural history—of madness. It parallels Rousseau's praise of origins, or, for that matter, the attempt by French revolutionaries to become Roman republicans. This is a historicism that takes as axiomatic a belief in the virtue of origins, and in this regard Pinel, like many doctors at the end of the Enlightenment, is a follower of Rousseau.

Pinel's neoclassicism is hardly the grounds for modern medical thought, though his philanthropic reform of the asylum began the development of more humane treatment of the mad. His theoretical thought is embedded in a matrix that sought to make Greco-Roman rationality a living presence. This is not altogether surprising, for one can argue that it was only during the Enlightenment that European thought began to approach the rigor and fullness of Greco-Roman philosophy and science, after the revolutions in mathematics and physics in the seventeenth century. Medical neoclassicism drew fully upon its origins with remarkable agreement, as is clear if we look at a pair of Pinel's contemporaries. For example, the use of the Greeks in the work of Doctor P. A. Prost informs the judgment he made of Pinel's work. Praising Pinel for his "moral reforms," this doctor criticized him nonetheless in the name of truths found in Hippocrates. With regard to mania Prost claimed that his own study of the endocrine system had showed him the presence of bilious mucous matter of dark color in the viscera of the mad whose autopsies he had undertaken. Black bile remained on the historical stage when empirical science, equipped with Hippocratic categories, could "confirm" Hippocratic readings of madness. But the rejection of Greco-Roman humors as causative agents also occurred when late-eighteenth-century thinkers recycled the passions theory of madness. For example, the very influential Joseph Daquin, in his *Philosophie de la folie* of 1791, coined the term *moral treatment* for dealing with the mad. With this, he proposed a therapeutic theory based on his renewed use of Ciceronian belief in the power of Stoic reason to cure madness (though Daquin also endorsed the belief that the moon causes insanity).[10] In short, medical discourse at the end of the Enlightenment was again using Greco-Roman concepts to define the mad self. These medical doctrines can be considered modern only to the extent our modernity still relies upon the same concepts—and an argument could be made to the effect that our somatic and psychological arguments about the nature of madness continue the debate between Galen and Cicero. This is not an argument, however, I wish to pursue.

It is more interesting for our modern concerns to see that what was modern in a narrow sense in the new philanthropic concern with madness was the belief that madness is in some sense a unique area of human experience. Literature pressed the claim that, however pathological or deviant madness may be, this singular realm is also a region of experience that may find some measure of commonality with normal experience. Communication with the mad, locked in their singularity, is not impossible. But because of the singularity of madness, it was incumbent upon medicine to find new methods or techniques for communication. The ancients were the prime model for doctors, because, to press my earlier point, many medical thinkers still felt that medical rationality had not yet at the end of the eighteenth century reached the standards set by classical antiquity. All these currents culminate in Pinel's *Treatise*, in which he showed a historical consciousness of the development of medical treatment. The *Treatise* is nonetheless a somewhat paradoxical work by the standards of medical practice that have appeared since the French Revolution. It is paradoxical in that it grants madness a singular voice while it makes singularity disappear in a reductive nosography that basically restates the Greek classification of madness. (But it is not clear that modern psychiatry has revolved this problem either.)

In Pinel's *Treatise* there is a lack of congruence between theories, taxonomies, and the mad patient's demand to speak. Pinel's psychiatric practice was conditioned by the necessity of allowing the mad to speak their singularity while attempting to analyze them in terms of universal categories. His practice also redefined the nature of the asylum. It was no longer conceived of primarily as a place of incarceration in which the spectacle of captive madness was offered as animal entertainment to the eyes of those reasonable enough not to be locked up. Pinel transformed the asylum into a clinical space in which the doctor had to treat each case as a singular example, a unique particular, endowed with a voice that can tell its own narrative. At the same time the doctor was also charged with the paradoxical task of describing the unique voice in terms of the reductive nosography that classified most cases as idiocy or dementia, mania or melancholy—the big four of antiquity.

Pinel was also a Ciceronian moralist. Accompanying his willingness to listen to the mad was a Stoic belief that passions are a, if not the, cause of insanity. Pinel makes this clear at the outset of the 1809 edition of the *Treatise:* "One would have no notion of what alienation is if one did not go back to find the most usual origins, or those human passions that have become very vehement or embittered by strong contrariety" (p. ii). The return to Cicero is part of the valorization of the origins of thought, and the parallel with Rousseau's historicism is clear in this regard. However, Pinel was also quite aware of the successes of natural history, of the discipline that Lamarck in 1802 baptized "biology," and he wanted to pursue a taxonomical systematics that would give him the same purchase on reality that natural history have given botany and zoology. And so, in addition to honoring singularity and praising reason for its power to overcome passion, Pinel called upon the psychiatrist to become a naturalist:

> The words of alienation, mania, melancholia, and dementia could be understood in the same sense as madness, delirium, extravagance, loss of reason, etc. that are used in the intercourse of civil life. In order to avoid any ambiguity I thought necessary to determine the physical and moral characteristics that serve to distinguish the first as maladies. . . . How can we understand each other if, taking Naturalists as our example, we do not designate each object by signs that are manifest to the senses and appropriate to distinguish it from any other? (1809 ed., p. iii)

This naturalist's credo is a demonstration of Pinel's faith in the semiology of natural history. Pinel wanted to find exterior signs that could reduce the "innumerable varieties" (p. iii) of alienation into four distinct categories of species that antiquity had defined. The foursome of the *Treatise* is more manageable than the hundreds of species that proliferate in the *Nosographie*. But the reduced number also points up even more sharply the problem of subsuming the infinite play of singularity under a limited taxonomic structure that is supposed to order the distribution of deviant traits. Pinel wanted it both ways: like Rousseau reading his own singularity and finding a universal history, Pinel wanted to respect the infinite complications of the singular voices of deviant passion while undertaking an extreme nosological simplification.

The logic of his neo-Hippocratic position allowed him to overlook what might be considered to be a procedural impasse. Pinel separated diagnostics and etiology and considered them as entirely separate issues (and this practice continues in contemporary psychiatric nosographies, such as the widely used psychiatric manual called the *DSM*). According to Pinel's view of etiology there is no fixed or even especially predominate causal relationship involved in the causation of madness. The causes of madness are nearly as numerous as the cases themselves. Once Pinel has discussed etiology, his next move is to place the case in question in one of the four categories with no regard for the causes he may have found leading to the madness. The second edition of the *Treatise* gives a great deal more consideration to causes of madness. Here they are logically considered prior to diagnostic categories. Causes of insanity include everything from heredity and living conditions to all manner of the passions, including those he calls the spasmodic, the debilitating, as well as the gay and expansive emotions. Singularity gets its due with gusto. It is also essential to note that Pinel did not include organic disorders as a major cause of madness, and this for empirical reasons. He could not find lesions in all or even in a majority of the cases of madness for which he did an autopsy. Moreover, he reasons that a doctor need not presuppose lesions as a cause because moral treatment has cured a good many of the insane. The burden of empirical proof, in Pinel's eyes, lies on those who believe there are always organic perturbations that cause madness—such as the iatro-mechanical school.

With regard to psychological or "moral" causation of madness, one can argue that Pinel showed either great naïveté or extreme sophistication. His separation of etiology and diagnosis set up an order of explanation that is different from the usual modern model of disease that makes of etiology the determining factor for diagnosis. This model is central to our understanding of organic disease: one is diagnosed as having tuberculosis because of the empirical presence of the tubercle bacillus *Mycobacterium tuberculosis*. In other words an indifferent number of species of bacilli cannot cause the same clinical entity. This is of course a nineteenth-century model for understanding disease, but, in refusing to identify cause and syndrome, Pinel rejected in advance this model for mental illness:

> One would fall into error if one were to believe that the diverse species of mania are due to the particular nature of their causes, and that it becomes periodic, chronic, or melancholia according to the fact that it owes its birth to an unhappy love, domestic troubles, religious devotion pushed to fanaticism, to religious terrors, or to events of the Revolution. (1800 ed., p. 14)

Pinel is not thinking in metaphors taken from microbiology—a science yet some decades in the future. He is taking his understanding of human experience largely from literary sources and trying to find some way to fit this understanding to a reductive taxonomy, inspired in this attempt by both Greek medicine and the Enlightenment naturalists who had shown that order could be found in the infinite profusion of flora and fauna. This aspect of Pinel's way of considering madness has continued to the present, and, for our present understanding, it is important to sort out what are the presuppositions involved in this analysis.

The literary understanding of madness included not only classical sources, but increasingly the writings of Enlightenment authors such as Goethe and Rousseau. Their works had defined new discursive possibilities for communicating through madness, and this is, it seems to me, the most important parallel to be drawn between literature and medical practice: Pinel's moral treatment turns on giving the mad a voice, the singular voice that literature had valorized, and on allowing the voice to tell its unique narrative. Every mad person has his or her "historiette," as Pinel put it in the 1809 edition of the *Treatise* (p. 344). Once heard, these "little stories" could then be categorized and inscribed in records. Pinel was probably the first administrator to keep statistical records of the types of cases he dealt with and of the results of treatment. But this rationalization of record keeping is secondary to granting the mad a voice and listening to their stories. Moral treatment could occur once the medical listener had entered into the inner distance between rational self and the self lost in alienation, for then the doctor could hope to find a therapeutic relationship based on an appeal to the remnant of reason—moral reason—that had not succumbed to passion. The belief in the Stoic will was fundamental, but so was the belief in a rational self still surviving as part of the relational self in each patient. Shakespeare and Descartes as well as Rousseau and Goethe all contributed to this belief.

The rapport between madness and literary understanding is a leitmotif in Pinel's work. For not only does literature provide a structure for knowing what madness is, but madness in turn is the source of elaborate literary and artistic forms. English novels, Pinel says, demonstrate the passions of the English and confirm the diagnosis of their natural melancholy. In turn, the passions nourish the novel and the arts in general, so that "chagrin, hatred, fear, regret, remorse, jealousy, envy" work to destroy the fabric of society—and, once channeled through sensibility, these passions give rise to the works that allow us to recognize their destructiveness (1809 ed., p. 27). Here we find the equivocal relations of cause and effect between literature and madness that Tasso and Rousseau, himself a novelist, had also described. Novels can cause madness by corrupting the imagination, thus inflaming the passions. But one can understand this mental alienation because literature is there to describe it, diagnosing, so to speak, what it had produced.

An enchanting cliché floats before our eyes in this identification of litera-ture and madness: novels drive young men and especially young women mad. Whatever be the empirical truth of this statement—and it has been repeated as a certainty by several centuries of doctors and moralists—per-haps at the end of the Enlightenment a truth emerged in this platitude. Lit-erature has the capacity to alienate the imagination in some way that is akin to going mad. At the same time, this hopefully temporary alienation offers a form of knowledge about the precarious relational nature of the self. And thus Pinel listened to his charges as if they were characters in a novel. In addition to fitting them into a nosological tableau, he also makes of them characters in a moral drama, soliciting narratives, arranging stories, and analyzing madness like a literary critic. The mad tell tales, and in their story is found the knowledge of their insanity—all that was needed was a theory of hermeneutics, a lack to which the romantics, and then Freud, would be sensitive. Hamlet is about to return as a medical syndrome.

Pinel's literary analysis was not lost on the younger generation of doctors who assimilated Pinel's practice—and rejected it. In *De la folie* the brilliant young doctor Georget (1797–1825) summed up the next generation's views about Pinel, and his followers like Esquirol, when Georget dismissively said that they "committed this serious error; they made up novels rather than pathological descriptions."[11] By midcentury positivism was in ascendancy, and the search for lesions returned, renewed by the successes of pathologi-cal anatomy. History is continuity, but there are moments when we have the sense of an ending. In Pinel we sense the end of some two thousand years of discourses about madness whose major themes we can find again, in postromantic psychiatry and psychoanalysis, only when we have dug beneath the surface and looked for the hidden presuppositions therein. On the surface there is a unity of Western culture that ends in the writings of Philippe Pinel.

Neoclassicism came to an end having developed, with Pinel, a literary semiology for the understanding of the passions, drawing upon novels, but also upon neoclassical moralists like La Bruyère or Chamfort, and their studies of *caractères,* as well as upon their Greek predecessors, such as Theophrastus. Yet this use of literature left no legacy of literary understanding, nor increased respect for the imagination. Neoclassical medical psychology ended with an affirmation of the moralist's traditional distrust of the powers of the imagination. Trying to stay abreast of new developments, Pinel wrote the following in the 1809 edition of his work:

> Imagination, this function of the understanding that it is difficult to maintain within just limits—sometimes even for the most moderate man endowed with the healthiest reason—often gives, in civil life, rise to so many scenes that one wonders if it could not become the source of the most fecund of illusions, the deviations and the extravagant opinions that mental alienation manifests? Imagination brings together or confuses diverse incomplete sensations, called forth by memory, in the form of more or less incoherent tableaux, more or less true, false, or sad, more or less in conformity with existing objects, or bizarre or fantastic objects, and sometimes presents the most monstrous and melancholic totality. (Pp. 112–13)

In describing the power of the imagination to overturn the senses, Pinel dramatizes the imagination as a character in a conflictual scenario who defeats the equally dramatic principle of empirical reality. This is a circular drama, for the multiple signs of madness are all deduced so as to be an illustration of the general truth that Pinel had enunciated about this treacherous faculty in the first place. Or, as Georget might have observed, this is the semiology of a *littéraire.* And Balzac and Stendhal were, in fact, more enthusiastic readers of Pinel than the next generation of doctors.

The Last Neoclassical Discourse in Madness: Hölderlin

The historian's interpretive prism determines whether the historian sees Pinel as the last major Greco-Roman doctor or the first practitioner of modern psychiatry. With different prisms we can also view our interpreter of

Rousseau, the mad poet Hölderlin, as the last Enlightenment writer in madness or the first modern to have foundered on a madness that seems to spring from his impossible desire to return to origins of thought, to the origins of logos. It is instructive for an understanding of the end of the Enlightenment to suggest this comparison between doctor and poet and then to see how the poet interpreted his own madness. There is, I believe, a parallel between Pinel, founder of the modern asylum, and Hölderlin, the writer who strikes me as the founder of modern prophetic discourse. Both poet and doctor announced the modern era by returning to the origins of Greek medicine and thought—the doctor in triumph, the poet in loss.

For our history of discourses in madness, no writer can more fittingly and emblematically conclude the first part of this study than Hölderlin, the poet who went mad on history. In an early poem Hölderlin saw in mad Rousseau the god of the coming time, the prophet of the return to origins of plenitude. But most of Hölderlin's work charts the dissolution worked by his desire to return to the fullness of origins that are forever beyond the grasp of the present. The pre-Socratic doctor and philosopher Empedocles appeared to Hölderlin as the emblematic figure for his frustrated quest: Empedocles, half-mad in his longing to be a god, found that the only way to deal with his passion was to throw himself into the flames of a volcano. In Hölderlin's version of Empedocles' suicide one glimpses a clue that might explain Hölderlin's desire to embrace madness, if that is the way to describe his case: madness is the volcano that vindicates the poet who longs for the presence of the gods manifested in the presence of divine logos.

What clearly is the case for Hölderlin is that memory is the source of anguish in a world in which one longs for origins. His fragmented memory of the past witnesses negatively to the fullness to which the poet aspires. In one version of the poem "Mnemosyne"—memory—Hölderlin recalls, in lines reminiscent of Paracelsus, the laws of the world and the way all things must enter, as in dream, into prophecy, but end in dissolution:

> Und immer
> Ins Ungebundene gehet eine Sehnsucht.
>
> (P. 212)

[And always into the unbound goes one's longing.]

A theory of madness is enacted here, since every boundless yearning for the past, for its "laws," sweeps the seeker beyond limits and into that which has no connection and no limits. Desire for the past alienates the poet from the present moment; so that as the poet yearns for the plenitude that might fulfill his yearning, the past, he only encounters his own dissolution. The fall into the volcano is thus a fall into time that sweeps the poet away into the decadence and madness that Rousseau saw as the essential working of history.

Memory is a source of torment. It is not so much a faculty allowing one to revive the past as a power enabling one to live its ongoing death. Under the stress of yearning, memories flood the present and recall the dead, the classical heroes, and notably the mad hero Ajax through whom the mad self stepped into history on the Greek stage:

> Am Feigenbaum ist mein
> Achille mir gestorben,
> And Ajax liegt
> An den Grotten der See,
> An Bächen, benachbart dem Skamandros.
> An Schläfen Sausen einst, nach
> Der unbewegten Salamis steter
> Gewohnheit, in der Fremd', ist gross
> Ajax gestorben
> Patroklos aber in des Königes Harnish. Und es starben
> Noch andere viel.
>
> (Pp. 213–14)

[Beside the fig tree my Achilles has died and is lost to me, and Ajax lies beside the grottoes of the sea, beside the brooks that neighbor Scamandros. Of a rushing noise in his temples once, according to the changeless custom of unmoved Salamis, in foreign parts great Ajax died, not so Patroclus, dead in the king's own armour. And many others too have died.]

Hölderlin's neoclassical mind is drawn back to Ajax and is moved by our forgetting the hero, the hero who died when struck down by the rushing in his head, and then was left alone, with only memory to preserve him. But memory is coming apart, and the classical world is dying even as Hölderlin struggles to revive it.

In the final confused lines of this third version of "Memory," in what really is a magnificent example of borderline discourse, Hölderlin evokes the city of memory, Mnemosyne:

> Am Kithäron aber lag
> Elevtherä, der Mnemosyne Stadt. Der auch als
> Ablegte den Mantel Gott, das abendliche nachher löste
> Die Locken. Himmlische nämlich sind
> Unwillig, wenn einer nicht die Seele schonend sich

Zusammengenommen, aber er muss doch; dem
Gleich fehlet die Trauer.

(P. 214)

[By Cithearon there stood Eleutherae, Mnemosyne's town. From her, when God laid down his festive cloak, soon after did the powers of Evening sever a lock of hair. For the Heavenly, when someone has not collected his soul, to spare it, are angry, for still he must; like him, here mourning is at fault.]

A number of readings and translations of these lines are possible, for in his tormented struggle with memory and dissolution Hölderlin came close to inventing his own syntax and symbolic system—but logos does not allow such inventions. Whence the anguish produced by the search for an idiolect to mediate singularity. In Hölderlin's case it is the singularity of the writer who would express his receptivity to the divine message coming from the origins of language, from the original logos. After a fall into some two thousand years of history perhaps only a new language can grant the poet this receptivity.

The heavenly forces to which Hölderlin refers in the poem are angry with whoever cannot gather himself together, collect himself, and find a center for his being. Without this gathering together of the self—gathering together is another meaning of *logos*—then there is no saving of the self. The self is outside the confines of logos, and to this self "mourning is at fault," for the self cannot mourn without the connections made by language. It is as if the "Open" that Hölderlin described in the poem "Rousseau" is as much a place of dissolution and madness as of revelation—and perhaps this is the great danger of prophetic yearning. Hölderlin's inverse symmetry with Pinel—of a patient with a doctor—is manifest at this point. The neoclassical doctor returned with assurance to his historical origins for the confirmation of his ongoing rationality, whereas the mad poet finds in the return all the contradictions of singularity. Like Tasso and Rousseau, he is unique, alone, waiting the revelation of the divine in a language nobody else can understand—and finally the poet knows the fall out of history that is madness. The self has broken apart in this attempted return and cannot find even the consolation of mourning. Completed as the poet was about to make his break with sanity, Hölderlin's poem on memory is the beginning of Hölderlin's experience of madness. Madness is beyond sadness and mourning; it is beyond the mediating logos that, in revealing the origins of the divine, might have given Hölderlin's self a foundation and a way of holding itself together. Mad Ajax has no place in the city of memory. Like him, like Homer's Bellerophon, Hölderlin found himself alone, excluded from the historical community. In Hölderlin's twisted syntax resonates the fear of being abandoned outside of history, outside of the community of shared logos. Hölderlin's experience of insanity is lived in effect through the Greek understanding of madness. This poetic experience of dissolution produced the last major neoclassical discourse in madness that, in its historicism, is a seminal discourse for madness in modern poetry.

Part 2

The Modernity of Madness

Intermezzo: A Conclusion to Classical Madness and
an Introduction to Modernity

In order to introduce the orientation that I now take in this study, and to help any readers who begin reading this study here for its considerations of modernity, I offer this intermezzo of commentary to situate us historically. For a general understanding of the development of medical psychology, it is important to be aware that the medical theories of the Enlightenment outlasted the literary neoclassicism of the eighteenth century. Some doctors remained convinced of the validity of iatro-mechanical medicine, for this doctrine could still draw upon the successes of physics to propose that human beings should be treated as machines run by systems of fibers and tubelike nervous conduits. Versions of the Enlightenment's iatro-mechanical theories also continued to survive because they offered a handy simplification of medical problems. In the absence of a coherent theory of disease, doctors often looked for universal mechanical principles to explain all disease, including insanity.

For example, Doctor Pierre Pomme published, in its sixth and final edition in 1804, his three-volume *Traité des affections vaporeuses des deux sexes* (Treatise on the vaporous affections of both sexes). The theoretical basis for insanity proposed by the work can be given in one sentence, or as Pomme wrote with some irritation about the failure of his theory to be universally accepted: "I repeat for the sixth and last time that the proximate and immediate cause of nervous or vaporous maladies must be attributed, not to the slackening of fiber, or to its weakness, but rather to the tension of this fiber and to its shortening" (pp. xii–xiii). A more influential English version of this theory was developed in the work of Cullen's student, the Scotsman John Brown (1735–1788). Brown had an international success, and *Brownianismus* served as the basis for the development of romantic medicine in Germany well into the nineteenth century. According to Brownian medicine, asthenia and sthenia—excitement or the lack thereof—rule over sick fibers. This binary opposition seems to have appealed to the dialecticians of romanticism. These later mechanical theories, with their taut and slack fibers explaining every conceivable mental and physical illness, seem today to be caricatures of the creativity that had gone earlier into the creation of "mechanical man," that physiological composite of forces and fibers that post-Cartesian medicine devised.

I bring up these examples to point to the continuities to which we must be attendant if we are to understand the ideological and scientific paradoxes that underwrite the discourses that lead from the Enlightenment to our modernity, if *modernity* is still a meaningful term today. Galen and Hippocrates did, in the nineteenth century, cease to be part of the medical curriculum—but only in the nineteenth century. In spite of the demise of Galen and Hippocrates, I am going to argue that the Greek experience of madness as a rupture in logos remains a hidden bedrock upon which we continue to elaborate many of our discourses on madness. In the second half of this study I shall deal with the specifically modern discourses that have often been erected or superimposed upon this cultural bedrock.

To understand these developments it is also necessary to keep in mind that the Enlightenment reprise of Greek thought occurred in a context in which a new understanding of the natural world was emerging. The Enlightenment began the naturalization of the concept of human community, which meant that we began to understand ourselves as part of a total ecology, at one with the entire realm of nature. An Enlightenment naturalist such as Buffon could announce in his *Histoire naturelle* the "humiliating truth" for humanity that mankind must classify itself as part of the animal kingdom; and that man is an animal whose reason may not even be as reliable as the instinct of other animals. This change in classification is a first step toward redefining logos and the relations constituting the human community. But it is a step that a naturalist like Buffon himself could hardly accept—as witness the panegyrics he made about mankind's superior place in creation. Relevantly Buffon uses the same hyperbolic terms of praise that we have seen in the atheist logophile La Mettrie's fear of animality. Even after God was banished from knowledge, language seems to have been promoted to take his place, which in effect assured the continuity of a vision of logos. It is probably safe to say that we have hardly completed the steps that would lead to a naturalizing of logos.

The Enlightenment's naturalizing of the human community was a first step toward the evolutionary theory of a Darwin and the positivist understanding of human beings as organic beings about whom there is nothing that cannot be explained by the laws of physics and chemistry, and, consequently, derivative sciences like physiology and neurology. The naturalizing of the human community did not eliminate the humanist belief in the supremacy of human logos, since it often seems to coexist with the belief that humanity is a natural community whose existence does not represent a break with nature. This is clear in the romantics. And even Freudian psychoanalysis often seems to embody this dual attitude according to which the human animal is part of nature, though also a very sick animal because it is forced, through language, to be a product of culture. And our most "postmodern" explanations of madness show that logos returns to affirm our belief in human specificity. The contemporary use of, say, cybernetics or linguistics may appear to present novel ways for describing madness, and in a sense they are; but as explanatory paradigms for madness the new models also present permutations on the belief that logos defines the human community to which we must belong if we are not to wander alone, like Homer's Bellerophon, on the fields of melancholia. In different guises language remains the human animal's access to the community that allows that fullness of being we call, hopefully, sanity. So the question remains as to whether we can define humanity primarily through logos and still view humanity as part of the natural world.

I recall, in summation of my preceding argument, that there has been that a great unity in our tradition's understanding of madness, in spite of failed attempts during the Renaissance to recast medical thought and in spite of a tendency during the Enlightenment to reductively explain madness as a question of dysfunctional, mechanical physiology. This is not to say that I see European discourses on madness as based on a single, unitary view of madness. However, it is clear that the Greek view that madness is a rupture in logos continued and continues to orient thought about madness even when Greek thought is not explicitly called upon. And for that reason, if the reader of this second half of the study wants to peruse quickly the most salient part of the preceding for a background, I recommend therein the first chapter's sections on Greek tragedy, medicine, and the pre-Socratics.

In the first half of this study, I have dealt, to the extent that it makes sense, with medical and literary discourses separately. This separation allows one to see the parallels between medical and literary discourse, and to see where literature has contested medicine and where it has contributed to an era's knowledge of madness. I shall continue this procedure, and, in dealing with literary texts, for the most part I shall make no rigorous distinction between texts written by the supposedly insane and writings representing madness, though written by the supposedly sane. I say for the most part, since I do offer some considerations here about the problems involved in interpreting a text of feigned insanity and a text written in an asylum. However, I have also endorsed the idea that some distinction in principle of sane writers and insane writers is rendered nugatory by the fact that literature can enter into madness, whether written by sane folk such as ourselves or by the Marquis de Sade, because literature has much in common with those forms of insanity that desire to negate the real. Madness and literature spring from the same imaginative capacity to entertain present worlds that do not (really) exist. And this is complicated all the more by the fact that madness can represent sanity, as well as vice versa; or as Hamlet shows, madness feigned by the mad is the most deviant of all.

Moreover, in literature as in life, we see that the mad inhabiting reality and the mad found in fictions live and experience their insanity in conformity with the explanatory paradigms that their era uses to understand madness. Medicine and literature offer models for madness to which the mad usually conform because they have no other way to give shape to their madness. They have no other way to reintegrate their experience into forms of reason, language, or logos, that will allow them to represent their madness to themselves as well as to others. In this respect literature has often offered more insightful knowledge of madness, or what the mad make of their madness, than medicine. Literature and medicine are sometimes, but not always, at one in the understanding of madness, and we shall also see that literature and medicine have an antagonistic relation as often as they have a relation in which they share axioms of understanding for explaining madness. This theme dominates our considerations of modern discourses on madness, but it is not unique to the postromantic era. No writers ever despised doctors more than did those insane rationalists of Augustan England, Swift and Pope.

The second half of this volume is a study of modern discourses on madness, beginning with the German romantics and going through what is now frequently called our own postmodern era. I do not wish to engage in polemics about the meaning of terms such as *modern* or *postmodern*. In their most neutral sense they are relational terms, with the semantic weight of "now" and "post-now." The amount of naive polemical energy they have generated is undoubtedly in inverse proportion to the precision with which they are used. However, when properly circumscribed, they can be useful. In this volume *modern* refers to medicine that has broken with the Enlightenment as well as with the Hippocratic and Galenic thought that was the dominant body of medical thought into the nineteenth century. It also refers to the medical naturalism that, in the wake of the development of histology, cellular biology, microbiology, and pathological anatomy, is the basis for today's medicine. Modernity in medicine evolves rather directly from these movements, though the development of modernity in medical psychology cannot be so clearly defined. This distinction will occupy us presently.

Modernity in literature can also have a negative and a positive definition. Like medicine, modern literature has, in negative terms, broken with its explicit tributary relationship to the Greco-Roman tradition. A positive definition is more difficult, since modernism has often been, from the romantics to the present, a self-conscious quest for foundations that would grant literature an ontological and epistemological status that it lost with the demise of neoclassicism. That quest for a ground to literature often led to an exploration of the Greek roots of our literature: Joyce rewrote *Ulysses,* Cocteau *Oedipus Rex,* and so forth. Seeking foundations, the modernists hoped to find transcendental myths in those works that lie at the origins of our culture. Paradoxically, modernity implies a break with the past, but modernity has also been suspicious that we have only deluded ourselves about breaking with the past.

With regard to madness and discourses thereon, the literary modernist might say that we have never really broken with the past and that there are more continuities in our thought and discourse on madness than we often allow. The comparison of literature and medical psychology then becomes quite relevant, for it can be argued that movements as diverse as psychoanalysis and medical psychology drawing upon cybernetics and linguistics represent a reprise of Greek models. To which I add that, in part, this continuity between Greek thought and modern psychology is by default, since medical theory about madness has really made no radical, disciplinary break with the past, such as has occurred in medicine dealing with organic diseases. The explanation of mumps and measles is, therefore, of a different logical order than the explanation of schizophrenia. There is not yet a microbiology for the psyche, or mind, or soul, as one prefers. More on this presently.

From our perspective, modernity begins with romanticism, which, in Germany, formed the last great cultural synthesis in our history, when doctors and writers, philosophers and scientists, all shared much the same conceptual framework and worked, with surprising unanimity, to found such enterprises as psychiatry and embryology, modern poetry and the science of history. I also begin with German romanticism because it established the conditions of possibility, to use a Kantian formulation, for the development of psychoanalysis. Psychoanalysis incorporated into its understanding of madness many of the concepts developed by romantic doctors—romantic in the philosophical sense—whose legacy to Western thought has lived long beyond the general oblivion to which history has consigned these early nine-teenth-century medical thinkers. An outgrowth of romanticism, psycho-analysis may not be a science, but its historical importance for a modern understanding of madness should not be underestimated. If romantic doc-tors are among the more obscure figures populating the history of medicine, their offspring named Freud is a pop icon of whom medical history has no better-known exemplar.

This study of romanticism is a prelude to understanding how our modern understanding of madness is dominated by two medical discourses, psycho-analysis and psychiatry. The term *psychiatry* was invented by a romantic doctor, but modern psychiatry owes far less to romantic medicine than to somatic and positivist medical thought that began to develop, in Germany and France, with the demise of neoclassical medical philosophy. As I sug-gested in the previous chapter, the rejection of the theories of the neoclassi-cal psychiatric reformer and theorist, Philippe Pinel, began taking place practically in his lifetime. Essential to the development of modern psychia-try was the development of the materialist monism characterizing the exper-imental medicine of a Claude Bernard. My thesis here is in fact that psycho-analysis can be understood as a reaction to the positivist psychiatry that attempted to make all mental disturbance an effect of lesions, which is to say, part of pathological anatomy. Psychoanalysis brought back a literary understanding of madness in reaction to this reductive medical thought. However, positivism prompted, by reaction, one development in modern lit-erature: much modern poetry proposes to explore madness in direct defiance of the medical doctrines that would reduce the mad poet to a sick oracle produced by disturbed anatomy. In the twentieth century psychiatry has not incorporated the more simpleminded doctrine of mental causality found in earlier positivist psychiatry, but it remains the case that, in its elab-oration of new diagnostic criteria for madness, psychiatry is still viewed by many modern poets as a dangerous enemy to be overcome. Modern diag-nostic categories can reductively devalue a poet's madness as thoroughly as the positivist's reduction of poetry to an anatomical dysfunction.

After dealing with positivism, and then the differences between psychia-try and psychoanalysis, I discuss the way that modern poets have been obliged, in the twentieth century, to live their madness in terms of both par-adigms. After this analysis of modern literary representations of madness, in the final chapter I turn to the recent contemporary scene, which, for lack of a better term, I am willing to call postmodern. Superimposed upon psychia-try and psychoanalysis, we find that much recent thought wants to conceive madness as a disturbance of information flow, on the model of a cybernetic dysfunction, or, analogously, as the breakdown in the functioning of the linguistic system that literally constitutes the mind or self. This kind of thought, often called postmodern, is a development of therapeutic analysis that appears to owe little to modern medicine. Here we find a medical psychology that wants to reconcile cybernetics or linguistics with our modern paradigms for madness, as usually elaborated by psychiatry, though it draws but little upon modern pathological neurological research. As I suggested, I think one can see in these postmodern developments a return of an updated version of the Greek doctrine of logos: mind is once again conceived as part of a transindividual "system," such as language, that is at once the foundation of culture and society and of the individual mind. Analogous to the Greek concept of madness, then, insanity is conceived as a perturbation in communication, an exclusion from a community based upon a shared language. Thus madness is lived as a rupture with the great ambiance of logos in which we all are immersed in our normal life, when our mind exists objectively as a point in the public matrix of language and information flow.

Postmodern literature parallels the contemporary theoretical understanding of madness by using or even anticipating the cybernetic and linguistic versions of logos to which I have just alluded. Viewing madness as a break in circuitry, or a collapse of logos, literature vindicates its own knowledge of madness in order to show that insanity is a societal problem that may destroy us, or even at times to show that our models for understanding madness are somewhat mad in themselves. This is especially true of the feminist reaction to the determination that madness is a rupture with logos. To illustrate this very important reaction in literature to medical psychology, I have selected three French women writers whose work enacts the most radical feminist revolt against patriarchal logos. Their desire is precisely to break with logos—by which I mean reason and its codifications in language—that has always excluded them as women in any case. Psychosis becomes, ambiguously to be sure, a condition of liberation when psychosis is lived as a break with a logos that has denied women's existence and hence always made of women psychotics for being women. In this postmodern context, belief in the gender determinations of madness determines, I believe for the first time, a mode of discourse that intentionally wants to be madness.

These are some of the issues that will engage us in the following pages. I again make no claims to demonstrate some exhaustive thesis. By proposing that our modern understanding of madness is largely derived from the two, somewhat antagonistic, medical discourses of psychiatry and psychoanalysis, I think I propose a useful overview of our cultural and intellectual history that can make sense of two centuries of conflict between doctors and poets. For that conflict involves two centuries of writers, novelists and poets, who have defined their often deviant being by opposition to the imperial claims of positivist and psychiatric medicine—and sometimes by calling upon and sometimes by rejecting psychoanalysis. Much of what we call poetic modernity takes on its full significance only if it is read in the context of this conflict, a conflict that valorized poetic madness as myth, and made myth into the science of psychoanalysis. Finally, by proposing that much of our cybernetic postmodernity is an attempt to reintroduce an understanding of logos into our discourses on madness, my argument suggests that the unity of our culture is sometimes never greater than when it is least apparent. Heraclitus said "psyche esti logos"—the mind is logos. Perhaps we are still saying some version of the same.

Chapter 6

The German Romantics and the Invention of Psychiatry

Psychiatry against Kant

The German doctor J. C. Reil (1759–1813) gave us "psychiatry" when he decided there should be an *iatros,* or doctor, for the psyche. This fusion of Greek terms is one of the lasting contributions of romantic medicine, which was largely German. However, if subsequently German psychiatry has often dominated the development of psychological medicine, later psychiatry owed little to the romantic movement. As we shall see, romantic medicine sets the historical stage for the development of that literary phenomenon known as psychoanalysis—or so I shall interpret it. For in German romanticism there existed a moment during which medicine and literature looked upon each other as complementary discourses, and this moment was continued on, perhaps unknowingly, in the development of psychoanalytic discourse. By the end of the eighteenth century, moreover, both literature and medicine were coming to accept the vitalism that replaced mechanical physiology. Both poets and doctors accepted the idea that life must be explained by some vital principle that is not reducible to the mechanistic laws that govern the interactions of inert matter. And, what is perhaps the defining trait of German romanticism, both literature and medicine saw vitalism as part of an interpretation of nature as an unfolding whole or a *Ganzheit* that provides the ultimate context for romantic scientific explanation. The belief that nature is a total system, with correspondences maintaining between all its parts, was largely foreign to the empiricism of English medicine, or the rapidly developing positivism in France, which would soon dominate medical research in Europe.

In the word *psychiatry* are wedded gods, souls, illness, and a science of the inner space of the self for which there should be a special doctor. Vitalism suggested that the vital life force of a psyche needed a new medical doctrine. Through a series of metaphors propped up by medical definitions, romantic psychiatry proclaimed the existence of a self that mechanical man had lost in the eighteenth century and that late neoclassicism had attempted to find by listening to the singular self of mad voices in both literature and in the clinic. One should not overestimate romantic originality in the discovery of a vital self: the romantics often appear new because they proclaimed their originality. In opposition to the French reformer Pinel and his followers, the romantic psychiatrists insisted, in hyperbolic fashion, on the break they had made with the past. However, they continued to use Greek nosography, their vitalism was a century old, and they insisted on using Christian beliefs as psychiatric concepts. Their tendency to use proclamation for proof meant that their French and English contemporaries could dismiss their doctrines as unfounded assertions having little respect for basic epistemological criteria. It is noteworthy that the romantic doctors were writing at the very moment that François Magendie (1783–1855) was founding modern experimental medicine.

Romantic psychiatrists were little interested in physiology or pathological anatomy. They preferred to press into service a wide range of traditional ideas to form doctrines to explain the psyche. Not only the vitalist Stahl, but thinkers as diverse as Jakob Böhme, and his mystical iatro-chemical theories, or Paracelsus, and his vision of correspondences between the micro- and the macrocosms, were called upon to mount a reaction against the Enlightenment, and especially against Kant. Reaction, reprise, and some little innovation characterize their doctrines. Most fundamentally, the romantics were united in their reaction to the new Kantian rationalism that now dominated European epistemology. Like the romantic poets and philosophers, the psychiatrists were largely united in their attempt to overcome the limits placed on knowledge by the philosopher Immanuel Kant (1724–1804). Kant's critiques of practical and theoretical reason had drawn up the limits of knowledge in terms of a rational empiricism. Romantic medicine, poetry, and philosophy were united in a common concern and drew upon the same sources for much the same reasons: to overcome the limits of Kant's rational empiricism, and in so doing, to proclaim that God, the soul, and the inner world can be subjects of meaningful discourse.

Kant had banished these subjects from the realm of knowledge. According to Kant, knowledge is a relation maintained by a subject to an objective world. This relation excludes any knowledge of what Kant called the noumenal world—such as the depths of the self or soul. In limiting our possibilities of knowledge to the objective phenomenal world, the epistemological revolution Kant effected was far-reaching. The romantic reaction is understandable. The world about which meaningful propositions may be uttered was suddenly quite truncated, even if, pious philosopher that he was, Kant left faith unto its own devices. Facing the Kantian revolution, the originality of the romantics lies not so much in their systems as in their attempt to open vistas on the self that Kant had placed on the other side of the legitimate boundaries of knowledge. The romantic reactionaries drew upon an array of largely past concepts to forge the new doctrines about the psyche. This maneuver characterizes the works of the three most important romantic psychiatrists: Reil, who brought to medicine the idea that the psyche has depth; Johann Christian Heinroth, who reintroduced the theological dimension of guilt into madness; and Karl Wilhelm Ideler, who introduced a temporal dimension into the development of madness, while allegorizing the passions in terms of theatrical conflicts that constitute the dynamics of insanity.

These three doctors were active, successively, from the end of the eighteenth century well into the nineteenth century. Taken together they represent the full range of reaction that went into the creation of romantic psychiatry. The themes and concepts they shared with romantic writers is remarkable. To both the poet and the doctor, madness offered a key area of experience that allowed them to get around Kant and to find a privileged realm of experience that is larger than the one delimited by critical reason. Madness offered poets a royal way to truths beyond rational empiricism. It could be argued that, historically, the poets led the doctors to this royal road into the inner depths that Kant had declared beyond the purview of reason. But because the doctors offer a clear condensation of anti-Kantian views, they will come first in our order of exposition. And because the books of these obscure, but important, doctors are nearly inaccessible (except for the medical library of the Library of Congress few libraries in the United States have them), I shall give the doctors the preponderance of exposition.

J. C. Reil and Rhapsodies about Madness

An early romantic, J. C. Reil is also a representative of the philanthropic movement that worked to reform the treatment of the insane throughout Europe at the end of the Enlightenment. Reform is a relative notion. Reil's philanthropy recommended intimidation as well as theater as forms of therapy, and some of it resembled torture by our standards. His principal treatise, *Rhapsodieen über die Anwendung der psychischen Curmethode auf Geisteszerrüttungen* of 1803 proposes various therapeutic procedures while it theorizes that the self has hidden depths hiding the fantasies that erupt in madness. In writing these *Rhapsodies upon the Use of the Psychic Cure*

Method for Mental Disturbances, Reil borrowed from Kant to dispute Kant. The metaphor of psychic depth is a topographical image that derives from Kant's description of the subject. Kant called the inner world of the noumenal self a "thing in itself," a *Ding an sich* that is unknowable in rational terms. The Kantian formulation stakes out a world about which the philosopher can say that it is known to exist, but about which nothing meaningful can be said. This formulation was an invitation for a search for access to the unknown. One solution was to propose that the full self can be spatially located as beyond or perhaps literally under the phenomenal self that can be empirically observed.

In his earlier *Von der Lebenskraft* (On the life force) of 1795, Reil accepted the idea that the mad have a singular experience. He wanted in fact to turn the doctrine of the singularity of the self into a generalized diagnostic concept. This entailed rejecting the Kantian idea that phenomena are perceived through the universal categories of the understanding. In defense of singularity, Reil claimed that the ground for mental illness lies outside the representations that, according to rational empiricism, are the grounds for knowledge. Every individual has his or her own harmony, and "Thus every individual has its own health."[1] Illness is outside the realm of empirical regularity, and so singularity becomes a paradoxical universal category for mental illness, paradoxical because it would seemingly lead to the conclusion that there is no universality in illness.

In his medical *Rhapsodies* the description of madness defines mental illness as a syndrome that is always specific to the singular individual:

> So long as a human being is healthy, the nervous system gathers together in a central point the parts that are stretched out through the entire organization. In this way the many *[Mannigfaltige]* are tied to unity *[Einheit]*. However, the hinges of the connection can come off. The whole can be dissolved in its parts, and every drive and gear *[Getriebe]* can begin to work for itself, or hook up with another, outside the common focal point, in a false hookup. A body is like a church organ; sometimes these parts, sometimes those parts, are playing, depending on how the stops are pulled. Sometimes, as it were, whole provinces become rebellious; one must forgive me this metaphorical language that one cannot dispense with in psychology. (1803 ed., p. 63)

Reil's tropes bespeak an attempt to define the singular, the nonuniversal, and hence the nearly ineffable workings of a self that lies beyond the limits imposed by the categories of rational empiricism. What is curious is that this description borrows from what it wants to contest. The image of perception's organizing the many in unity is Kantian. To contest Kant, he seems to use an image of machines, drives, and gears taken from mechanical physiology. The image of madness as political rebellion is classical. But the syncretic stew cooked up here is Reil's.

Reil was nonetheless a doctor, and he wanted to show other doctors what caused the mad self to fall into a singular disjunctive state. He did accept the Kantian view that the objective world bombards the subjective self with sense data, so madness is a rupture between inner and outer worlds. Reil's reliance on the dichotomy of objective and subjective realms, separated by a metaphysical wall, shows that he had hardly begun to get around Kant. Armed with this Kantian premise, Reil's relational notion of madness, defined as the lack of congruence between inner and outer world, is the essential notion that is presupposed by all other romantic perspectives on insanity. The realm of subjectivity—psyche—finds itself walled off, and in this disjuncture inner and outer forces can besiege the inner self. Reil's *Rhapsodies* presents analyses of the perturbed inner realm in which forces from the deep, outside of the rational realm of Kantian categories, can spring forth and create disjunctures. When the self is besieged from within, "Jeder Kranke ist ein Subject eigner Art" [Every patient is a unique type of subject] (p. 244). And psychiatry is obliged to be the science of the absolute particular.

Madness effects a unique disclosure: it shows the subject without a mask (p. 51) and grants a view into the depths of psychic space beyond the Kantian phenomenal self. A Freudian topography of the self is prefigured here when Reil describes the process by which, as representations go astray, the self becomes a place of revelation and discovery. This can occur when the temperature of what Reil calls the "soul organ" fluctuates, which causes the fluctuation of the patient's "normal receptivity to exterior objects."

> [T]he propagation of sensations then deviates from the laws of association. The hinge of the connection comes off, individual gears work for themselves, constellations *[Nebelsterne]* push up out of the depths, and a world becomes visible to us about which we had no idea that it was at hand. (P. 115)

Reil again uses figuratively the language of materialist physiology in his confrontation with Kant—in this alternation between imaginary neurology and trope he also anticipates Freud. In madness, the machine is unhinged, and an unknowable noumenal world appears on the inner stage of consciousness where empirical representations are normally present. This means that in some sense one can speak, at times, of representations that are not necessarily accompanied by consciousness of them: the self can entertain "Vorstellungen ohne Bewusstseyn." Reil probably took his notion of the unconscious from Leibniz—the notion had been gaining currency throughout the eighteenth century—but his postulation of the unconscious is neces-sitated primarily by the fact he must explain the presence of ideas to the self that the self cannot rationally know. He must explain how representations can exist that are not allowed by the conceptual categories that Kant made a part of the understanding. To this end Reil theatricalizes madness. He pre-sents the self as a stage upon which, with or without consciousness, the self functions as a representing power, to translate literally Reil's *vorstellende Kraft*. Madness creates an inner metaphysical theater to which the self is an unwilling spectator, when not a willing participant therein. Or madness can produce the disjuncture between the self as spectator and the irrational rep-resentations in which the self is an actor. Madness is much like a dream.

In this regard Reil anticipates modern psychiatry by giving precedence to the inner dimensions of madness rather than to a semiology of exterior symptoms. This interiorization of madness on a metaphysical stage also promoted the romantic identification of madness with dream. Before Freud, Reil saw in dreams a privileged way of explaining the nature of deviant states of mind. Like madness, dreams are an inner representation for which there may be no signs in the outer world of objectivity. Dreams occur with-out rational consciousness, and they seemingly have the same capacity for delusion as madness.

That madness, like dream, produces metamorphosis is not for Reil, as for many romantics, necessarily a favorable state of affairs. For many of them delusion was not deception; and the logic of the anti-Kantian stance meant that it was almost inevitable that many romantics declared that madness and dream are superior to the exterior world: they are superior to that impoverished empirical world known as only so many phenomenal repre-sentations exterior to the self. Thus the romantic doctor G. H. v. Schubert elaborated a philosophy proclaiming that only in dream and madness is revealed the true inner self. Dream offers the ontologically superior state in which, as Schubert put it, the dreamer is at once the observing subject and the observed object—and ergo Kantian oppositions are overcome. Or, as Philippe Lersch put it in his classic study of romantics and dream, dream became a superior science.[2]

Madness is representation; therefore, Reil thought that theater could be a form of therapy. By acting roles or watching theatrical representations, the mad should experience alternative representations that were designed to capture their attention and bring them back to reason. In practice, however, the historians Singer and Underwood note that Reil also used near torture by scaring the patients with his theatrical therapy (*Short History of Medi-cine*, p. 501). One may doubt the benefits of dramatized terrorism, though it was consistent with the view that representations might, if dramatic enough, replace other representations.

The doctrine of representation led to what I call the speculum view of madness. *Speculum* is the Latin word for mirror, and in modern medicine it is a probe allowing perception of the body's interior. It also supplies the point of departure for a later psychoanalytical notion, or Lacan's mirror stage in human development. According to Reil's theory, when the doctor looks into the patient's mind, he sees that the mad look upon an inner mirror and find doubles that they take to be "real" representations; or, in confusion, they doubt real representations and take them to be false doubles of what in fact are real phenomena. The mirror notion lies behind Reil's basic description of madness and the confusion it produces in the mad when they can no longer trust their representations: "Either we doubt our personality or mistake our self *[Ich]* for a stranger; we attribute foreign qualities to ourselves, or we transplant our own circumstances onto others" (pp. 73–74). Lost in a mirror play of images, the mad take phenomenal appearances as deceiving representations, or false images as real ideas. In the mind's theatrical world, reality and appearance cease to be differentiating notions, for, as Descartes once discovered, when one cannot distinguish the image from the mirror, there are no criteria for the differentiation of the real and the hallucinatory. And locked behind a metaphysical wall, Reil's mad can observe nothing else, except the speculum that constitutes the mad self in the first place. The poet's traditional wonder about that rhyming pair *Sein und Schein*, being and appearance, has become the basis for a clinical description.

Heinroth and the Theological Dimension of Romantic Madness

By theatricalizing madness and establishing a proto-Freudian topography of the self, Reil opened the way to the further developments in psychiatry undertaken by J. C. A. Heinroth (1773–1843), who is usually taken to be the second most important of the romantic psychiatrists. Notably, after the secular theorizing of the Enlightenment, Heinroth reintroduced religion into considerations of madness. Kant had relegated religion to the realm of faith, a conceptual move that banned it from the realm of knowledge. Religion could be an object of knowledge, but not a subject. Part of the romantic reaction to Enlightenment empiricism was, not only to press forward to find access to Kant's noumenal realm, but also to restore religion to an epistemological position from which it could speak with certainty. In his attempt to integrate religious thought into medicine, Heinroth was apparently the first to coin *psychosomatic* to describe an organic dysfunction that has a psychic origin.[3] Psychic origins of somatic disturbances included a wide range of causes, for Heinroth brought back sin, guilt, and damnation as ways of understanding deviance. A Leipzig medical professor, Heinroth published in 1818 his *Lehrbuch der Störungen des Seelenlebens; oder, der Seelenstörungen und ihrer Behandlung* (Textbook on the disturbances of soul life or soul disturbances and their treatment). In it Heinroth tried to get around the Kantian revolution by historicizing our understanding of self and madness. Turning to Schelling's views about the history of consciousness, he borrowed a philosophy of historical development to buttress psychiatric theory. According to Heinroth, mind develops in history as a phylogenetic development (or consciousness in general) that in turn allows ontogenetic development. In other words, the individual mind develops in function of the general history of consciousness. The individual mind, like the collective mind, undergoes stages of development, first of self-consciousness, then of reason, and then of the moral sense, all of this development opening finally, in romantic fashion, onto the infinite or the *Unendlich*.[4] Sounding like a Christian Hegel, Heinroth equated reason with the light of revelation. Man is reasonable only insofar as he is reasonable, that is, stands in the light of revelation. This tautology is meaningful insofar as we usually stand in sin, which means that, in this reprise of medieval theology, we usually stand in madness.

In evaluating this Christian historicizing of consciousness, historians have looked upon Heinroth as another precursor to Freud. One need only replace the concept of sin with guilt to see that Heinroth's view of insanity is a prototype for Freud's view that psychosis is an adaptation to excessive guilt. But, as the Church taught, guilt is a fundamental part of sin, and Heinroth can also be situated in the Western tradition that sees madness, in a theological interpretation, as a result of the Fall. Calling passion the equivalent of sin, Heinroth brings back the Christian Stoic views that makes madness an intrinsic part of human desire. As Borges might have said, Heinroth makes Cicero and Augustine into Freud's contemporaries.

In the context of the romantic period, what is important is that, in defiance of the Enlightenment principles of rationalism, Heinroth made sin and guilt into a medical categories. He did this sleight of hand by using the Kantian notions of objectivity and subjectivity to explain sin and passion in metaphysical terms describing perception. To this end he also put forward the view of madness as a speculum. Sin and passion are experienced as inner representations seen in the self's inner mirror. Passion sets up a deformed image in the inner mirror and inevitably produces a delusion: thus the inner image produced by passion is an erroneous representation. Victims of their passions, the insane, in their delusions, are trapped in false images and are continually deluded about the objects that these images represent.

Heinroth's psychiatry also uses the concept of the unconscious to get around the limits that critical reason had imposed on knowledge. In historicizing the development of consciousness, Heinroth says that the development of self in time unfolds as an unconscious dimension. For *Seele*—spirit, soul, or self—is a power that develops through self-determinations of which it is not conscious: "[D]as Seelenleben bestehet, auch unbewussten Weise, aus nichts als solchen Acten" [The life of *Seele* consists, also in a unconsciousness way, of nothing but these acts] (p. 174). These self-determining stages of development had already been described by Schelling in his theories of the unconscious development of mind, and Heinroth extends the philosopher's theory to include the insane as well as the rational mind. He locates the genesis of madness in a realm of unconscious thought wherein there is an etiology unfolding in time. The necessity of temporal dynamics to explain madness means that Heinroth refuses to accept the idea that an innocent person is suddenly catapulted into madness. There is a theological side to this argument, but, in strictly medical terms, Heinroth established the notion that there is a hidden etiology to madness. This etiology presupposes a temporal development to all madness. For Heinroth, this development takes place unconsciously in the noumenal realm wherein the soul threads its way between sin and guilt. But the temporalizing of etiology is hardly dependent upon this theological context.

Heinroth's is theistic medicine. His thought should be distinguished from the rational dialectics of a Hegel or even Schelling. But the ultimate effect of Heinroth's concept of temporal development was to secularize sin, making of it a dynamic concept for understanding the avatars of a self that develops in time. Heinroth himself contributed to this secularizing by propagating Enlightenment ideas about the relativity of madness to reason. He accepted that madness is relative to a historical context. His historicism is reflected in his belief that the relation of reason to unreason is rooted in the history of culture:

> [O]n the whole madness carries in itself the color of its era *[Zeitalter]*, of the character of the people and of their relation to their culture. Antiquity had its metamorphoses, the Middle Ages its demonology, and modern times also has its spirits *[Geistersche]*. Nordic madness is constituted in one way, southern madness in another. (Pt. 1, p. 294)

In contradiction to his theistic propensities, Heinroth's recognition of relativity is part of a secularizing process that denies the absolute truth of any religious determination of madness as well as any diagnostic procedure that fails to account for cultural norms. At once theistic and relativistic, Heinroth seems emblematic of the entire German romantic movement and the way in which it ushered in our modernity by trying to retrieve the Middle Ages.

Romantic medicine also ushered in a crisis in the diagnostic knowledge of madness. Heinroth continued to separate etiology and diagnostic nosology or taxonomy as he, in eclectic fashion, accepted the basic Brownian categories that classified all illness in terms of asthenia and sthenia. This was a simpleminded dichotomy that simplified therapy by decreeing that everything could be cured by either excitation or sedation. The crisis in diagnosis was evident in the proliferation of clinical entities that Heinroth, along with many others, invented to describe types of madness. Coexisting with the unitary principle that madness is sin was Heinroth's nosological tableau that wanted to reconcile all previous tableaux, from Cullen to Pinel. Taxonomist Heinroth invented three orders of disease, with three genera and variations, giving rise to some fifty-two species of madness, ranging from the recently invented "nostalgia" to more classic species such as *furor poeticus* and *paranoia catholica*. Heinroth reserved four species, with four modifications, for poets alone, such as the famous *melancholia metamorphosis*.

Later psychiatry had nothing but disdain for these taxonomies (though the ease with which we have recently created new clinical entities should cause us some hesitation about our scorn). In 1904, the most influential of all psychiatric nosologists, Emil Kraepelin, looked back on Heinroth and "his school" and commented with scorn that all Heinroth and his followers had done was to propose that "mental disease resulted from a moral transgression, from a voluntary surrender to a life of sin."[5] Kraepelin's harsh dismissal of Heinroth was typical of reaction to Heinroth's work after the mid-nineteenth century when positivist psychiatry turned its back on the cultural components of madness. With its refusal of cultural determinants, positivist psychiatry continued what earlier mechanistic medicine had already attempted to do: banish guilt and affects from the sphere of official medicine. Machine man was subject to religious delusions, but guilt feelings were not quite a medical issue.

If modern psychiatry rejected Heinroth, psychoanalysis seems to have profited from the way that, with his nearly medieval sense that the struggle between good and evil can destroy the self, Heinroth reinscribed allegory into psychological medicine. In Heinroth's work allegory is the essential trope for describing the essence of mental disturbance. Much as in Freud's later scenarios of self, Heinroth describes a self composed of abstractions that are engaged in conflictive dramas:

> If we consider the main forms of mental disturbance, madness and melancholia, we find they are characterized by entirely opposing characters, in that in melancholia the mind has lost the world, and has become a self [Ich] that feeds on itself; in madness, on the other hand, it is, as it were, torn out of itself, and against itself it floats in dream images and the airy forms of phantasy. (Pt. 1, p. 383)

That much of this vocabulary has become a seemingly naturalized part of our psychological language games should not hide the allegory that Heinroth unfolds. The self is personified and then placed in an allegorical drama in which it can lose a world or be thrown against itself. The self is an allegorical agent for a drama unfolding on an inner metaphysical stage, though this is not the only allegory Heinroth uses. With expansive ambition, the eclectic doctor also annexes physics and continues the allegory with metaphors from dynamics:

> We find here [in madness] the traits of two opposing physical principles: centripetal or contracting force, that is, the striving to lose oneself in the minimum of a center point and thus gradually to disappear in nothingness; and the centrifugal or expansive force, that is, the striving to extend oneself out into infinite distance, and thus also to disappear into nothingness. (Pt. 1, p. 383)

The allegory draws on mechanics to make of the self a dynamic locus of forces. Specifically, it prefigures the kind of allegorical discourse that Freud relies on in his borrowing from mechanics and kinetics to discuss the self and its dynamic organization. Perhaps Heinroth's example points up the way "dynamic" models of self often end up being an allegory that parasitizes other discourses, usually successful scientific disciplines. Successful disciplines furnish tropes that, by analogy, seemingly justify or naturalize the allegory.

Ideler and Allegories of Drives and Instincts

Heinroth gave psychiatry a model of unconsciously unfolding processes that lead to a loss of world in madness. In ways unknown to themselves the mad lose themselves in sin, and this process can never be perceived by mere introspection of the phenomenal self. This view of the unconscious was criticized by the most influential doctor of the next generation, Karl Wilhelm Ideler (1795–1860), who nonetheless did much to continue the allegorization of medical discourse about madness. Ideler's manner of criticizing the notion of the unconscious is of interest for seeing how the romantics trafficked between medicine and literature. In initiating a debate about whether the self is an unconscious drama, or whether it is constituted by a conscious relation to itself, Ideler asked how one can know the unconscious. Is not insanity a conscious state? In his *Grundriss der Seelenheilkunde* (Outline of mental therapy) of 1835, he asked what is the nature of the deviant intent that characterizes sin and madness. For a phenomenology of consciousness, Ideler turns to Shakespeare's *Richard the Third* and the soliloquy in which Richard ruminates, at the play's outset, on his intent to become a scoundrel by setting Clarence and the king against each other:

> To entertain these fair well-spoken days,
> I am determined to prove a villain,
> And hate the idle pleasures of these days.

(1.1)

In these lines is manifest the "hidden self-knowledge" of every evildoer who, with consciousness, overrides the moral law—and scorns the voice of conscience. Evil and insane intent are present to consciousness. Therefore, asks Ideler, is Richard's intent to be explained by some abstract "evil principle" such as the unconscious, or is his insane bitterness to be explained by the fact that he "found himself curtailed in the pursuit of his interests?" (pt. 1, p. 124). Ideler's use of a literary text, to criticize Heinroth's use of allegorical abstractions such as the unconscious, points toward the potential for conflict that will erupt when poets begin to confront psychiatrists who claim mastery over states of mind. In Ideler's example, Shakespeare offers a model for knowing madness. In effect, literature is used as a hermeneutics of consciousness.

By introducing a literary text as an exemplar, and proposing literary analysis to obtain knowledge of madness, Ideler melds together here psychiatry and literary criticism, which sets out another strategy of psychoanalysis. This hermeneutic model is not without ambiguity: does literature provide special knowledge for the doctor; or does the doctor use his science to make sense of the text?

The interesting precedent is that literature is used to criticize a medical doctrine, for Ideler is convinced that literature offers knowledge about madness: not the contemporary romantic literature that he scorns, but classics such as Shakespeare, Cervantes, and, by now, Goethe. This, too, is not without ambiguity. Literary knowledge is subject to interpretation. Literature is also a hermeneutics of experience. However, that relation also demands interpretation, both of literature and of its relation to experience. What we saw earlier as Shakespeare's demonstration of the need for hermeneutics to understand madness comes to the fore here, and it seems accurate to say that this need was integrated into psychiatry by the romantics. This is a most important precedent for the hermeneutics developed by psychoanalysis.

Ideler came from much the same background as Heinroth. He was a teacher at the psychiatric clinic of the Friedrich Wilhelm University in Berlin when he published the first part of his *Grundriss* in 1835. Three years later he published a second part. Very little of these tomes is given over to directly discussing literature or hermeneutics. In fact, this work offers, in some eighteen hundred pages, a mixture of incredibly banal platitudes describing allegorical encounters produced by strife among the soul's faculties. These allegories appear more modern than Heinroth's, for Ideler describes madness in terms of conflictive situations in which drives—*Triebe*—and passions are opposed to each other within the metaphysical framework provided by Kant's description of the mind's faculties. Ideler's drives are nonetheless allegorical personifications: drives become characters acting out roles on the self's stage. In spite of his interest in literary models Ideler does not seem to realize that he is writing allegory. He offers the perhaps too familiar example of a theoretical mind inventing a theory or a language game in which abstract entities become personifications that act out roles predetermined by their own character traits. Freud did much the same thing when he discovered that the libido always wants to have sex.

In the first part of the *Grundriss* Ideler sets forth his dramatis personae. His drives are mainly ethical categories that have been transformed into qualities or intrinsic properties of the conscious self. They read like a list of the virtues of the ideal conservative, neo-Kantian Prussian. The self that Ideler describes has religious drives, inner and outer freedom drives, the drive to truth, to honor, as well as to mastery, social and imitative drives, and, finally the well-known drive that leads to love and the love of humanity—the *Trieb der Menschheit* that Ideler presumably observed among his fellow Prussians. Opposed to these drives stand the passions, like an army of so many desires for sickness set agonistically against drives for health:

> [S]o long as they [the passions] have not completely repressed the other mental drives, the latter will struggle against them and through this bring the mind into a state of revolt that can be recognized by the disturbance of the

understanding; on the other hand, if the struggling interests can be stifled, then they no longer disturb the mind's calm and thus do not influence the use of reason [*Verstandesgebrauch*]. (Pt. 1, p. 546)

The allegory is classical, indeed Ciceronian, though the key terms for mind and understanding—*Gemüth* and *Verstand*—show that Ideler updates it with Kantian terms describing the self and its faculties. Finally, to round out the allegory of struggle, Ideler introduces the concept of repression, or *Unterdrücken*. In this allegorical context the term has decidedly modern resonances.

Psychoanalysis is again prefigured in this allegory of drives and passions waging war on each other with successful repression leading to a victory of morality. Ideler also offers another link in the continuity running from classical philosophy to psychoanalytical thought in his attempt to frame a unified concept of madness. Madness is the result of "misrelations" caused by raging passion. In madness all physical and psychic appearances—phenomena in the Kantian sense—are produced through pathological incongruities that are so many signs that passion has been victorious. The incongruities take the three forms of affect, representation, and somatic disturbance: for they are revealed "im Gemüth, im Vorstellungsvermögen und in den körperlichen Functionen" (pt. 2, p. 201). In effect, one single cause for madness can thus manifest itself in three different areas of symptomatology.

In the conflict between the drives and the passions the mad person is again likened to a stage on which a drama is enacted whose result is "truth." Madness acts as an agent of revelation not unlike a poetic faculty. It does sound strange to read Ideler, much more the neo-Kantian than his predecessors, propounding a doctrine about the truth-value of madness, but madness offers him, too, a way of loosening the Kantian straitjacket of rational empiricism. In madness, truth comes to the fore in a new light, for example, the truth of desire:

Here madness, which tears away the veil of falsification, has not really brought forward any change of the mind, but rather brought the truth to light. For it is not to be denied that many morally correct people become lascivious when mentally ill. This is explained simply by the natural power of the sensual instinct that, during healthy days, is reined in by our feeling of duty and by decorum, but which does not let itself be stopped by these from appearing at times during sleep in lustful dreams. (Pt. 2, p. 205)

Lust and duty are of course a traditional opposition, renewed by Freud after romantic psychiatry renewed the medical use of allegory. Ideler seconds the general romantic belief that madness and dream reveal a truer inner realm than the one phenomenally perceived in the light of the diurnal reason of critical empiricism. In this joint role, madness and dream, two sides of the noumenal world, are valued because they are the agents of revelation of some higher—or lower—order of truth, be it truth repressed or truth hidden in some noumenal realm. Truth is thus made conscious.

In Ideler a reevaluation of the imagination and fantasy is central to his interpretation of madness. Ideler was at one with the poets in decreeing that fantasy is the faculty that allows one "to make perceptible, to embody all of one's representations, whether they contain concepts or feelings, and then to perceive them in that form concretely and clearly in consciousness so that they attain completely clearness, light, and sharp delineation just like so many perceptions [Anschauungen]" (pt. 2, p. 430). This seems to mean that fantasy can produce representations that cannot be distinguished from any other form of perception. Using fantasy, madness has the same power to produce representations as dream and art. Once the will, another character in the allegorical cast, loses its power to serve the understanding, fantasy takes over as the chief director of the inner play. And as "fantasy turns loose passion in an empty pushing forward and longing. . . , consciousness is lost in a passive watching of mad images [Wahngebilde]" (pt. 2, p. 242). Madness produces this inner cinema in which passion may scorn fantasy as an illusion, but fantasy offers compensation for the disjuncture between objective reality and the inner stage of representations. So passion uses the power of fantasy to create representations that can satisfy its desire. Offering a magical realization of passion's wishes, fantasy causes the insane to be indifferent to objective representations having no relation to their passions. Freud's later theory of psychosis is contained here in the description of madness as the creation of a world that is sufficient unto itself. Madness is a compensatory world that fantasy, like an artist, creates to replace the real world.

With this allegorical bent, psychiatry found itself engaged in philosophical debates about the difference between delusion and art, madness and ideal. It rejected Kant's belief that his favored faculty, the understanding, should be able to differentiate between hallucination and objective images, though Ideler waffles on this point. The refusal to follow Kant suggests strange consequences. For the idea that fantasy offers gratification for reality's deficiencies logically entails that one's greatest desire is to be deceived—which is to say psychotic—or at least lost in poetry. Art and madness, understood as representations created by fantasy, are both compensations for a lack that desire cannot fill. Freud and Lacan will reason in the same way. Following this reasoning the conservative Ideler ends up sounding like a radical romantic apologist for madness when he writes that every true passion has a poetic potential and is capable of setting afire the poet's spirit. For every passion is a form of nostalgia or longing: "Every unsatisfied passion is now, according to its deepest essence, nothing other than such a longing [Sehnsucht], which in the worst of cases can silence every remonstrance that the understanding brings against it" (pt. 2, p. 431). Romanticism gives us a legacy in which the self is dominated by nostalgia for an intuited plenitude, by a longing for totality, or the Lacanian "lack" that is the modern version of romantic finitude. And these all are interlinked in passion and madness, as well as the poetic imagination. Romantic psychiatry shows its most profound affinity with romantic art in the characterization of madness as a permanent state of *Heimweh*, of nostalgia or a longing to return to plenitude. This description of longing can serve as a résumé of the central theme of romantic aesthetics.

Romantic Aesthetics: The Text as an Allegory for the Psyche

The world of German romanticism was the last time, in our history, where doctors and poets, philosophers and scientists—often one and the same person—shared a unity of thought. Virtually all the themes found in the romantic psychiatrists and their views of madness are embodied in the literature of the romantics. What is most striking about psychiatry and literature is their representation of the self. For both it is a space described by allegory. Allegory is the standard literary and psychiatric technique for the romantic exploration of madness, and, through madness, a description of the psyche. One should probably speak of a new literary genre in this respect: the romantic space of narration is an allegorical space representing a dramatization of the psyche. Often this space is the stage upon which are acted out the disjuncture of representations that characterize madness. This disjuncture had to be acted out by allegorical characters, for the romantics believed, as Schlegel put it, that the metaphors characterizing the self must be *shown* allegorically, and not abstractly represented. Since the inner world is not directly expressible, it can only be shown indirectly by allegorical figures.[6]

In German romanticism any number of texts, from a great variety of writers, could illustrate the construction of this irrational narrative space that depicts an allegory of the self. I shall limit myself to four writers: Eichendorff, Tieck, Novalis, and Hoffmann. They are clearly four of the most important in the creation of the type of text that enacts an allegory of psychic space. And unlike the romantic doctors, they are easily accessible and continue to play a role in our sense of the possibilities of literature. Each of these writers can bring a different accent to this common project of inventing the allegorical self and, taken together, offer a rather complete introduction into the problematics of madness and romantic literature.

The allegorization of self, the mad self, that literature shared with psychiatry, is well illustrated by one of the defining romantic tales, "Zauberei im Herbst" (Enchantment in autumn) by Joseph Eichendorff (1788–1857), and so, for purposes of illustration, I turn first to Eichendorff. Eichendorff is the writer whose poetry gave the most lyrical expression of romantic longing, nostalgia, and all that is summed in the pathology called *Sehnsucht*. Dramatizing the pathologies generated by the lack and longing to which his poetry gives ideal form, "Enchantment in Autumn" (1808) creates an allegorical space that ambiguously represents the mad self by enacting the allegory that the self holds up to itself as in a mirror or speculum. The narration creates the space of madness as it exists in a noumenal world outside of the objective coordinates of space and time. Space and time are the most basic Kantian categories that the mind uses to have rational knowledge. To get around Kant, fantastic romantic literature had no firmer goal than to bend, when not transcend, these basic categories.

Eichendorff's story begins as an objective third-person narration in which a restrictedly omniscient narrator tells a tale about a knight. The knight, named Ubaldo, went astray one day and encountered, on his hunt, a strange hermit who gave him shelter in a mysterious cave. In the night Ubaldo heard the hermit lamenting his sin and guilt. In subsequent visits Ubaldo notes that an "earthly longing" is perceptible in the hermit's need for redemption. Ubaldo persuades the hermit, who has come to visit Ubaldo and his wife, to narrate the tale of his life. The hermit tells, in a first-person narration embedded within the main narration, a tale that begins with the hermit's decision not to go on the first crusade. The hermit preferred to stay with a beloved girl who, however, was the fiancée of his best friend. Wandering one day, the hermit encountered the girl, who declared that she loved him, and not the friend. Later, led by a strange bird, he caught a glimpse of the girl unclothed. Filled with mad desire, he wandered until he ran into the friend—whom he threw off a cliff. The hermit begins to narrate his happiness with the girl and also her strange death when Ubaldo interrupts him, calling the hermit by his name Raimund. He tells him that he, Ubaldo, was the friend, that his wife was the girl, and that this is all pure fantasy on Raimund's part.

Crying that all is lost, Raimund flees the castle. Objective space and time seem to disappear, for Raimund suddenly finds himself wandering on a fall morning, exactly like the one upon which he left his castle years before. Returning home, Raimund finds the same bird of years before. His breast filled with the same longing, he discovers that Ubaldo's blood-covered face is looking down at him from a window. The voluptuous maiden of years ago rides by, smiling at him: "And lost in madness went poor Raimund following the sounds [of the hunting horns] into the woods and was never ever seen again." With this final convolution the story seeming designates itself as Raimund's madness. But the narration has told the tale as if he were a participant in it. The allegory presents itself as speculum for a demonstration of how the mad self is split into an actor and a spectator. And it ends with the demonstration that the world of longing is the world of eternal loss, of madness that destroys, for the insane, the world of empirical reality.

Desire is omnipresent in Eichendorff's allegorical space that must lie beyond the realm of objective representation. Only music can bridge the gap between the two (and the role of music in madness would merit a study unto itself). In this tale, the sound of music or simply the peal of bells reverberates in some space beyond madness, but these sounds can enter the text. Bridging the chasm between objective and subjective, music is a correlate for a desire that can never be satisfied, even in expiation after the hermit Raimund has abandoned his castle:

> [T]hen soared up again detached well-known sounds out of the woods in my loneliness, and dark voices in me played them back again in answer, and in my most inner being I was frightened by the sound of bells of the distant church, when they came to me on a bright Sunday morning from over the mountains, as if they were looking for the old, quiet kingdom of God, of my childhood, in my breast, that was no longer present there.[7]

Symbolic bells are an objective correlative for an inner longing, perhaps for a return to childhood. But childhood, as Freud was to show, is gone, and what remains is its absence in the present, a never-present that determines the present and its pathologies.

The subject of the story is thus at once a character and an allegorical space in which psychic functions are allegorized in their disjuncture. The narrative shows from the exterior that Raimund goes mad, and yet the narrative itself is the allegory of inner insanity. Ideler's romantic psychiatry would have attributed this madness to a fall, for Raimund has fallen into sin, or perhaps adulthood—for adulthood and guilt are often synonymous in the romantic view of time and its inevitable process toward alienation. After Rousseau temporality always involves a loss of origins and plenitude—nature in the case of society, and the mother's breast for the individual.

As an allegorical space dramatizing this loss, the story *is* madness, though Eichendorff's play with rhetorical techniques shows that a narrating intelligence is at work, allowing the reader to view from within the space of the story and without. The first part's limited third-person point of view respects space and time. The second tale, embedded in the first and told from Raimund's first-person point of view, is a fantasy in which months may be lived as days. And the final narration is related from an omniscient third-person viewpoint that brings the reader onto the inner stage of fantastic representations. Given the same degree of credibility as the first part, the final narration seems to enact "objectively" the fantastic, and thus shows the power of madness to create a world that can replace the world of reality, the world of Kantian objectivity. The tale becomes a world of madness, coinciding in part with a character's insanity, yet remaining larger than the character's world, as the story allegorizes the disjunctures worked by fantasy in madness.

In short, the world of mad fantasy is produced by the disjuncture between the phenomenal and the noumenal, between the objective and the subjective worlds. The fundamental disjuncture is represented by the dream effects that the text imitates, as well as by the suggestion that somewhere beyond normal space and time lie inner depths out of which spring longing, lust, and fantasy. The mirror effect also produces the disjuncture. Raimund is mirrored by the text as if in a speculum that reflects images of him, taken from the outer world, but seen in the interior world in which he acts out his madness on the inner stage of his own desire. Finally, sin coincides with the etiology of madness, for the split between objectivity and subjectivity is due to the guilt that tears the inner world apart, so that it is no longer in contact with the world represented at the beginning of the story. Perhaps the major difference between a romantic psychiatric description of insanity and this allegorical enactment of madness is that, in this early romantic tale, the reader finds little compensation created by fantasy. Raimund's insanity is horrible. His psyche is torn apart by a lustful longing that his atonement cannot repress.

Madness as Dream

The dream effects in Eichendorff's story are found in many other fantastic tales, and it is accurate to say that many romantic texts use dream effects to circumvent the Kantian coordinates limiting our knowledge of reality. A dominant romantic strategy, opposing madness to rational empiricism, was to annex madness to dream, and to proclaim the epistemic superiority of dream—and hence the superiority of madness as knowledge. We have all been sensitive to the possibility that dream has its own rhetorical system, ever since Freud placed it in the foreground of psychoanalysis. But the difficulties of knowing through dream are great, as can be well illustrated by one of the best-known proponents of dream as knowledge, the engagingly mystical Novalis (1772–1801). Poet and theorist, in his medical theories Novalis proposed that every disease is in some sense a mental illness, since mind is always in correspondence with the totality of being. This theory of totality also imbues his almost programmatically anti-Kantian novel *Heinrich von Ofterdingen* (1802). In its rejection of rational empiricism, the novel puts "inner contemplation" on the same level with experience as a way to knowledge. With regard to dream, the novel's first chapter gives the most famous literary "proof" that dream has the capacity to give access to a world superior to the world of empirical experience. The novel's hero dreams of a blue flower, a "hohe lichtblaue Blume," that symbolically represents the superior world of inner ideals. Only in dream can Heinrich have access to a superior vision, a vision whose only difference from madness is that, as Heinrich says, in the dream he sees his vision so clearly and so brightly.

Heinrich sees the blue flower in all clarity, but it is a clarity that never goes beyond that of an unspecified allegory. Novalis did not finish the novel, perhaps because he could find nothing in empirical reality that corresponds to what a dream image represents. He found nothing that condensed into itself so much that its meaning could never be specified. The meaning of the novel's dream remains an open allegory. Or, alternatively, the blue flower represents something beyond the limits of language, a showing of desire for which Novalis could find no conceptual expression that would necessarily limit the meaning by pinning it down. The romantics all took the blue flower as the supreme image of an allegory that pointed beyond the phenomena that mere language could describe. Or beyond the rational . . . the blue flower.

Novalis formulated for romanticism a program, but other writers enacted it. Above all, they equated dream with madness, or vice versa, and then looked for the rhetorical strategies that would allow the realization of dream texts. Eichendorff's work was part of this movement, but the most influential inventor of fantastic madness drawn from dream sources was undoubtedly Ludwig Tieck (1773–1853). A major influence on Poe, Tieck has been curiously neglected by the Anglo-Saxon world. Yet this early romantic deserves as much credit as any for creating the narrative rhetoric capable of transposing the irrational rhetoric of dreams into literature. If dream is a narrative form, and if dream can be said to have its own rhetorical devices—devices that are the underpinnings of psychoanalytic hermeneutics—then Tieck's work should at least be studied for its role in borrowing rhetoric from what Freud saw as our private nightly psychosis. Borrowing the rhetoric of madness from dream, Tieck puts it in public purview in fiction and creates therewith a plausibly intelligible discourse. In his originality Tieck's work clearly precedes in this regard the elaboration of psychiatric or psychoanalytic concepts. One of his earliest tales, "Der Blonde Eckbert" (The blond Eckbert), can demonstrate this claim.

A résumé of "Der Blonde Eckbert" shows that Tieck foregrounds the devices Freud later called condensation and displacement—the use of a single image for multiple symbolizations and the use of an image to symbolize something other than what it appears to symbolize. The story's protagonist Eckbert lives in seclusion with his wife Bertha, only occasionally visited by the friend Walther. Wanting to reduce the distance between his friend and his wife, Eckbert asks Walther to listen to his wife's tale of her life. This opens the type of framed tale that Eichendorff also used for narrative embedding: Bertha tells in first-person narration that, as a girl, she ran away from an unhappy home and was taken in by a bizarre old woman with a dog and a bird that laid eggs containing jewels. After some years of serving the old woman, Bertha took the bird and jewels and ran away. She met Eckbert and has been happy ever since.

The friend Walther casually reveals that he knows the dog's name. Bertha is upset, becomes ill, and Eckbert, growing angry, finally kills Walther, only to return to his home to find that his wife is now dead. Eckbert encounters a new friend, but, one night after telling his sad tale, Eckbert finds that the new friend looks like Walther. Eckbert runs away, only to enter the same landscape that years before Bertha had fled. Unable to decide if he is now dreaming or if he only dreamed that he once had a wife, he suddenly hears the old woman of Bertha's past asking for her bird and jewels. She declares that she was both Walther and the new friend. Moreover, she declares that Bertha was Eckbert's half-sister. Eckbert collapses, guilty of incest, and now quite mad.

Tieck draws upon the irrational articulations of dream narrative to narrate the etiology of psychosis. The tale begins as a seemingly objective story in which representation respects the empirical coordinates of space and time. Time seems to unfold in linear fashion, and the story is set in a referentially real place, the Harz Mountains. But the narration already contains condensations that disguise desire. The wife is also a sister, and Walther is also an old crone that one could interpret as a hidden or displaced mother. The narration slips away from the rhetoric of objectivity to engage the reader in a first-person narration whose images are insane: what is the meaning of a bird that lays eggs with jewels? The first-person narration then gives way to an even more disjointed dream narrative, in which the narrator himself may be present to himself as his own double when Eckbert kills Walther, finds his wife dead, and wanders in a landscape that seems to mirror a projection of the inner world. On the inner stage of representation the condensations of characters as doubles rejects the law of the excluded middle and other logical principles. With the suspension of logic, Eckbert attends to an allegory of his own madness as he wanders into the area of interdicted desire. The tale is finally an enactment of dream and psychosis, for there is no real distinction between the two in this fantasy enactment of incest.

The representation of psychic projections through doubles is one of the discoveries of romanticism, though one might just as well call it an invention. In the development of the self there is often no distinction to be made between invention and discovery: what can be imagined to be part of the self can usually be discovered in the self, once belief, in some sense, attaches to the invention. This imaginative invention can become part of the way the mad live their madness in confirmation of whatever explanation of madness their era offers them: the mad can believe they are sleeping with devils as easily as they can all believe that they want to commit incest. The romantics, with their speculum concept of the self, discovered madness attaching to a double, the double that is at once oneself and other. The belief in the double springs naturally from the speculum view of the self as a inner stage upon which one watches the images that are oneself. If these images detach themselves from the self, then one can watch oneself wander into the world—in dream become madness. The double is also a form of condensation that creates the hypersymbolization of dream and madness. For doubles also collapse structures of identity so that finally everything is everything else: Bertha's tale of flight is also Eckbert's tale of flight, each allegorizing the other in a dream in which the collapse of identities reflects incestuous desire. Or, if we follow up the Freudian development of this theme, we see that all desire is a double of the original desire: all desire is a form of incest—and hence the grounds for our daily madness, whether in dream or psychosis.

Hoffmann and the Need for Critical Irony

The romantics worked to get around the limits of critical rationalism. However, they soon wanted to get around the limits they had imposed upon themselves when they made the self accessible only to dream and madness. The impulse to break open the hermetic self, lost in its mirroring on the stage of dreams, was quickly felt. This impulse animates the rhetorical dimension that is used to counter constant irrational fantasy: the dimension of irony. Much has been written on romantic irony, and hopefully the following comments will enlarge upon that discussion by showing how irony is related to the romantic exploration of madness. From our perspective, romantic irony can often be understood as the attempt to communicate around the closed stage of irrational representations and dream rhetoric found in romantic fictions. Irony offers broader meanings, but it is double communication, affirming and denying, and pointing to an intelligence beyond the madness of the text, to the intelligence capable of the ironic judgment.

Also interesting for our argument about modernity is the idea that romantic irony begins the modern separation of science and literature. After the second generation of romantics, irony became a frequent strategy of writers who wished to show their distance from the pathology and deviance attributed to them by those stern taskmasters, medicine and philosophy. Or, as the century progressed, irony was increasingly used by poets to affirm positively the value of their pathology in the face of reductive medical definitions and philosophical rationality. In anticipation of the next chapter, I note that from Hoffmann on, through Poe and Baudelaire, and well beyond, irony becomes a rhetorical ploy that allows the writer to confront and affirm lack and longing, as well as the pathology that ensues from this lack and longing. Irony is then a form of self-affirmation that grants the mad a position of superiority over those nonironic philistines, such as doctors, who see the deviant simply as deviant. The reason for the poet's disdain for science, beginning with the later romantics, seems clearer when placed in this context: with irony the poet can affirm madness and yet communicate in objective terms with ironic tropes that escape the grasp of any reductive rationalism. Doctors are not ironic, especially positivist doctors, and neither was Kant.

The mad master ironist was E. T. A. Hoffmann (1772–1822), a figure who dominated nineteenth-century literature. Hoffmann is well known for having introduced the doppelgänger into world literature, though his fellow romantic Jean Paul deserves equal credit. But no writer combines in quite the same measure equal parts irony and madness. The aging Goethe rejected Hoffmann's work for its "sick" qualities, for its *Verirrungen,* or craziness. But Freud saw in it the fundamental exploration of the uncanny, and Dostoyevsky paid the ultimate compliment by perfecting the creation of the insane inner vision of the doppelgänger in his novel *The Double.* For his creation, Hoffmann drew upon the doctors, for he was a reader of Pinel and Reil, and used the psychiatric texts in order to reflect upon them in irony. In this he continues a tradition that begins with Swift and Diderot, if not with Rabelais. In Hoffmann one finds the example of a mind that in constant irony conflates psychosis and literature. Hoffmann offers the example of a writer who at once accepts medical notions about madness, subjects them to ironic manipulation, and in turn elaborates discursive practices that a later generation of doctors as well as poets could utilize—Ideler and Heinroth, Poe and Baudelaire, to offer key examples.

Hoffmann's earliest work on madness used Diderot's *Rameau's Nephew* as a springboard. Following Diderot's demonstration that the insane artist is capable of seducing reason with a mastery that humbles both medicine and philosophy, Hoffmann framed in his "Ritter Gluck" (1809) an experiment with the power of madness to determine the real. Hoffmann's "Knight Gluck" is a mad musician who believes that he is the great composer Gluck. In his capacity for mime, for the empty imitation of pure form, the knight bears the same relation to Gluck that Diderot's nephew bears to his uncle, the composer Rameau. The insane mime can enchant reason by representations that bear the same relation to the real that an ironic trope bears to an unambiguous statement: the mime enacts one thing while purporting to express something else. One must get beyond the surface representation to find the "real" that is represented. According to Diderot's mad mime, the ultimately real is found in the mechanical fibers that direct the muscles that beat in imitation of art. Hoffmann's knight, on the other hand, says that his madness comes from his inner depths—the depths that romanticism had recently brought to light. His madness springs from a pure inner psychic space, somewhere beyond the "ivory portals" leading to dream. In this kingdom of dreams, "im Reiche der Träume," is found truth, the eternal, and the ineffable.[8] The knight narrates that in making a voyage into the inner king-dom of dreams, he was tortured by pain and anguish. Upon awakening from the trip he found that he continued to be observed by a great eye, one that accompanied him even when he subsequently went to listen to flowers singing. Among the flowers he found, within the calyx of a sunflower, an eye looking at him. The eye is his own, like an exteriorized speculum. The eye seems to represent the power of vision that is necessary to transform the knight into an artist in insanity. But it also appears that an eye looks at the eye here with an irony that points up the incongruous nature of the speculum image used to explain inner representation: if I represent myself to myself, must I contem-plate my eye on the mirror of inner representation?

In irony Hoffmann uses Kant's establishment of a line of demarcation between subjective error and objective truth. This is the rationalist line of demarcation between madness and reason, and the line is increasingly blurred in later tales such as the first story of the collection called *Die Sera-pionsbrüder* (or *The Serapion Brethren,* published in four volumes in 1819–21). The key story, "Der Heilige Serapion," or "The Hermit Sera-pion," is the tale of an insane hermit whose creative madness is a form of inventive poetry.[9] The hermit binds together great knowledge with an extra-ordinary talent for writing: "[A]ll that he wrote was animate with a fiery fantasy, with a special spirit that looked into the deepest depths" (4:28). Serapion's most notable poetry consists in the creation of himself. In the nineteenth century he becomes a fourth-century hermit who settles in an imaginary Theban desert. The story's narrator Cyprian is a representative of psychiatry. He reads Pinel and Reil and, armed with their theories to explain the monk's idée fixe, goes to see the mad anchorite. Using therapeutic tricks learned from the psychiatry books, Cyprian falls upon the insane Serapion, and, in a great burst of reasoning, he demonstrates the irrationality of a belief that defies empirical reasoning. Cyprian's appeal to moral reasoning would have been approved by Pinel or Kant:

> I called out in a loud voice . . . "Awaken from the destructive dream that is stifling you, throw off these detestable garments, give yourself back to your family that is made desolate by you, and who is making legitimate claims upon you once more." (3:31)

But Serapion, the hermit, has not, in his insane vision, lost his capacity to reason. In the dialectics of reason in madness, Hoffmann introduces an ironic variant on that motif by renewing the use of logic in the service of madness. Serapion is a sharp logician who uses the tools of reason to defeat the attack on madness by critical reason. First, Serapion reasons that any hermit would know that he should reject Cyprian as an emissary of the devil: since the time of Saint Anthony, it has been part of the ascetic's situation to be tempted by Satan. It is, so to speak, part of the logic of the ascetic's situation that he be tempted to believe that he is not logical. However, with appropriate irony, Serapion concedes that Cyprian is a mere human reasoner, albeit an illogical one. For if Serapion is mad, then it is by definition illogical that Cyprian should try to convince him with reasoning: "If I am truly insane, then only a crazy person can have the illusion that he can talk me out of the idée fixe that has produced my madness" (3:32). For if such moral reasoning were possible, then there would be no mad on the earth. Turning to the basic Kantian categories for fixing empirical reality, Serapion notes that time is relative and that proof about space quite difficult. To wit: if Cyprian maintains that the present time is the nineteenth century, centuries after Serapion's martyrdom, and that the space they occupy is in southern Germany, then Serapion will have no choice but to believe that Cyprian is insanely mistaking a Theban desert for a German woods. And what could he say in answer to that charge? Very little, as a good reader of *Don Quixote* such as Hoffmann might ironically prove.

Serapion's mad logic aims at showing that assertions and counterassertions cannot prove anything about time and space. The Kantian categories are useless for determining sanity, since any appeal to time and space already presupposes the shared rationality that is based on these categories of perception. The circularity of rational empiricism does not invalidate it, but Serapion's logical demonstration points up the limits of appealing to evidence when two points of view do not share any grounds as to what constitutes evidence. The consummate irony of this demonstration is evident in the way that Hoffmann uses reason to demonstrate the limits of reason— and to show that madness can use reason in the creation of what Wittgenstein called, in musing on the madness that often threatened him, the *Weltbild,* or worldview of shared assumptions. Hoffmann's irony affirms that a mad worldview can function quite well to create a framework for interpreting all of reality with a coherence that defeats the would-be psychiatrist. Cyprian, in recognizing his defeat, can only lament, "With all my wisdom I stood in confusion, in shame, before this madman" (3:33). Serapion creates a world parallel to Cyprian's, with total coherence. He would be, in his insanity, the supreme artist, if only he had not lost his sense of doubleness, of ironic duplicity, which, for Hoffmann, is the foundation of romantic art.

In Hoffmann's work madness creatively uses literary devices to stage its pathologies—the same devices that theory uses without ironic self-consciousness. His version of the double, for example, is a model for the creative projection onto the exterior world of what is created on the inner stage of representation. One might say that madness is mimesis transformed into reality. When the projected double is seen, belief in the double is insanity—as one sees in the novel *Die Elixiere des Teufels* (1815–16), a work in which Hoffmann himself seems to have lost control of the power of doubles to mimic madness. The projection of a double can also resemble a literary performance that, in underscoring a commonality of literature and madness, complicates the task of sorting out literary and insane fantasies. I offer a superb example of this mimetic madness as narrated in Hoffmann's "Don Giovanni" from the *Phantasiestücke.*

In this story a narrator is awakened from slumber at an inn at which, strangely enough, Mozart's opera is about to be performed in a theater that is somehow attached to the inn. Having watched the first act, the narrator discovers that one of the opera's characters, Donna Anna, has been in the loggia with him for most of the act. She tells the narrator, in Italian logically enough, that in his own music he has understood the magical madness of eternally yearning love. She then leaves him. Later, after the performance, he returns to the loggia to meditate on Don Juan, on his yearning and the "lustful madness" that he feels he could ignite in Donna Anna. In the midst of this meditation on art and madness, desire and yearning, at two o'clock in the morning, he feels an electrical breath glide over, accompanied by perfume and music.

The story ends with a brief epilogue taking the form of a midday conversation of local burghers who say that the singer playing Donna Anna's role died at two o'clock in the morning.

The epilogue is set in objective empirical reality—the world we usually agree upon in public consent. But the preceding narration has been viewed through the narrator's subjectivity as he interacts with the world created by Mozart—with a strong suggestion of the influence of dream. From this perspective Hoffmann asks the reader to view art as a literal double: during the performance the narrator felt so strongly his double in Don Juan that Donna Anna, the fictional object of desire, entered his world. In its doublings mimesis alters subjectivity so that the mind becomes an objective space, the space of art—or mind enlarged by another subjectivity. In this series of doubles Donna Anna enters into the loggia as the literalization of what is ordered by mimetic logic: the fictional character can be separated from the living actress, as in dream, insane hallucinations, and the works of desire that we call operas and stories.

Hoffmann's work implies ironically that the literary space of representation is analogous to a space of madness in which representations split themselves into doubles, which can then allow one double to appear like an objective presence. "Don Giovanni" ends with the actress's death, since the dissolution of the self in death is the only limit to this mirror play of doubles. It is something of a platitude that absolute yearning must end in death, but Hoffmann has enlarged the context in which this platitude has meaning. From his romantic perspective, longing for what lies beyond the possible explains the need for art and the origins of insanity. Psychosis and poetry are forms of compensation, produced by what a doctor like Ideler called fantasy. The need for mimesis to compensate for deficiencies creates a new self, one invariably ready to fall prey to psychosis, unless irony offers the bootstrap with which the ironist pulls back from the edge. In Hoffmann, and the romantics in general, this drama created by the constraints of finitude can be represented henceforth in a text that is an allegory for a psyche whose fundamental relation to itself is to recognize its desire and its lack.

After the romantics the psyche and literature could be identified as two sides of a new type of allegory. For this allegory, psychoanalysis would create, in a new allegorical hermeneutics, a literary criticism commensurate with old and new heroes embodying doubles of the self: Narcissus, Oedipus, Hamlet, and Hoffmann's own Sandman, the hero allegorizing the self fissured by the uncanny. But before analyzing psychoanalysis, historical accuracy requires that we study the invention of our literary modernity and its rebellious praise of folly that arose in the face of the victorious positivist psychiatry that dismissed romanticism as rubbish. After romanticism, nineteenth-century medicine usually preferred scalpels to allegories.

Chapter 7

Pathological Anatomy and the Poetics of Madness

The Background to Positivist Psychiatry

A new chapter in the history of discourses on madness began when medicine demonstrated it could account for a mental disease using the findings of pathological anatomy. Probably the earliest example of this medical determination of a relationship between a physical condition and a psychic state occurred when Antoine Bayle (1789–1858) showed that general paralysis was correlated with chronic meningitis. No real theoretical knowledge was involved in Bayle's demonstration of the correlation in his thesis of 1822.[1] He did not know that syphilis is the ultimate cause of this then prevalent mental illness. The doctor simply showed the constant presence of a pathological organic state accompanying a pathological mental state. However, the demonstration of the regular correlation of a mental pathology with an organic lesion strongly suggested that an organic explanation of all mental illness was possible. In explaining madness in the eighteenth century, mechanistic medicine had made its rather weakly defined lesions a matter of faith. But Bayle's correlation seemed to promise the positive reduction of mental phenomena to a correlative function of organic phenomena—in this case of an inflammation that could be easily recognized. As a diagnostic principle, correlation had come into its own, and, with this, an affirmation of the materialism underlying German somatic medicine or French positivism. The demise of neoclassical medicine was assured by this kind of discovery that led to the elaboration of the positivist belief that pathological anatomy is the basis for all medicine. In this chapter we shall examine this belief, with its consequences for discourses on madness and, especially, the poets' reaction to the consequences of positivism.

Bayle's discovery was part of what the historian E. H. Ackerknecht calls the transformation of the medicine of symptoms into a medicine of lesions.[2] This medicine was embodied in the first half of the nineteenth century by the French physician François Broussais (1772–1838), whose basic medical doctrine was that all disease was a matter of inflammations. Reversing Brown's polarities of sthenia and asthenia, Broussais invented a universal syndrome in which all disease resulted from the augmentation or loss of organs' *contractilité* (or, roughly, resiliency). The necessity of studying an organ's state meant that the autopsy room was the ultimate place for diagnosis, for only there could the doctor see if an augmentation or loss had occurred that had led to the patient's dying of Broussais's universal malady, gastroenteritis.[3] Alterations of tissue were correlated, if not identified, with disease. (This theory led to the therapeutic mania for leeches as a panacea for reducing inflammation.) In other words, the principle of correlation was not yet the basis for a modern medicine, even if this principle is used today as a criterion for causality. In the early nineteenth century, the principle was established as a descriptive guide to what might be the case. It is "really" the case that general paralysis, the mental disease called paresis, is accompanied by inflammation of brain tissue. In a strict sense, however, this is not the "cause" of the mental perturbation: several decades had to elapse, and the invention of microbiology had to occur, before the spirochete responsible for that inflammation could be identified as the causal agent.

Outside of the sphere of romantic medicine, nineteenth-century writers— mad and sane—faced in medicine an increasingly imperial science for which the principle of correlations provided a simplifying logic to account for much mental phenomena. This was true for "normal" medicine as well as short-lived sciences such as magnetism and phrenology, or for the nascent disciplines such as pathological anatomy and positivist psychiatry. These sciences were guided in their initial development by the correlations they could establish between phenomena. Some were more successful than others. Less successful, for example, was Gall and Spurzheim's phrenology that promised to correlate somatic features, or bumps on the cranium, with mental phenomena. Nor was the notion of correlation exactly the same as ours, for the nineteenth-century doctor usually wanted to *see* with his eyes these correlations: hence Bichat's refusal to use a microscope in classifying tissues in histology. The positivist doctor wanted palpable correlations that point to a relation between organic forms and human comportment, such as lesions his scalpel could reveal in the cases of attested mental aberration.

The search for correlations accompanied the materialism and early positivism of medical research, such in the work of first important experimental physiologist, François Magendie (1783–1855).[4] Having recognized the motor and sensory character of the anterior and posterior spinal roots, Magendie then undertook some fifty experiments in 1826 to prove that fluid is normally present in the brain. Seeking meaningful correlations, he looked for a relation between cerebrospinal fluid and the faculties of the intelligence. To this end he measured the quantity of the fluid in people in possession of their reason, and then the amount found in imbeciles and in the insane. Finding experimental subjects at the Salpetrière asylum, his scalpel revealed that the cadavers of idiots and the insane have greater than normal quantities of cerebrospinal fluid, though differently disposed. Apparently a "genius," recently dead at an old age, had less fluid (*Emergence of Experimental Physiology*, p. 185). This rigorous materialism, with its use of quantification, sought correlations between the body's condition and mental phenomena. It is not far from the viewpoint that reduces poetic genius to a question of a few grams of spinal fluid.

Increasingly under the influence of physiology and pathological anatomy, psychiatry gave up the idea that its task was to look at exterior symptoms and to draw up nosological tables. Rejecting reform neoclassicism and the romantics, psychiatry took its task to be the study of pathological physiology in order to correlate mental states and afflicted tissues. Not all psychiatrists were strict somatic materialists, since, as Ackerknecht notes, in a reprise of an earlier ideology, many of the psychiatrists in Germany became *Somatiker* because they were convinced that the immortal soul could not become diseased.[5] This recycling of seventeenth-century controversies about madness and the soul occurs, however, in a context in which materialism has begun to dominate medical debate.

Two corollary principles underwrite, not only the new medical doctrines about mental illness, but also a growing consensus about psychic functioning. First, medicine became, as propounded by the positivist Claude Bernard (1813–1878), resolutely monist in its materialist approach to pathological phenomena. Second, again according to Claude Bernard, the separation of the normal and the abnormal was no longer conceived as an ontological divide between two realms. Rather, the normal and the pathological were integrated as relative positions involving the same natural processes. The normal and the pathological are expressions of the same natural laws that all physical phenomena obey.[6] There are no "abnormal" laws. For the history of psychiatry as well as physiology—and an understanding of deviance in general—this elimination of the opposition between the normal and the abnormal is an anti-Cartesian revolution: medicine is rid of any dualism. Disease in not a struggle between good and evil principles, or any other polarizing opposition. As Bernard observed, in nature there is nothing troubled or abnormal since everything takes place according to natural laws, laws that are by definition always "normal" (see *Le Normal et le Pathologique*, p. 62). Physiology, pointing the way for psychiatry and, later, psychoanalysis, defined the pathological as a relative variation from the norm and thus as a part of a natural continuum that contains the norm. The abnormal is something of an extension of the normal.

Moreau and a Materialist Poetics of Madness

Psychiatry embraced the materialist monism that seemed to guarantee the success of physiology and pathological anatomy, though it was largely a pious hope that such a monism would provide a reductive model for explaining mental illness. But materialist monism provided a model for mind and deviance that allowed nineteenth-century poets and doctors to share a consensus even when they shared nothing else, except a belief in the other's deviance. Yet all was not conflict between doctors and poets. For example, a somatic doctor like Jacques-Joseph Moreau (1804–1884) undertook medical research that led both to new theory and to the elaboration of a materialist poetics, which we will find in the case of Moreau's friend, the poet Charles Baudelaire. To explore the organic unity of mind and body Moreau undertook some of the first drug-oriented psychological experimentation. These experiments open onto our future belief in transforming consciousness, for these were some of the first experiments that suggested the possibility of cultivating a poetics of madness by the transcendence of ordinary consciousness through drug-induced alterations. Usually using hashish, Moreau induced euphoric states of consciousness that could be identified with poetic experience. Materialist monism makes all psychic experience a matter of physical states. Moreover, materialist that he was, Moreau also subscribed to the romantic view of madness as revelation. From this perspective, madness and poetry are defined as psychic states, and any means is as good as any other for changing the brain and producing those revelatory states of consciousness that could also be identified with poetry or madness. Baudelaire could only agree, and it is instructive to bring to the foreground the medical materialism that poets like Baudelaire accepted even when they revolted against purely rational attempts to explain their madness.

Moreau was a materialist who believed that the unity of physical and psychic phenomena were demonstrated by using a physical cause—hash, in this instance—to induce at will the fantasy or dream state that Moreau identified with madness. Having experienced madness from within, Moreau logically reduced, in his *Hashish and Mental Illness,* madness to a single experiential state:

I use interchangeably the terms delirium, madness, and mental illness to designate mental disorders. I am not unaware of the many differences that distinguish . . . from the point of view of symptomology and treatment, delirium, as it is precisely defined, and madness; but from a psychic point of view we have to admit that these differences just do not exist. The causes, the symptoms, or the exterior signs may vary; the intrinsic psychic phenomenon is the same, essentially, in whatever form acute or chronic, partial or general, the mental illness presents itself.[7]

Moreau's monistic reduction of madness to a single "psychic" unity is a moment of equal interest for the history of psychiatry and of poetry, for in taking this step he in effect decrees the experience of madness to be a unified aesthetic phenomenon. From our contemporary viewpoint an objection will inevitably arise, for who today trusts the notion of unity? The notion allows the conceptual sleight of hand by which the madness and aesthetic experience are equated as one state of consciousness. And the notion of consciousness itself is also so amorphous that any unification based on "experience" allows any conscious experience to be abusively equated with any other. But such logical quibbling overlooks the power this identification has had in allowing us to believe poetry can be a transforming power of "consciousness."

Moreau's views of consciousness were based on introspection, that most radical empiricism. He claimed that under the influence of drugs, especially hashish, the mind can behold itself as if in dream. Though Moreau admitted that the truly insane rarely have the capacity for self-reflection, Moreau made of his delirium a self-reflecting condition. In a self-mirroring reflection the mind can experience the nature of insanity, or, if one prefers, the "meaning" of insanity. By this Moreau meant that one can experience directly phenomena that are hidden normally from the medical observer. It may not seem entirely logical for Moreau to have identified his hallucinations with those of the insane whom he treated in his medical practice. But Moreau was not a timid soul. Having viewed his own delirium, he was ready to assert, "To understand an ordinary depression, it is necessary to have experienced one; to comprehend the raving of a madman, it is necessary to have raved oneself, without having lost the power to evaluate the psychic change occurring in the mind" (p. 17). Understanding acquires the romantic meaning of authenticity here: understanding must include direct experience in a moment of ineffable empathy. If most psychiatrists would refuse this demand, it is nonetheless characteristic of the next few generations of writers for whom madness is a privileged experience to be known from within.

Moreau's monistic view of mind resulted in no clinical tableaux, but rather in a poetics of experience in which the knowledge of madness is defined as the coincidence of lucidity and unreason—of which poetry is a primary form. Knowledge entails an "expansion" of self, to use the spatial metaphor Baudelaire coined in his sonnet "Correspondances." Moreau's debt to poets fond of drugs, to those *haschichins* with whom he associated, underlies the quotation he uses to open his major book *Hashish and Mental Illness*. He gives credit on the title page to the poet Theophile Gautier for proof that we desire madness to overcome the limits imposed by culture, or, more precisely, that "the aspiration toward an ideal is so strong in man that he tries to release the bonds that keep his soul within his body." To release these bonds the doctor or the poet can induce insanity through artificial means and know the expansive delirium of the normally body-bound mind. In brief, medical experimentation with drugs validates and is validated by the poetic "expansion" of the delirious mind in the quest for the knowledge that mind can have of itself.

Griesinger and the Positivist View of Madness

Moreau's was not, however, the dominant view among doctors, for the beauty of going insane was lost on most of the medical world. The positivist current in psychiatry was usually not allied with the poets. In the case of Wilhelm Griesinger (1817–1868), the most important midcentury psychiatrist in Europe, we find a positive hostility toward literature and its claim to know madness. In contrast to Moreau, Griesinger was the imperial type of scientist, unwilling to concede authority to any discourse but medical, and positively forbidding that his readers give heed to the poets and their views of madness. His *Mental Pathology and Therapeutics* (as his *Pathologie und Therapie der psychischen Krankheiten* of 1845 was translated in 1867) established itself as a standard textbook in its various editions over a twenty-year period. This textbook shows an interesting difference from eighteenth-century attempts to establish a separate medical discipline dealing with the mad. As in those attempts, Griesinger wanted to show that psychiatry was a separate medical discipline; but by 1845 he had to demonstrate that psychiatric thought was also on a par with pathological anatomy, physiology, and, by now, neurology. In fact, Griesinger wanted to be considered a neurologist, though there is nothing in his psychiatric treatise that made any contribution to neurology. (Psychiatrists' desires to be neurologists have rarely to date led to any major contribution to neurology; perhaps only Charcot could be counted as a scientist who made contributions to both disciplines.)

Griesinger illustrates for a history of madness a recurrent conceptual problem. He accepted the materialist monism of positivism as the basis for this thought, and yet relapsed constantly into the terminology of psychic dualism or mentalism. There is an ongoing inconsistency in his textbook: he declared that all mental illness *must* be due to an organic lesion, but, in his discussion of concrete cases, he fell back on the nosological descriptions and etiologies that his predecessors had codified, especially Pinel and his disciple, Esquirol. Griesinger knew that he should not have recourse to a priori categories. He accepted that the principle of correlations obliged him to show an empirical relation between pathological anatomy and mental disease; and that his task was to relate mental processes and their pathologies to the realm of biological necessity.

Positivist psychiatry developed at the same time that biology, as an all-encompassing theory of life processes, began to exist. In fact, the patron thinker of positivism, Auguste Comte, was also a primary theorist of a unitary science known as biology. And so the question of lesions for nineteenth-century medicine was a different question than for the mechanical science of the eighteenth century: the positivist belief in lesions is part of a faith in the regularity of biological processes, in the existence of physiological norms, and in the operation of laws governing one natural realm. But it was not clear how to reconcile this unitary vision of nature with the disparate clinical entities that Griesinger inherited as the baggage of traditional nosology. For, quite simply, no clinical entity, neither melancholia nor mania, had ever been shown to be part of a realm in which natural law holds sway.

Griesinger's psychiatry faced other conceptual problems. His descriptions of syndromes suggest that madness is an unfolding process, having a temporal dimension—and the Freudian school was willing to salute a precursor in the Griesinger who describes the etiology of madness in terms of the many causes that fit together to give the patient a unique life history. Or as Griesinger wrote in his textbook:

> Very often the germs of the disease are laid in those early periods of life from which the commencement of the formation dates. It grows by education and external influences, or in spite of these, and it is but seldom that the abnormal psychical irritability attains either gradually or through scarcely noticeable intermediate stages to an evident disorder of mental function. More frequently there are a greater number of psychical impressions and bodily

disorders, by the successive influences or unfavorable combinations of which the disease is developed. It is then not to be ascribed to any one of these circumstances, but to them as a whole. (P. 130)

This description, presenting madness as a unitary form, is belied by Griesinger's refusal to pursue the idea that the human subject always has a unique life history. Rather, in practically the same breath he declares madness is a general organic affliction: "After extensive observation and comparison, we find that the etiology of insanity is in general none other than that of any other cerebral or nervous disease" (p. 131). The psychiatrist and the neurologist in Griesinger are not in agreement about the causes of madness, and the psychiatrist felt obliged to give into the neurologist or pathological anatomist.

Griesinger was struggling to reconcile two levels of description, two orders of causality, or, as Wittgenstein would have observed, two types of language game. Moreover, there was a quandary here for the practicing doctor who took this seriously. Without seeing lesions, the doctor had to determine if madness exists in his patients. This diagnosis meant that, once the doctor determines that madness exists on the basis of mental states, he must assume that "irritations" have been working directly on the brain. To cover all bases the doctor had to suppose that there are direct internal irritations—idiopathic—as well as secondary or symptomatic sources of irritation. After irritation, Griesinger says that the brain is subject to three types of receptivity to morbid states: anomalies in the circulation within the cranium; nervous irritation of the brain; and, finally, deficient nutrition "and excitation of the brain in consequence of dyscrasia (general anaemia, etc.)" (p. 132). This discourse is essentially circular: irritation can result in irritation, metabolic disorder is metabolic disorder. These statements of identity may be true, but they demand an opened cranium to see if they are true in any meaningful sense. And they do not open up new ways of finding criteria for understanding mental disorder.

Griesinger was not a fool, nor obtuse. He wanted to find a way of speaking of mental life with the same vocabulary that one uses to describe physiology and neurology. These disciplines had given him a model showing how science should be done. This model prevented him from framing questions about cultural influences on madness: education, upbringing, social relations. Culture was at most a predisposing circumstance for madness. Science meant establishing correlations with visible phenomena and limiting the variables that could count in the correlation. It is not always easy to see the variables in a soul warped by neglect, or a mind destroyed by hatred.

Knowledge for Griesinger demanded that he work with the immediately visible—as the reader sees vividly in the dramatic descriptions of pathological anatomy in the forth part of his textbook. These descriptions suggest that Griesinger wanted to compensate for his lack of innovation by making lesions palpable. With scalpel in hand, he went to the postmortem arena to look for those correlations that he was obliged to forget when, in describing mental states, he culled through the works of his predecessors and repeated the descriptions of mad types whose behavior alone classified them as insane. It was without relish that Griesinger took on the role, in his textbook, of the purveyor of those outlandish types that oblige the psychiatrist to be a bibliographer of the systematically absurd. The cataloging of the bizarre had been a primary task for psychological medicine since the Renaissance, but Griesinger wanted to relinquish that joyless task and be the pathological anatomist who could derive visible insight from the craniums of the insane:

> Whoever attends not merely to the symptoms of disease, but also to the abnormal organic conditions from which the symptoms spring, will readily admit that in insanity the observation of postmortem appearances is a department of psychology of the utmost importance. . . . Here . . . is to be found the basis of a true diagnosis—that is, an anatomical diagnosis. (P. 410)

The doctor should be able to see, for example, the "opacity, thickening, and hypertrophy of the arachnoid" that is, Griesinger claims, visible in every form of insanity of long duration. He, or rarely she, should see that mania is more often accompanied by lesions than depression. It is probably with regret that Griesinger had to deal mainly with living patients.

Reason has become a question of visible anatomy. Experience and sanity are read as a visible correlation of the ventricles' condition with the amount of blood in the brain. It is with more than some interest that we in turn can correlate this materialism with the anger with which Griesinger positively forbade having recourse to the poets for a knowledge of madness. His own positivism could, with irony, be taken as a poetics of madness, for his work leads to Moreau's obvious conclusion that one need merely change the material conditions of the body to change the nature of consciousness. And if drugs do not suffice, one could try changing anatomy—or at least cultivating one's diseases, like warts on one's face, as the poet Rimbaud declared the poet's task to be a few years later. Positivist monism, with its materialist image of the mad body, was in fact accepted by those poets for whom madness was a necessary condition for poetic experience.

However, positivist medicine gave poets little choice in the matter of their madness, since medicine decreed that hereditary factors were responsible for madness: hereditary determinism created a materialist basis for tragedy in the second half of the nineteenth century. Griesinger himself relegated hereditary influences to the role of a "predisposing factor" for madness, though later materialism made of inheritance the predominant factor. Positivist views of inherited madness were not the same as modern views of genetics. Nineteenth-century views of inherited disease patterns are partly a product of statistical correlations, and mainly a product of ideology. To understand the ideology of genetic determinism, let us briefly consider the role it played in psychiatry. In the genesis of this ideology none was more influential than doctor Benedict Morel (1809–1873). His doctrine of degeneracy as a cause for non-middle-class behavioral patterns—such as madness—owed its success as much for its consonance with original sin as to any overlap with the Darwinism that was then giving biology its unity as a science. Medicine elaborated a doctrine of genetically caused deviance and then applied it to the poor, the hungry, and the exploited. Degeneracy became a nearly universally accepted doctrine. It was convenient in that it allowed bourgeois medicine to justify the appalling conditions of the working class by pointing to their congenital depravity. In Morel's work a version of Lamarckian biological determinism dovetails with bourgeois self-justification: like giraffes who cannot help having long necks because their ancestors preferred the leaves on the tops of trees, the degenerates of society are predestined to their alcoholism, crime, and insanity because their fathers were unhealthy. Inheritance offered a drama that writers utilized, with a sense of Greek tragedy, to show that fathers could bequeath a curse to their children. Naturalists, like Ibsen and Zola, welcomed scientific verification of their visions of destiny. Morel presents the interesting case in which a mediocre scientist was able to influence great writers.

The Context of Poetic Modernism

By the mid-nineteenth century, positivist medicine was dominant in Europe, though poets could draw upon romantic medicine for their own purposes. What interests us in this context are the poets who accepted the scientific claims of positivist medicine while rejecting its philosophical authority. This rejection was usually not due to philosophical differences about the nature of mind. By and large the postromantic poets accepted, often in spite of themselves, the doctors' materialistic monism. But, facing the imperial claims of positivist medicine, the poets reacted with ill-tempered or ironic rejections of science that often entailed proclaiming the superiority of madness over reason, or, more broadly, the irrational over science. The romantic irony we saw in Hoffmann would be one resource for these rebellious poets whose discourses on madness give birth to literary modernism. This modernism evolved with a constant affirmation of the rights of the irrational. To defend madness, their own true madness as well as madness they cultivated, poets tried to overload the circuits of rationality and to revel in the freeplay of the irrational joys of madness conceived as the supreme poetic experience. This reaction was especially acute in France, where positivism received its first philosophical imprimatur. After the romantics, French poets, often grouped together as "symbolists," are the most important for our understanding of the development of modernity and its exploitation of madness. Four names almost automatically impose themselves in this regard: Nerval, Baudelaire, Lautréamont, and Rimbaud. All exhibited in their lives various degrees of madness, and all turned to poetry to express the joys of insanity. Probably no other nineteenth-century poets can better advance our understanding of how poets in quest for modernity accepted positivist theories of madness in order to contest the authority of psychiatry. In their poetic works we find the confirmation that in the nineteenth century psychiatry was becoming the discipline that represented the police power of the state to repress the irrational.

A historical note is in order to situate the development of literary modernity. Literary modernity is born at the moment when medical modernity also comes into full-fledged existence. This was around 1857, when Flaubert published the first demonstration-novel of modernity, *Madame Bovary,* and Baudelaire published his hash-inspired tributes to superior madness in the poems in *The Flowers of Evil.* In the same year Morel published "Des caractères de l'hérédité dans les maladies nervreuses," though this essay on the inherited characteristics of nervous diseases is insignificant compared with the following year's publication of Virchow's *Cellular Pathology* or Darwin's publication a year later of the *Origin of Species.* Darwin's work is not medical, but, by definitively introducing temporality into the realm of nature, evolutionary theory created modern biology; and with this, it created the epistemological framework in which medicine worked henceforth as a regional discipline in biology. In fact, Darwin completed the development of science by which all aspects of life were subject to some regional discipline: from the scientist's point of view there was no province of knowledge that escaped the scientific method. And with the elaboration of positive scientific discourses, many other discourses lost all claims to truth-value as far as questions of knowledge are concerned—such as metaphysics and theology and perhaps literature.

As the nineteenth century unfolded, the poet found himself challenged to defend his existence. (Women poets had known that challenge for some time longer.) One way to meet the challenge was to deny that literature has a truth function or, alternatively, to declare that the epistemological function of literature is situated on a level beyond reason—reason as defined by positivist rationality. Both of these responses occurred, and both responses made the poetic text receptive to the irrational. In fact, they invited the cultivation of madness. Such an attitude on the part of the poet justified in turn the positivist attitude toward literature, which was to deny it any truth-value—such as when Griesinger declared that psychiatry must free itself from reliance on literary models.

The doctors wanted to take madness away from literature. Consider that, in spite of Moreau's admiration of the poets, he reduced madness to drugs; and that with no admiration, Griesinger reduced it to lesions. In effect, Moreau and Griesinger, our two model somatists, had de-allegorized madness and, with that, the functioning of the psyche. When madness lost its literary structure as a dramatic conflict of allegorical psychic forces, literature could claim no special privilege in knowing psychic life. Mind was reduced to a troublesome fiction when physiology, or later, biochemistry, became the ultimate discourse for speaking of that enigma, the conscious mind. The French writer Maurice Blanchot has summed up the situation of madness in this context by saying that positivist psychiatry imposed on mental alienation a status that "alienated this alienation."[8] Blanchot's paradox is a starting point for reading the modern poetic texts that want to defend the rights of madness to exist as literature.

Nerval and the Mad Poet's Knowledge of Himself

The first modern poet who, in response to modern doctors, offered his madness to public purview was Gerard de Nerval (1808–1855). Nerval was also a key figure for bringing the German romantics to a larger public, and he drew upon them to frame his own myth of himself. Nerval delved into his experiential states and, in reaction to his doctors, created a personal myth for his madness. In his work madness weaves intertextual constructs that relate themes taken from classical literature, the German romantics, and science and medicine. In his madness Nerval says he found that he had a layered self, with roots extending back in time, much as Cuvier's paleontology suggested the presence of time found in layers of rocks that are the repository of time past. This myth is directed largely against medicine, for, if Nerval admired his own psychiatrist, Emile Blanche, he believed that he was a victim of those doctors whose science aimed at dispossessing him of his insanity. For example, in a letter written in 1841, Nerval described with anger the doctors and commissaries around him as agents who watched to make certain that the "operative field of poetry" would not be able to extend itself out to the public thoroughfare.[9] Here Nerval defends the right of madness, which is to say poetry, to manifest itself as public revelation.

Doctors had a police function; and the task of the guardians of the asylum was to keep poetry off the streets. Nerval's reaction to this police function was to protect his madness by valorizing it as a revelation of knowledge. His major work for this epistemic allegorizing is the prose piece *Aurélia*, published in 1855, though the writing of the text occupied Nerval from 1842 to 1854, during several bouts of insanity. Centered on this insanity and the multiple strata of self that insanity revealed, the text narrates the way dream invades waking life. In dream the poet descends into the netherworld and finds access to an archeological recovery of lost layers of past existence and myth. In this dream state, madness is the same experience as poetry. Nerval asserts that this is not pathological, and he wonders why he ever described himself as sick:

> I don't know why I use this term of malady, for as far as I'm concerned, never did I feel better. Sometimes I believe my strength and my activity to be redoubled; it seemed to me that I knew everything, understood everything; imagination brought me infinite delights. Will I have to do without them now, upon recovering what men want to call reason?[10]

In *Aurélia* Nerval claims as his own an alterity that escapes medical diagnosis. This otherness is centered first on the loss of his beloved, who is at once an actress, his mother, the Great Mother, and Isis, to name her main incarnations at different levels in the psyche. This self's experience of otherness can be likened to a series of tests or ordeals that Nerval had to undergo to find a relationship to himself. And at the heart of the ordeal is the fear of the double who could replace him in his own relation to himself. Nerval's experience of alienation is informed by the fear that there lurks within subjectivity the double who is himself and yet who might usurp his role. With no apparent irony, Nerval lived his madness through the Hoffmannesque model that proposes that the inner stage of experience can result in a permanent split between actor and observer—who are the same self and yet other.

There is probably an intentional symmetry in the fact that Nerval, like other symbolist poets, pressed into service the medieval principle of analogy at the same time the principle of correlations was becoming the dominant epistemological principle in medicine. The principle of analogy is a powerful, if often deceitful, tool. Correlation is limited to empirical variables, whereas the principle of analogy can establish correspondences between all phenomena. Thanks to metaphor, analogies tie the universe together; and with such a principle the poets could surpass the scientists, with their limited correlations, in knowing the cosmos.

For example, Nerval finds, in the midst of mad euphoria, that he has begun to understand that objects around him have meaning and harmonies unknown to him until then:

> How could I have lived so long exiled from nature and without identifying myself with her? Everything lives, everything acts, everything corresponds with everything else. The magnetic rays that emanate from me and from others penetrate with no obstacle the infinite chain of created things; it is a transparent network that covers the world. (P. 81)

In discovering his alienation from the world of harmonious correspondences, remarkably, Nerval experiences his insanity in terms that are quite unoriginal. His knowledge of it is couched in terms of early-nineteenth-century scientific paradigms, such as theories of magnetism and the cosmology of the "great chain of being." These borrowed paradigms are used by him to create the myth of his divided self:

> I shivered immediately upon thinking that this mystery might be understood. If electricity, I said to myself, which is the magnetism of physical bodies, can take on the direction imposed on it by laws, then, by even greater logic, hostile and tyrannical spirits can enslave intelligent spirits *[intelligences]* and use their divided forces in realizing their goals of domination. In this way were the ancient gods conquered and enslaved by the new deities. (P. 81)

Madness speaks with a voice that organizes multiple discourses into an intertextual whole that should make manifest the correspondences—manifest at least to the poet to whom madness offers access to his inner world. Nerval concocts therewith a mystical materialism in which all interconnects with all. Electricity, magnetism, physics, myth, history, religion, nothing is extraneous. Nerval's madness creates a monistic vision in which scientific paradigms and myths unite in an overdetermination of correlations. This procedure produces a redundancy of meanings and analogies that is almost a parody of a monistic attempt to understand everything, all of life and nature, within one framework.

In Nerval's case madness is the excess of meaning. It is the operation by which everything correlates with the entire world, and everything is a double for everything else. Madness is the possibility of discovering an infinite amount of sense by applying the principle of correlation to every phenomenon. Cuvier had used the principle of correlation to reconstruct, from fossils, extinct species of animals whose existence had hardly been suspected before the nineteenth century. Nerval by analogy reconstructs monsters as he exhumes his past, finding there fossils that open onto the infinite meanings of the hidden history of the world. In describing Nerval as an alienated writer, Ross Chambers has pointed out that the status of literature today is bound up with alienated writing. Writing is alienated in the sense that it offers no immediate communication, only the possibility of interpretation.[11] Modern hermeneutics often seems a form of madness in its desire to establish an infinite number of correlations and analogies, and thus meanings. Modernity is born in the gesture by which madness generates knowledge— and I invite the reader to turn to Nerval's sonnets for an initiation in the kind of mad hypersemiosis that seems to have reached its culmination in the texts of recent vintage inspired by deconstruction.

Baudelaire and Materialist Melancholia

Historians of literary modernity often avoid an encounter with suicidal Nerval. They prefer to nominate Baudelaire–poet and ironic theorist—for the role of initiator of our literary modernity. Baudelaire was also on intimate terms with madness: before he died of general paralysis, he frequently induced hallucinations with drugs, probably to combat the morbid depression that he described in masterful terms in his poems. Baudelaire's own analysis of himself, as he felt insanity approaching toward the end of his life, was that he had been a hysteric: "J'ai cultivé mon hystérie avec jouissance et terreur. Maintenant j'ai toujours le vertige, et aujourd'hui 23 janvier 1862 j'ai subi un singulier avertissement, j'ai senti passer sur moi *le vent de l'aile de l'imbécilité* [I have cultivated my hysteria with terror and bliss. Now I am constantly suffering vertigo, and today, 23 January 1862, I felt pass over me *the wind of the wing of dementia*].[12] This was in part the ironic pose, hysterical perhaps in itself, of the poet who believed in his own singularity and felt that medical labels were for the ignorant—though he knew quite well that his final dementia could be adequately explained by pathological anatomy.

Baudelaire's deviance seeks to flaunt bourgeois cultural norms, through his active search for madness, for drug-induced delirium and "expansion" of consciousness. Thus, most pointedly, Baudelaire uses the taxonomy of medicine to denigrate it with an irony whose intent is to show the superiority of the ironic intellect over the misery of the material body. But the material body is the center of Baudelaire's poetic universe. An ironic anatomist, Baudelaire uses poetry to explore states of elation and depression that are rooted in the body. His poetry proposes a new concept of literature as essentially the experience of mental states that are coterminous with the material body. Like his friend, the psychiatrist Moreau, Baudelaire advocates experimenting on the body; for he is a poet who makes of literature an experimental act probing states beyond the limits of normal consciousness. Coleridge and De Quincey notwithstanding, this is a new task for literature. After Baudelaire, poetry is no longer simply a rhetorical structure that aims at communicating certain affects or an interpretation of experience. Rather, it wants to be *experience*. It wants to be the space into which one enters in order to experience elation and hallucination, depression and madness. Like the experimental psychologist, then, Baudelaire conceives the poet's task as the cultivation of mental states by transforming the body, and this by any means available: from sex and poetry to wine and hashish. The problem for the poet is to find the linguistic structures that can, in some unmediated fashion, serve up this experience. Baudelaire's work asks, with appropriate irony, "If a whore's perfume, a glass of wine, or a puff on a water pipe can transform consciousness, then why not rhymed alexandrines?" Baudelaire's was the ultimate materialist poetic credo.

Baudelaire did not unreservedly give himself over to madness, however, since poetry was also to be an antidote for the madness at its origins. The paradox is that madness should be an antidote for madness. In what I take to be a nonironic text like the sonnet "Correspondances," the poetic transformation of consciousness appears to be a balm for the self lost in the body's melancholy and hysteria. This sonnet calls upon the principle of analogy, drawing together all sensual realms, in order to convert the world into a domain of aesthetic bliss. In effect, it transcribes how drug experiences produce euphoria. After beginning the poem with a romantic description of nature as a sacred realm of divine correspondences—wherein nature is a temple of living pillars—Baudelaire uses the last three stanzas of the poem to demonstrate a materialist monism in which euphoria is the experience of the analogies obtaining among all sensations:

Comme de longs échos qui de loin se confondent
Dans une ténébreuse et profonde unité,
Vaste comme la nuit et comme la clarté,
Les parfums, les couleurs et les sons se répondent.

Il est des parfums frais comme des chairs d'enfants,
Doux comme les hautbois, verts comme les prairies,
—Et d'autres, corrompus, riches et triomphants,

Ayant l'expansion des choses infinies,
Comme l'ambre, le musc, le benjoin et l'encens,
Qui chantent les transports de l'esprit et des sens.

(Les Fleurs du mal, no. 4)

[Like long-drawn-out echoes mingled far away into a deep and shadowy unity, vast as darkness and light, scents, colours, and sounds answer one another. There are some scents cool as the flesh of children, sweet as oboes and green as meadows,—and others corrupt, rich and triumphant, having the expansion of things infinite, like amber, musk, benzoin, and incense, singing the raptures of the mind and the senses.][13]

The first quatrain ironically lures the reader into considering nature as a realm in which spiritual correspondences hold sway. This is not the nature of positivist science, nor is it a realm of universal analogy that Baudelaire believes in. The next quatrain and the two tercets quoted above show that the described correspondences are not found in nature, but rather in the experiencing mind itself, reflecting upon itself. On the model of the allegorization of text and self proposed by the romantics, this mind undergoes an experience—a poem, drug-induced euphoria, or manic elation—allowing the mind to spin out correlations unfettered by empirical limits. Melodious flesh, sweet-tasting sounds, visual odors, this is the experience of sensations in which all connects with all in a materialist ecstasy beyond the limits of ordinary reason.

The mind contemplating itself in this region is in a borderline state in which its experience alternates between extreme depression and expansive elation—the "expansion of infinite things" with their infinite correspondences. In *The Flowers of Evil,* whose oxymoronic title sets out the manic-depressive polarity of experience to be found within, Baudelaire transcribes moments of consciousness ranging between what he calls spleen and ideal. This polarity, oscillating between ironic reversals, celebrates the disintegration of self while vaunting the virtues of hallucination. I think, however, that the ultimate basis for Baudelaire's ironic search for insanity is his depressive madness that he would flee at any cost. Melancholy is the foundational experience of Baudelaire's poetic quest. As described in "Rêve parisien," depression is the experience of the quotidian that awaits the poet when he returns from ecstatic elation:

> En rouvrant mes yeux pleins de flamme
> J'ai vu l'horreur de mon taudis,
> Et senti, rentrant dans mon âme,
> La pointe des soucis maudits;
>
> La pendule aux accents funèbres
> Sonnait brutalement midi,
> Et le ciel versait des ténèbres
> Sur le triste monde engourdi.

(No. 102)

> [Upon reopening my eyes full of fire
> I saw the horror of my hovel,
> And felt, returning to my soul,
> The sting of cursed worry.
>
> The clock with funereal accents
> Brutally sounded midday,
> And the sky poured darkness
> Upon the benumbed sad world.]

Falling back into reality, the poet finds the Kantian coordinates of space and time to be agents of torture. Daily reality is experienced as depressive insanity, and only the elation of hallucinatory transcendence prevents suicide. Flowers plucked from evil and sickness—two meanings of *mal*—are brief antidotes. The ultimate *mal*, however, is the material body and its subjection to time, space, and all those natural laws whose degraded end products the scalpel could lay bare. Only Baudelaire could write a rhapsodic poem on a rotting cadaver.

Baudelaire's ironic poetics results in a dualism analogous to the dualism that positivist psychiatry could not overcome. The body is the locus of all natural processes, thus all pathologies. But experience is a mental state. It seems to be all the more dramatic in that experience denies or transcends the body, as in manic elation. Baudelaire and the modern poet's understanding of experience points to a problem in understanding madness, for the very notion of inner experience seems to escape a nosography that wants physiological signs to define madness. Madness thus introduces a disjuncture into the natural world that is prime material for the ironist, who, like Baudelaire, would throw the bourgeois rationalist into confusion by subscribing to his materialist science while undercutting it with his superior insight. For all his ironies, however, Baudelaire was ultimately the kind of materialist who, in Catholic despair, saw the body as the locus of the Fall. So his notion of experience ends up defining the body as a space of alienation. For Baudelaire and the positivist, the self is the way the body comes to experience experience. This is a strange notion, but one that describes the dualism that haunts literary modernity and modern psychiatry. Self and mind are unifying experiences, rooted in the material body, yet inner and invisible presences that seem to enjoy their own existence, especially in madness. And the ironist Baudelaire found a philosophy of irony ready-made in the somewhat illogical belief that the mind emerges from, but is distinct from, the material body.

These considerations of dualism anticipate our next chapter, but in this context it is relevant to point out that modern psychiatry came into existence when it broke with the physiology of the sort that Magendie founded and that Griesinger wanted to emulate. The founder of contemporary psychiatric nosology, Emil Kraepelin, needed mind as a separate scientific category so that psychiatry could have an object of study. He made that point when, in commenting on Griesinger, he declared that nineteenth-century nosographies tried to classify individual cases almost invariably on the basis of the external symptoms of insanity. These "fluctuating and interpenetrating" symptoms, as Kraeplin put it, could not be delineated and used as a basis for consistent classification. With self-celebration Kraeplin noted that the only useful distinctions in psychiatry are those based on the "mental condition" of the patient, by which Kraeplin meant inner experience. Inner experience became the object of medical classification—though with perhaps insufficient reflection on the epistemological conditions that permit definitions of mental conditions.

Kraeplin was ungenerous toward his predecessor, since Griesinger had set up conditions, in spite of himself, for defining experience. In reading Griesinger, one is obliged to overlook the description of the old types of madness such as melancholia, mania, monomania, or the newer types such as *folie circulaire* and nostalgia. Griesinger really wanted to find the total syndrome, the unified concept of Mental Illness that would underwrite all manifestations of insanity. To do this, he defined the self in experiential terms and then defined the central feature of madness to be a discontinuity or alienation of the "I," or *ich:*

> [I]n the great majority of cases, there appears in mental disease a change in the mental disposition of the patient in his sentiments, desires, habits, conduct, and opinions. He is no more the same; his former *I* becomes changed, he becomes estranged to himself (alienated). (P. 114)

Even the positivistic neurologist was obliged to use the phenomenological self or mind as part of the criteria for sanity—with which the rebel poet could only concur and then proceed to destroy the unity of the "I." The rational ego of classical philosophy is now embedded in a new matrix, in the physiological system of medicine. Yet a dualism persists in that it is the self as a form of experience that defines what is continuity, what is rationality, and what is pathology. Seemingly the poet need only change experience to change the mind. This belief points to the poetics of madness for several generations to come.

Lautréamont and Rimbaud: The Active Quest for Madness

This commentary on Griesinger and his successor Kraepelin sets up the medical context for reading poets like Lautréamont and Rimbaud, two poets who became icons for several succeeding generations of poets in revolt against rationality. Lautréamont and Rimbaud each launched an attack on rationality by denying or trying to destroy the continuity of the self that psychiatry postulated as the grounds for sanity. In denigrating scientific thought and rationality, they made madness into a positive achievement, an ultimate experience, that could be upheld as a goal for all those who, in revolt, wanted to overcome the limits of reason as represented by the newly prestigious science of biology, its related disciplines, and especially medicine. Their poetic works vary considerably, however. Lautréamont enacts madness in texts that mimic an adolescent dream of omnipotence, whereas Rimbaud describes, with differing degrees of irony, madness as an experience to be cultivated for supreme knowledge. Rimbaud also wrote visionary texts, especially the prose poems known as the *Illuminations,* that may be taken as suprarational demonstrations of the liberation granted by the experience of madness. I stress that in both poets, subsequent generations were ready to salute a young rebel who, more or less successfully, made of madness a poetic goal. Later expressionists, surrealists, beatniks, and numerous others are direct descendants of this pair. Themselves spiritual descendants of Rameau's nephew, they issued a call for the poetic exploration of deviance that defied the world of science, philosophy, and bourgeois values to justify why the self or "I" should not be alienated in radical discontinuity.

Little is known about Lautréamont (born Isidore Ducasse, 1846–1870) whose work *Les chants de Maldoror* (1869) became a breviary especially for the surrealist poets and painters. If we consider the poems of Maldoror in the context of positivism, they appear to be an exercise in discontinuity that proclaims a belligerent revolt against all the foundations of rationality: against God, logos, the human subject and all its achievements. These "songs" spew out torrential streams of abuse against God, the personal enemy of both the poet and of his omnipotent alter ego, Maldoror. The insults are a megalomaniacal revolt that proclaim the desire to destroy anything that hinders the poet's fantasy of omnipotence. The desire for omnipotence is a defining characteristic of most infantile fantasies, and it is probably accurate to say that Lautréamont is the most insanely puerile of poets.

It is a curious commentary on our desire for discourses on madness that Lautréamont's work is so widely celebrated, especially the deicide he wants to commit in his quest for total autonomy. Lautréamont considers God to be the symbol of all that can limit this autonomy. Therefore, the poet needs to kill God, the absolute otherness, or "the Great Exterior Object." God is identified with a nocturnal doctor, a surgeon perhaps, who can use his medical skills to get into the poet's world, by literally boring into his body and his skull. God, the embodiment of logos, sounds like a positivist psychiatrist in the following bit of insanity:

> At least it turns out that, during the day, everyone can oppose a useful resistance to the Great Exterior Object (who doesn't know his name?), for then your will watches over your own defense with a remarkable tenacity. But as soon as the veil of nocturnal vapors unfolds, covering even the condemned prisoners who are going to be hanged, oh! what anguish to see one's intellect among the sacrilegious hands of a stranger. An implacable scalpel ferrets about in its thick bushes. Consciousness [conscience] exhales a long death rattle of malediction, for the veil of its modesty is being cruelly torn asunder. Humiliations! our door is opened to the savage curiosity of the Celestial Bandit. I've not deserved this horrible torture, you, you hideous spy of my causality! If I exist, I am not another. I do not admit in me this equivocal plurality. I want to reside alone in my intimate reasoning. Autonomy . . . or else let me be changed into a hippopotamus. . . . My subjectivity and the Creator, that's too much for one brain.[14]

If God is a doctor, then reason is a scalpel, an assertion to which the positivist doctor might have given limited assent. The scalpel is the power of the father figure who can violate the physical brain in which is lodged the "I" that asserts its right to singularity. In this image the power of medical reason is contested, even as it is granted. God, or logos, is experienced as a total otherness whose presence is identified with the theft of subjectivity. This might seem simply eccentric—which it indeed is—were this not to anticipate a pattern of the modernist experience of madness from Artaud through Sylvia Plath.

This refusal of violation of self by the divine omnipotence of reason is not in itself crazy, and one inevitably asks if the empirical person Ducasse was insane. Whatever be the response, and it should probably be positive, a debate about the answer should not cloud the real issue: the *chants* aspire intentionally to the condition of insanity. The demented imagery and insane claims want to be taken as madness. To judge these exercises in delirium as any thing else is to judge them a failure in their own terms. Lautréamont's will to madness thus necessarily assumes the determinations of reason as defined by the scientific discourses of the nineteenth century, primarily by biology and related disciplines. In fact, Ducasse plagiarized scientific texts freely to parody their language and to invert their taxonomical categories. By subverting taxonomy, Lautréamont portrays himself as a singular animal outside of all categories. His singularity results in fantasies of insane bestiality. For instance, he mates with a female shark and encourages his faithful dog to rape a small girl. The blurring of categories reaches a high—or low—point in the narrator's self-portrait, an Arcimboldi-like accumulation of subhuman traits that demonstrate that his existence is incommensurable with the rational categories of science:

> I'm filthy. Lice gnaw on me. When pigs look at me, they vomit. Scabs and leprosy scales mark my skin, which is covered with yellow pus. I do not know the water of rivers, nor the dew of the clouds. On my neck, as if on a manure pile, grows an enormous mushroom with umbelliferous peduncles. Sitting on a shapeless piece of furniture I have not moved my members for four centuries. My feet have taken root in the ground and compose, right up to my stomach, a kind of perennial vegetation, full of ignoble parasites, which derive no more from plants, nor are they animal flesh any longer. Yet my heart beats. (P. 175)

With toads growing on him, the narrator occupies some undefinable position outside the plant and animal kingdoms. Conflating biological terms in a nonsensical way—a mushroom with "umbelliferous peduncles"—he seems to want to show that he has no place in the scientific ordering of the world. The question of the text's intention is problematic at these nodal points where the reader wonders if there is irony at work or if this nonsense is a mechanical reproduction of terminology like that found in certain schizophrenic discourses. One viewpoint may not exclude the other, though the determination as to what constitutes the meaning of insane rhetoric is singularly difficult—as we shall see again in our considerations of the modernist experience of madness.

What argues for the irony of this kind of *art brut* is that it uses, nearly systematically, a rhetoric that exploits the mechanical properties of language to create worlds that are outside of what is codified as the rational. Lautréamont's automatic use of comparisons forces language to create new worlds—which of course is what fiction has always done. But, in the historical context, by using language to compare anything with anything, the text apparently parodies the principle of universal analogy. And one is inclined to think that there is a referential dimension to these rhetorical operations that produce the semblance of a world through the mere mechanical application of grammar: the texts want to destroy the world of science and poetry itself.

In any case Lautréamont shows that the principle of analogy can use the combinatory possibilities of language to generate mad worlds through rhetorical play. The surrealists found this systematic madness to be the acme of poetic experience, for example, when Lautréamont sings the praise of a boy's physical beauty:

> He is sixteen years and four months old! He is beautiful like the retractility of the claws of raptors; or even, like the uncertainty of the muscular movements of the wounds of the soft regions of the posterior cervical area; or rather, like that perpetual rat trap, which the trapped animal always resets and which all by itself can continue catching rodents indefinitely, and can function even when hidden under straw; and above all, like the fortuitous encounter on a dissection table of a sewing machine and an umbrella! (P. 234)

The final simile is one of the most quoted in modern poetic discussions, especially by surrealists, though always out of context: for the encounter of a sewing machine and an umbrella on a dissection table takes place at the end of an automatically generated series of similes, based on scientific texts, that is part of Lautréamont's perhaps ironic rhetorical game. Structurally, however, little differentiates this from a schizophrenic word salad, a contention that André Breton would have undoubtedly agreed with.

The analysis of this insane rhetoric is further complicated by the play of textual voices. This presence of multiple voices in these "songs" enacts the refusal of the unified "I" that psychiatry had defined as the unified mind of sane experience. Lautréamont's voices are primarily divided between a first-person "I" who, as he says, sings of laughter, evil, pride, and madness; and a third-person "he" who wants to sing for himself alone while attacking man and God, "as when a swordfish drives his sword into the belly of a whale" (p. 169). The "I" refers to itself as a "he" in an alienating movement of self-objectification. This self-objectification breaks the continuity of the first-person self. Moreover, in his will to madness, the first-person "I" disassociates itself into several other selves or roles, including animals and animate objects. All of this refraction of voices, this disassociation of the self into scattered textual roles, parallels the programmatic disassociation of self that the young poet Rimbaud declared to be the necessary condition for poetic experience. The relational self comes apart, in a challenge to the doctors to find a way that one body could contain so many voices.

The dissociation of self is the basis for a potential poetics in Rimbaud (1854–1891). It has undoubtedly been the most influential program for madness as literature in recent history, for, unlike Lautréamont, Rimbaud was unquestionably one of the poetic geniuses of the nineteenth century. In refusing the limited identity of the phenomenal self, Rimbaud is perhaps the most important poet in our recent history, for his equation of poetic experience with the disorder of madness stakes out the conflict between science and poetry that we almost believe is natural. His commitment to madness is all the more perplexing in that it was undertaken by a teenage boy who gave up poetry upon becoming an adult. In rejecting the petit bourgeois culture of his elders, Rimbaud set out to create a utopian culture, through poetry, that would transform existence. In a letter written to Paul Demeny in 1871, a letter that was taken as a manifesto by later several generations, the adolescent Rimbaud showed his rejection of scientific rationality when he asserted that "I" is another, "je est un autre." This assertion has received much commentary, for it concords with the romantic belief that a "true self" is hidden from the ordinary workings of consciousness. But Rimbaud's declaration is as much an acceptance as a rejection of the psychiatric norm that the continuity of self must be part of a definition of sanity. He accepts it as a norm for sanity, but only because he wants to dissolve the empirical "I" as a prelude to his demand that the poet explore insanity.

Paradoxically, in *A Season in Hell* (1873) Rimbaud proclaims his respect for rationality and modern science. Science represents the "new nobility" from which unfortunately, for hereditary reasons, the poet is excluded "for all eternity." Hereditary reasons are basis for the judgment that Rimbaud sees science making of him: he sees himself subject to a total condemnation. Modernity is materialism and progress, he writes, again with so many ironies that they undermine themselves. Rimbaud's play of irony works to undermine any belief in a self behind a discourse that affirms that the poet has long been on intimate terms with madness, real madness, the kind they lock up, as he puts it. However, Rimbaud wants his poet, in playing with madness, to be a rival of the scientist. In the letter to Paul Demeny, Rimbaud declares the poet to be the "suprême savant"—the "ultimate scientist." But

Rimbaud's poetry, in *A Season in Hell* as well as in the *Illuminations*, often documents the failure of the poet to arrive at supreme knowledge through the dissolution of the self. His work, and perhaps his life, document the usually failed attempt to offer madness as the supreme form of knowledge. There is a confessional side to this poetry. But, unlike later psychoanalytically inclined writers, Rimbaud pursued his madness knowing with positivist certainty that his reason was tied up with his viscera; and that his body was the arena for his quest. The failure of madness was a failure to transform the body.

Let us first deal with Rimbaud's attitude toward science before considering the failure of his utopian desire to transform consciousness through madness. With savage irony Rimbaud affirmed the basic postulates of positive science and then used these postulates as recipes for finding access to madness, imitating but going beyond Baudelaire. His sarcasm can be perplexing, when, for example, Rimbaud seems to mock a writer like Renan who, after Comte, declared that his religion was the progress of reason, or in other words, the growth of science.[15] Rimbaud ironized at the expense of the dominant ideology, but it is clear that he did so without really rejecting its materialist axioms. At most one might say Rimbaud was sarcastic about the dominant belief that only science could accomplish anything meaningful, but sarcasm is finally the sign of angry acceptance. In *A Season in Hell* this caustic ironizing takes the form of derision as the poet looks at his century, its institutions and ideology, and its belief in such cherished notions as the people, reason, the nation, and science:

> Oh! science! they've corrected everything. For the body and the soul—our viaticum—we have medicine and philosophy—remedies of old women and arrangements of popular songs. And the diversions of princes and the games they forbid! Geography, cosmography, mechanics, chemistry! . . . Science, the new nobility! Progress. The world marches on! Why wouldn't it turn?[16]

With sarcasm Rimbaud identifies the new nostrums of medicine with old wives' remedies, while reducing philosophy to renewal of old songs. So we live in our "corrected" world with medicine as our viaticum, though yearning for some unknown experience that would have nothing in common with what one calls progress. At the same time this sarcasm recognizes the power of the myth of progress, the belief in which fostered many a nineteenth-century illusion about the perfection of things to come—a myth in which Rimbaud also clearly wanted to believe.

Rimbaud's letters spell out his ambivalent revolt against positivist hegemony. As I have suggested, this revolt takes the form of calling for the end of the unified self that is the precondition for positive knowledge. His letters prescribe the dissolution of this self as the necessary step toward a liberation of poetic experience in madness. There is no irony in the letters when Rimbaud describes the self as a potential receptacle for irrational forces that are larger than the self-conscious "I." The poetic self is larger than the rationally known self, and thus it is the poet's task to create the conditions in which "I is another":

> If upon waking copper discovers that it is a clarion, that's hardly its fault. That is obvious to me: I am an audience for the blossoming of my thought: I watch it, I listen to it. I give a movement of the violin bow: the symphony moves in the depths or suddenly leaps onto the stage. (P. 202)

In recasting the self, Rimbaud makes of the self-conscious "I" a spectator. This point of vision is distanced from the movement of consciousness that springs from sources outside of consciousness. The self is, perhaps like Hoffmann's narrator looking at an operatic stage, a spectator to an inner theater. The metaphysics underwriting the idea that the poet has an inner state of vision or perception is questionable; for, in demanding that the self be present to itself as a double, it makes of madness our normal metaphysical condition. But perhaps that is the point of Rimbaud's theatricalization of madness.

As Jacqueline Biard has shown, doubles proliferate throughout Rimbaud's texts, especially *A Season in Hell,* where scattered voices double what should be the central voice of the damned poet.[17] One voice belongs to the mad virgin who narrates the poet's adventures with gleeful sarcasm (and whom critics have wanted to identify with Rimbaud's companion, the poet Verlaine). The poet also judges himself, in a theater of recalled voices, when in "Delirium II" he recalls his bouts of insanity—in the text called "Histoire d'une de mes folies." Since theater is a key metaphor for this recurrent alienation, in dreaming of new histories, the poet stages the voices on the platform of the inner self. Or, in his "Alchemy of the Verb," echoing Rameau's nephew, Rimbaud declares himself quite simply to have been a spectacle born of defective physiology:

> I became a fabulous opera: I saw that all beings have a fatality for happiness: action is not life, but a way of ruining some strength, a form of enervation. Morality is a weakness of the brain. (P. 145)

In spite of the materialism decreeing that his madness is merely sickness, the poet also wants to believe that the disorder of his mad mind is "sacred."

Contradiction is the stuff of the inner theater born of a weakness of the brain, even if irony might allow some reconciliation of opposites.

Rimbaud's belief that he can cultivate madness—and perhaps become part of the sacred—depends on the somatic view of mind. Rimbaud meant quite literally that the poet should cultivate madness in a most materialist sense. Or as he put in the letter of 1871:

> The first study of the man who wants to be poet is complete knowledge of himself; he looks for his soul, he inspects it, he tempts it, he learns to know it . . . it is a matter of creating monstrous soul: like *comprachicos!* Imagine a man implanting and cultivating warts on his face. (Poésies, p. 202)

Like "comprachicos"—child thieves—the poet is a deviant who becomes a visionary seer by cultivating hallucinations, and this involves manipulating the body to change the "soul":

> The Poet becomes a seer by a long, immense, and well-reasoned-out *disordering of the senses*. All forms of love, of suffering, of madness, he looks for them himself, he uses up every type of poison in order just to keep the quintessence of it. Ineffable torture in which he needs all the faith, all the superhuman strength, in which he becomes among all others the great sick person, the great criminal, the great cursed one—and the ultimate Scientist! (Pp. 202–3)

After Moreau, after Baudelaire, Rimbaud wanted to push experimentation to its extreme point at which knowledge derives from the ineffable experience of sickness, crime, deviance, insanity. This nineteenth-century equation of deviant inner experience with superior knowledge strikes me as something new in our history, unless mystics, in their rupture with logos, are to be counted among the precursors to Rimbaud, the surrealists, and the beat generation. Mystics usually did not believe, however, that changing the cells in their brain would grant them transcendent experience. Rimbaud's cultivation of madness was an outgrowth of the materialism that finds the self to be that part of the body in which experience is known to itself. Wanting to cultivate warts on the soul is a logical, if paradoxical, expression of this view: if all is bound up in a materialist monism, warts must, in some sense, have experiential meaning. And one can "know" that meaning only by growing them.

Rimbaud seems at once very remote and very recent. We see in him a flower child and a belated utopian romantic whom we scarcely recognize, though perhaps both images are related as foreground and background to two centuries of attempts to use madness, deviance, and nonconformity to displace our worldview. For Rimbaud was also a utopian who believed, at various times in his young life before he gave up poetry, that the transformation of consciousness and experience would bring about, on some new morning, "Christmas on earth" (p. 150). In *A Season in Hell* he alludes to this morning, and texts in the *Illuminations* speak of a new democracy in which love would be reinvented. This hallucinatory utopia seems to have almost been within Rimbaud's grasp:

> Sometimes I see in the sky beaches without end covered by white nations in joy. A great golden ship, above me, waves its multicolor banners in the morning breezes. I've created all the fêtes, all the triumphs, all the dramas. I tried to invent new flowers, new stars, new flesh, new languages. (P. 151)

Is this recollection from *Illuminations* a form of utopian madness? With its past tense, it is clearly one of several adieus to literature punctuating Rimbaud's work. Every movement toward a utopian madness, toward some materialist transformation of the conditions of existence, seems to be accompanied by a farewell on Rimbaud's part. The adieu marks the failure to go beyond materialist science and the bourgeois culture whose ideology Rimbaud cannot ever really shake off.

The narration of Rimbaud's failure also concludes his Dionysian elegy, "The Drunken Boat," his portrayal of a child rushing to the liberation offered by a dive into the sea of experience. Represented as a boat revolting against its moorings, the child learns that every revolt, every attempt to plunge into the depths of the sea-self, will play itself out as a journey that goes astray. In the first part of the poem, having gone through a utopian experience of vision in the depths of dissolution, the child-boat must lament his incapacity to bring back to other children the wonders he has experienced. Finally, the boat must return home and sail under the watchful guard of the prison boats that protect the rationality that secures the commercial port. The bedraggled child poet laments his misery in the final stanza:

> Je ne puis plus, baigné de vos langueurs, ô lames,
> Enlever leur sillage aux porteurs de cotons,
> Ni traverser l'orgueil des drapeaux et des flammes,
> Ni nager sous les yeux horribles des pontons.

> [I can no longer, swimming in your languidness, oh waves,
> Follow in the wake of the merchant ships bearing cotton
> Nor move through the pride of banners and flags,
> Nor swim by under the horrible eyes of the prison ships.]

Madness, utopian or otherwise, runs into the prison boat, the synecdoche for all the institutions of incarceration that began proliferating in the nineteenth century. Rimbaud was never a dupe about where madness might take him, and the final stanza of "The Drunken Boat" is the most powerful tragic lamentation about the failure of madness, in its struggle against institutionalized limits, that I know.

The struggle announced here is emblematic of struggles to come. It also is suggestive of the differences between psychiatry and psychoanalysis that we shall analyze in the next chapter, for psychoanalysis would refuse to reduce insanity to a question of lesions, nor would it refuse meaning to madness. But toward the end of the nineteenth century, the image given by Rimbaud's accepting the basic premises of positivist medicine, in order to use them to cultivate deviance, is the dominant image we take away from this moment in our cultural history when psychological medicine was granted a police power it never had before. The poets were not the only deviants threatened with incarceration, but they were the primary deviants for whom the expression of their madness was conceived as a challenge to those psychiatrists who had power over them. Positivist medicine was more that just a medicine based on a rather mechanical materialism, it was a medicine that believed in its political rectitude. It believed that it was a, if not the, bastion of rationality. Facing these imperial claims, the poets sought to fight back by blowing up the bastion from within. We have not yet seen the end of these counterattacks, for they continue, I think, in the drug culture of today that has, in many ways, inherited the legacy that the nineteenth-century "cursed poets" bequeathed us. Not every punk rock singer is a Rimbaud, but many seem to accept the same suicidal views promoted in the name of revolt. The question remains open as to whether we should keep building the prison ships that Rimbaud saw as the main arm of psychiatry and that we continue to believe will promote social sanity.

Chapter 8

Modern Determinations of Insanity: Psychiatry and Psychoanalysis

Contexts for Modern Medical Discourses on Madness

The conflict between positivist medicine and the poets' cultivation of madness sets up, in a direct way, the conditions for the next important development in our discourses on madness. In dealing with psychoanalysis and psychiatry, I shall here discuss a development in which literature, taken in a large sense, and medicine propose two different discourses. To contextualize this development, we must recognize that twentieth-century views of madness have been largely derivative from the thought of two medical men: Emil Kraepelin and Sigmund Freud. The first is barely known outside of medical circles, the second is a household term of use and abuse. Questions of fame aside, what this development means is that we think about madness either with the nosology of medical psychiatry or with the dynamic concepts of psychic conflict proposed by psychoanalysis. These two bodies of thought are not the same, however much they sometimes overlap, and however much even the educated public confuses psychiatry and psychoanalysis. But it is essential to keep the two straight. On the one hand, Kraepelin's psychiatry undertook a reorganization of positivist medical thought about insanity that developed in the nineteenth century, and his work still provides the basis for the present classification of mental illnesses in our medical schools. On the other hand, Freud's thought represents the return of literary ways of theorizing about madness in terms of symbols and allegories. Thus, in a very real sense, Freud's psychoanalysis continues the work of the poets, especially the romantics, against the positivist doctors. I say this fully cognizant of the fact that doctor Freud himself started out hoping to create a branch of medical science that would ultimately be a part of neurology. But, most succinctly, Freud's work has nothing to do with neurology.

Present trends in neurology studying the neural mapping of memory may someday buttress Freud's doctrine that successful repression is central to a sane psyche, but nothing in psychoanalytic thought today makes psycho-analysis a part of neurology—or really of medical science. Freud (1856–1939) reluctantly relinquished using biology as a source for metaphors as his career advanced, though he always believed biology might be some ultimate court of appeal. Kraepelin (1856–1927) never had cause to doubt that he was a medical scientist. During his career as a German medical professor he never ceased working on the system to which contem-porary psychiatry largely owes its foundations—though from the point of view of modern neurology it might appear that psychiatric thought has done little more than psychoanalysis to advance neurological science. Neurology has made great progress in this century, and medical applications have been quite fertile. In fact, each time some aspect of mental illness has become a province of pathological neurology—such as general paralysis, epilepsy, Alzheimer's syndrome—it has ceased to belong to the domain of madness. Psychiatry and psychoanalysis are not the only disciplines that deal with madness, and it is with regret that I do not include a more varied sampling of schools ranging from ego psychology to existential psychiatry. However, I feel justified in that Freud's psychoanalysis and Kraepelin's type of psychi-atry have been the dominant discourses in the twentieth century. They have provided the basic paradigms with which we speak of madness, and most other psychological disciplines can only be understood insofar as they have accepted either psychiatry or psychoanalysis—or, like antipsychiatry, have developed as a reaction against them. It is noteworthy that psychiatrists sometimes claim neurology as part of their discipline, though the converse is more likely to be the case in the future, especially if pathological neurology continues to demonstrate ever greater capacity to explain mental anomalies.

In fine, the psychiatric understanding of madness is still largely tributary to the categories Kraepelin elaborated in successive editions of his textbook of psychiatry—the *Lehrbuch*. It is remarkable that much of the nosology this book proposes is still the basis for contemporary works like the *Inter-national Classification of Diseases* of the World Health Organization or, more used by the American medical profession, the *Diagnostic and Statisti-cal Manual of Mental Disorders,* the famous *DSM* that makes headlines as it is regularly revised and clinical entities are invented, updated, or dis-carded. This relative nosological stability suggests that, whatever be the new drug therapies for madness that have proliferated in the past few decades, the theoretical understanding of madness has remained rather static for the past ninety years or so. For better or worse, the major innovation in theo-rizing about madness in the twentieth century was made by Freud, his fol-lowers, and the various schools that Freud's thought has engendered.

The contemporary positivist may object by noting that Freud's thought is not scientific. I would agree. I consider psychoanalysis to be a literary language game, perhaps a mythic language game, not far from what Wittgenstein saw in it. Or if one prefers, it is an allegorical discourse that purports to represent the human self. It seems indisputable that Freud uses literature, both its themes and its techniques, for knowledge. In this regard Freud is on the side of the writers who have contested the hegemony of medical discourse, and, in spite of himself, Freud can be considered as part of the modernist revolt against psychiatry, a revolt led by poets and seconded by psychoanalysis. To understand this revolt, psychiatry and psychoanalysis will concern us in this chapter, and then we shall give consideration to this century's legions of modern, mad poets in the next.

To complete this introduction to the context of our modernity, it is essential to recall that medical modernity did not begin until a little over a century ago. And by medical modernity I mean a change in our view of medical history as well as any medical advance such as the discovery of the causes of specific diseases. At the end of the nineteenth century, as gadfly sociologist Bruno Latour has observed in his book on Pasteur's "revolution," the history of medicine became irreversible.[1] Until the nineteenth century—and even into Griesinger's work—history was reversible in the sense that any medical doctrine of the past might be called up from the past and pressed into service in some sense or another. Especially after the revolution in microbiology, or emblematically after Pasteur, the history of medicine assumes the shape of linear unfolding that condemns to relative oblivion most of the doctrines propounded in the history of medicine's attempts to deal with what have been considered pathologies. When, in the nineteenth century, the doctrine of spontaneous morbidity became an object of antiquarian interest, the great works of medical history ceased being edited except for literary and philological interest, such as Littré's edition of Hippocrates. The past of medical thought became an irrevocable past, and no doctor ever since has felt obliged to consider or even to know Galen or Boerhaave's opinion on gall bladders or fevers.

It is in this context that we must place the development of psychiatry. One can argue that it is the medical discipline for which no revolution occurred. Psychiatry never acquired a general theoretical model for the pathologies it deals with. Nothing analogous to pathological anatomy or microbiology yet exists that can serve as a model for a psychiatric understanding of madness, even if psychiatry must draw upon both of these disciplines and others as well. For all the speculation that has recently occurred about the relation of genes and dispositions to madness, the history of psychiatry has not been marked by any rupture that allows us to speak of a premodernity. In this respect psychiatric theory about psychosis and schizophrenia is different from all other medical discourses. Of course, historians of psychiatry usually want to find in their history a moment of rupture that marks the moment when psychiatry achieves the same full-fledged scientific status that we grant to endocrinology or neurology, but I do not yet see that moment in the history of psychiatry. So when I say that Kraepelin's work is the basis for modern nosology, I am not suggesting that some conceptual revolution has taken place in his work. And this despite the fact that Kraepelin himself, quite cognizant of the changes characterizing the nature of the history of medicine, tried to create a medical history for psychiatry that would grant psychiatry the same status as other medical disciplines. The very title of his history of his discipline, *One Hundred Years of Psychiatry,* published in 1918, shows the amount of time Kraepelin allotted to the history of psychiatry as a "science." He accepted the idea that psychiatry began with Enlightenment rationalism, and he was willing to grant Pinel the role of the first important precursor to the scientific treatment of insanity. True scientific investigation of madness really began with Griesinger, though Kraepelin believed psychiatry achieved full scientific status only with the arrival of his own generation at the end of the nineteenth century. Successive generations of psychiatrists have turned Kraepelin's assessment of himself into something of a truth, for they have continued to use his categories as the basis for much of our modern classification of madness. Once the medical historian has replaced Kraepelin's syndrome of dementia praecox with Bleuler's later notion of schizophrenia—or the schizophrenic disorders of the *DSM*—then Kraepelin's *Lehrbuch* looks rather contemporary.

Kraepelin's Classifications of Madness

Kraepelin's work brings together many nineteenth-century currents and amalgamates them into a more or less tidy system. "Enfin Kraepelin vint . . ." [At last Kraepelin showed up . . .], wrote the young psychoanalyst Jacques Lacan in his doctoral thesis on paranoia in 1932. Lacan's play on words parodies the famous comment by the neoclassical poet Boileau about his precursor Malherbe, the poet who came at last to put an end to baroque excess. With irony characteristic of a psychoanalyst, Lacan pointed up that Kraepelin was our modern neoclassicist who put an end to the nosological excess of nineteenth-century psychiatry. This classical impulse, if we can now speak of a classical system for psychiatric classification, was based on criteria for madness as defined by mental states. As we saw earlier in Krae-pelin's critique of Griesinger, these criteria should not depend on external symptoms or problematic inner lesions.

Kraepelin respected the materialist monism of his predecessors. In fact, he took over many of the theses of positivist medicine when he tried to find organic causes of mental illness. But the basis for understanding is not etiol-ogy, since the causes of madness cannot be determined with any precision. Therefore, Kraepelin proposes to understand madness in terms of fixed syn-dromes, or nosological entities, that are not causally defined. These syn-dromes describe internal states that evolve in time—and they thus allow some regularity of prognosis once a proper diagnosis has been undertaken. In a sense Kraepelin renews Hippocrates and the Hippocratic belief in the regular processes that can be identified as a clinical entity. However, Krae-pelin's rich descriptions of types of insanity show that he saw madness, not unlike a Moreau or a Baudelaire, as a form of inner experience that can be interpreted at times as an inner world. In postulating the experience of the inner world as the basis for understanding madness, Kraepelin insisted that earlier nosologies had failed to recognize the inner self. These systems were "complicated unduly by the fact that attempts to classify individual cases were based almost invariably on the external symptoms of insanity; these fluctuating and interpenetrating symptoms simply could not be delineated and used as a basis for classification." To which he adds with reference to his own codification: "Only gradually did there emerge from this confusion distinct classifications based on the mental condition of the patient and cor-responding apparently to identical causal conditions" (*One Hundred Years*, p. 116).

Kraepelin's appeal to causality here is an article of faith—positivist faith to be sure—for he knew that, without identifying causal agents, he had not fulfilled his own expectations for a positive science. But nothing in his data really justified his assumption about causality. His belief that a uniformity of causal conditions produces a uniformity of effects is simply an a priori axiom. Kraepelin's dilemma with causality has repercussions for a psychia-try that wants to be phenomenological in its understanding of madness and still respect medical axioms about etiology when explaining insanity as a disease. In organic maladies the same microbes always produce the same diseases; but the analogy with disease that justifies the term *mental illness* founders on a forced comparison when the psychiatrist evokes causation. Kraepelin himself waffles:

Profound changes have marked the development of our theory of the physical causes and bases of insanity. Though our attitude toward the influence of psychic forces on the development of mental disorders has changed but slightly, our assessment of their importance has fluctuated. While the old psychic school [i.e., the romantics] assigned them a dominant role, the somatic school tended to consider them unimportant. Popular opinion steadfastly championed the important psychic influences in the etiology of insanity, and even Griesinger held that they were generally more decisive than physical injuries. Today we have apparently arrived at a clear cut definition. We know that frequently so-called psychic causes—unhappy love, failure in business, overwork—are the product rather than the cause of the disease, that they are but the outward manifestation of a pre-existing condition, and finally, that their effects depend on the most part on the subject's anlage. (P. 132)

Though Kraepelin's reversal of causal relations here may seem resolutely modern, the word *Anlage* that the translator slips in shows that Kraepelin's work also wants to appeal to hereditary determinism.

The German word is a scientific import meaning "constitution." *Anlage* effects a circular sleight of hand by which the cause of a malady is declared to be a hereditary disposition to the disease. This is clearly proved by the fact that the patient has the disease. This explanation is another variant on the abusive use of deductive logic based on the a priori principle of causality: it boils down to saying, "You have x proves that you (were caused to) have x." The parenthetical deduction can be easily left out. Freud's dissatisfaction with this kind of magic causality is clear throughout his work, such as when he dismissed "disposition" *[das Dispositionelle]* as a causal explanation; disposition, says Freud, is always of less interest that what the analyst really finds in a real case history.[2]

This is not to argue that there is no hereditary disposition to madness. But Kraepelin's causal determinism is an article of faith that has no rigorous empirical dimension showing a causal linkage. In effect anlage is a kind of genetic curse that has more to do with the gods than with what we today think might be the effect of a defective gene. And today, when looking for the chromosome on which madness is encoded, one should recall that the circular curse of heredity has often appeared to be buttressed by statistics that "proved" an a priori belief in causal necessity. In any case, Kraepelin did change his mind about relative causality. After Charcot seemed, in the late nineteenth century, to have demonstrated the nonorganic basis of hysteria, Kraepelin recognized a larger "psychic" component in mental illness. Of course, as Freud recognized, a seemingly irrefutable proof that psychic stress has a role in the etiology of mental illness was given by the Great War

and the mental disturbances that battle trauma created. However, Kraepelin's work was largely completed by the time of the war. The final edition
of his manual in 1927 was a collaborative enterprise.

Kraepelin's phenomenology of madness evolved over a long period of
time. Some historians think it reached its "classical" formulation in the fifth
edition of the *Lehrbuch* in 1896, but most prefer the sixth edition of 1899
when, as Paul Bercherie describes it:

> In 1899 he [Kraepelin] went all the way and decided to group together
> "demential processes" and "fantastic paranoias" by creating the unified
> framework of *dementia praecox*. Correlatively the concept of *paranoia*
> found its modern meaning and now covered only non-hallucinatory
> chronic delirium. . . , whereas *manic-depressive madness* took in all non-
> disassociative forms of critical psychoses *[psychoses aigües]* that thus man-
> ifest in their loss of virulence *[décours]* an integral restitution of the earlier
> personality.[3]

The sixth edition was translated by A. Ross Diefendorf for American doctors in 1902 as *Clinical Psychiatry* (and revised in 1907), which speaks to
how rapidly Kraepelin's system was disseminated throughout the non-Ger-
man-speaking world (with the notable exception of the French, who have
resisted the *Lehrbuch*'s taxonomy until the present day). In this most
influential textbook, Kraepelin was pessimistic about curing the insane. Part
of his pessimism springs from his views of causality. He classifies causality,
in a priori terms, under the general categories of interior and exterior
causes, and by exterior causes he means organic causes such as cortical damage. Interior causes would include hereditary factors. The opposition of
inner and outer parallels the current distinction of exogenous and endogenous psychoses. Dementia praecox, or our schizophrenia, is classified as an
exogenous psychosis, since Kraepelin believed that it arises from inner self-
intoxication, or as *Clinical Psychiatry* phrases it, as a "severe disease
process in the cerebral cortex."[4] There is no discernible empirical reason
why Kraepelin thought the cerebral cortex is involved in dementia praecox,
and Kraepelin himself admits that he had found few cerebral lesions in the
cases he had studied.

Later, in his *Lectures on Clinical Psychiatry,* Kraepelin avoided questions
of etiology and causality in favor of the phenomenology of individual cases
presenting the syndromes that make up Kraepelin's taxonomy. These lectures, translated in 1904, offer a vivid picture of the doctor as teacher, lec-
turing before an amphitheater, transforming madness into spectacle before
a class of medical students and young doctors, much as Charcot had done.

Our recurrent theme of the theatricalization of madness finds illustration in this teaching context in which the mad were brought forward to illustrate the drama of the insane—and to fit them into a taxonomical pigeonhole. For instance, after displaying a patient whose confused rantings include the beliefs that "Napoleon was used for uncleanness by Catherine I in Russia" and that Napoleon "got the testicles and penis of new-born children to eat, and so was turned into a hermaphrodite who could let himself be used by men," Kraepelin observes that this paranoidal form of dementia praecox presents some difficulties:

> [T]he senselessness and incoherence of the delusions, expressed with a complete absence of emotion, show that we have to deal with a state of mental *weakness*. The automatic obedience, the confusion and indecency of the patient's talk, and the quite senseless playing with assonances [as in echolalia] remind us of what we have observed before in cases of *dementia praecox*. We last met with entirely similar disturbances in our last patient.[5]

Underlying this theatricalization of madness, of studying the roles of the mad as they play them out, is the taxonomical impulse that considers classification to be the hallmark of understanding.

Classification entails making comparisons to find an ordered series. Etiology is forgotten here: it is the series of tableaux vivants that counts for the doctor who, in composing a clinical tableau, was charged with ordering the irrational as a series of recurrences. Kraepelin's classification is a continuation of the belief in taxonomical ordering that found successful expression during the Enlightenment in Linnaeus and other naturalists; and crazy application in the proliferating medical nosographies of a Cullen or a Pinel. But more than taxonomy is involved in this theatricalization: the theatrical presentation also speaks of the power that has accrued to psychiatry. The doctor has the power to oblige the insane to perform for a public. The power of medicine is on stage here.

From the preceding discussion it might be inferred that clinical entities are little more than shifting focal points that highlight recurrent, but variable, aspects of mental disturbances. This is not the case. Kraepelin and his followers believed that, as they continually combined taxonomical entities, they increasingly revealed in positive terms the types of madness that exist in nature. The belief that clinical entities were "discovered" by Kraepelin means that in the fifth edition of the *Lehrbuch* the psychiatrist was launched and under way to truth in nature; and in the sixth edition he did something akin to arriving at a new continent. Or, to give a precise example: Kraepelin's taking Morel's notion of dementia praecox, from roughly 1860, and combining it with Kahlbaum's catatonia (1874) and Hecker's hebephrenia (1871) resulted in the discovery of a "disease." Though Bleuler's term *schizophrenia* came to be preferred over *dementia praecox* by the psychiatric profession, Kraepelin presumably discovered a real entity that, in some sense, had not been named or even known before.

The problem is that the epistemology of botany or physiology is applied by psychiatry in a way that does not recognize that metaphorical linkings are being used to cover up the failure to provide positive criteria for psychiatric "species"—other than those found in the rather murky attempt to characterize mental states. As an amateur naturalist I have come to expect that my favorite plants and birds will change genus or family every few years or so, for higher levels of taxonomic classification reflect the changing criteria of systematics. But each species itself usually remains a rather permanent entity. Since Darwin we have a theory to explain why species appear and disappear in history, but, while it exists, a given species has positive traits that have often been identified for centuries. In its classifications psychiatry seems to act as if it were dealing with species, but then treats its diseases as changeable categories that are more like higher levels of organization. It is probably only an extended metaphor that allows clinical entities to be treated as if there were some systematics that could account for them. What is to the point here is that those cases classified by psychiatry, unlike plants and birds, find it very relevant as to how they are classified: when modern poets find their anguish reduced to one more case of dementia praecox or schizophrenia, it is likely that their anguish will even be greater.

Psychiatrists and clinical psychologists will at this point probably be ready to point out that this critique fails to take into account the research going on today that delimits clinical entities on the basis of various types of tests, often using drugs. I am perfectly willing to recognize the value and, indeed, the necessity of this modern research looking for recurrent characteristics; but I feel obliged to quote in this regard the Michel Foucault with whom I am usually not in agreement. Foucault has suggested that classical psychiatry was in the thrall of an essentialist view of mental illness:

> Side by side with this "essentialist" prejudice and as if to compensate for the abstraction that it implied, there was the naturalist postulate that saw illness in terms of botanical species; the unity that was supposed to exist in each nosographical group behind the polymorphism of the symptoms was like the unity of a species defined by its permanent characteristics and diversified in its subgroups: thus dementia praecox was like a species characterized by the ultimate forms of its natural development and which may present hebephrenic, catatonic or paranoid variants.[6]

Foucault's elegant critique of "essentialism" charges that much of psychiatry relies on what many critics would see to be a premodern epistemology: the search for essences in nature. What is perhaps more serious is that an essentialist understanding of madness offers little grounds for therapy—and indeed Kraepelin found little hope for curing most of the mad.

The net Kraepelin cast to catch the mad is of course larger than one syndrome. In the translated version of *Clinical Psychiatry* his taxonomy is divided into thirteen categories: (1) infectious psychoses, (2) exhaustion psychoses, (3) intoxication psychoses, (4) thyroigenous psychosis, (5) dementia praecox, (6) dementia paralytica, (7) organic dementia, (8) involutional psychoses, (9) manic-depressive insanity, (10) paranoia, (11) general neuroses, (12) constitutional psychopathic states, and (13) defective mental development. To adjust these categories to more modern terms, the book's recent editor Carlson suggests that we see in Kraepelin's taxonomy "divisions that we today include under the following headings: organic conditions, mental deficiency, schizophrenia, affective disorders, the neuroses, and the asocial personality disorder" (pp. viii–ix). Whether one agrees with Carlson or not, it is clear that Carlson is participating in the kind of taxonomical recasting that characterizes the history of psychiatry. Psychiatry is a special language game, as also illustrated, for example, by the earlier mentioned Bleuler, who redefined "dementia praecox" as something that is not really dementia nor precocious, and then said that in psychiatry "we might as well regard the original meaning of the terms . . . as irrelevant."[7] And so dementia praecox, our dominant mental illness, was defined by Bleuler as a group of psychoses, at times chronic, that can stop or retrograde at any time, but that do not permit a full *restitutio ad integrum* (p. 9).

In this history of changing terms, Bleuler's comment is instructive. Of course etymology does not necessarily weigh on the meaning of a scientific term, whose meaning often depends entirely on the context in which it is used. However, the historical nature of psychiatric concepts means that each concept carries with it a genealogy. Given the historical nature of the evolution of the self, that genealogy often demands understanding before one thinks that a clinical entity exists where there is really only a history— the history of a linguistic token used in a language game whose rules are transformed in history. The doctor may think that he or she has discovered a disease, when a deflected meaning of an old term is only patching up our ignorance. *Hysteria* is famous in this respect: a term designating the wandering uterus of Greek medicine, it made its way into late-nineteenth-century medical language games to describe Charcot's theatricalizations, only to disappear in the *DSM,* and then to reemerge in postmodern psycho-analysis. Hysteria is indeed a wanderer.

What I want to stress is that discourse on madness, when reduced to a taxonomy, becomes a language game or a form of discourse that feeds as much on its internal dynamics, often generated by history, as on an entry into the world of experience. What we mean by madness escapes easy definition, since it is linked to determinations of language, and, in its histor-ical evolution, language is beyond our control. This is a difficult, if essential, point to grasp. Our understanding of madness is marked by the same his-toricity that characterizes the historical emergence of the self and of the structure of consciousness. These structures often seem to exist because they have been defined to exist. Perhaps this historicity of understanding explains why it is so difficult to cast new theories for understanding madness, since psychiatric concepts are derivative from language games that are more pri-mary than the theory and determine them in ways hard to understand. Psy-chiatric concepts must derive from language games defining, for example, what we mean by self, consciousness, reason, and the irrational, and these notions often function as givens that derive from historical development. In addition, we seem to be powerless to change discourse that allows us to think about changing discourse in the first place: this is the bind of historic-ity. All our concepts seem to implicate each other in a conceptual web that we cannot take apart. Any single concept implies all the others. Dissolution of self, for example, can only have meaning when it is set against an under-standing of self, the integration of self, and some notion of consciousness as it functions with a grasp of itself. These notions have all evolved historically, and if we pinpoint the Greek beginnings of these notions, that does not mean that we are easily empowered to change them. If Greek tragedy and Greek medicine determine much of what we mean by madness, what are we to make of that fact?

The Foundations of Psychoanalysis

The historicity of madness and self is not highlighted in psychoanalysis, any more than in psychiatry, but Freud's work does effect a historical return. It borrows structures from theater and allegory that show us the workings of Greek thought present in our own. Psychoanalysis returns to a literary understanding of madness that stands in opposition to the "scientific" understanding of madness of Kraepelin and his successors' work. Freud wanted very much to be recognized as a scientific thinker and felt that he could gain acceptance for psychoanalysis only if it were recognized as a scientific paradigm. Freud's desire has little to do with what he actually accomplished. In drawing upon a long history of thought about self, consciousness, and mental illness, Freud reintroduces a literary understanding of the self. And this historical return occurs at the very moment when psychiatry seems to have denied literature a role as a form of knowledge. It is not by accident that, in the universities today of the English-speaking world, Freudians are found today largely in the social sciences and departments of literature, whereas the medical schools of the same universities have no Freudians on their psychiatric staffs.

Before turning to Freud the mythologist, Freud the scientist merits commentary. Educated in a scientific milieu at the forefront of medical research, as a young man Freud did work in neurophysiology. In brief, he was immersed in the major issues in neurological research. As Peter Amacher has shown in his study of Freud's neurological education, Freud studied in a milieu in which the parallelism of organic and psychic processes was an accepted axiom—though no empirical demonstration of any positive sort had proved this parallelism. Freud worked with Theodore Meynert, who did important research on the cerebral cortex. Meynert, sometimes more influenced by the romantics than by experimentation, equated cortical activity during dreaming with the same activity found during amentia, the latter being a syndrome characterized by hallucinatory states. Meynert's thought is exemplary of the kind of ease with which scientists could slip from one side to the other of the mind-body dualism when dealing with mental pathologies. Causes for amentia had to be localized in the "cortical mechanism," but they could be either physical or psychological in origin. Amentia could spring from anything as diverse as overwork, old age, homesickness, masturbation, fevers, childbearing, or alcoholism. Comparing Meynert and the young Freud, Amacher notes:

> When he [Meynert] gave his lectures on amentia in 1890, his student Freud had already begun the treatment of similar disorders, some of which he regarded as having physical causes and other mental causes, by working with the mental processes rather than with their physical concomitants. This was not inconsistent with Meynert's theory of concomitant mental and nervous functioning, although it was a radical departure from Meynert's and the orthodox ideas of proper therapy. Freud's innovation gave psychoanalysis an appearance very different from Meynert's psychiatry, but behind this appearance lay some very significant resemblances.[8]

It is revealing that in the *History of the Psychoanalytic Movement,* written in 1914, Freud makes no mention of this Meynert-influenced work, preferring instead to note that psychoanalysis began with the doctrine of repression as the foundation-stone upon which all his thought rests. Among medical scientists, only Charcot, with his work on hysteria, is mentioned in this book as having had an influence on Freud. Perhaps Freud was repressing the memory of his successful *Doktor-Vater.* Clearly, by 1914, Freud had distanced himself from the medical community that, by and large, did not accept him.

Kraepelin, the scientist, was the author of one book that he constantly rewrote in recasting his systematic taxonomy. *Litterateur* and theorist, Freud was, by contrast, the author of innumerable writings—papers, essays, studies, monographs—in which from his student days until the end of his life, exiled in London, he constantly reformulated theories and hypotheses. *An Outline of Psycho-Analysis,* written toward the end of his life, in 1938, is as rich as any work for an introduction into psychoanalytic theory—though written some forty years after Freud had published with Breuer their *Studies on Hysteria* (1895). This latter book was the work that founded psychoanalysis. It did so by investigating the sexual repression that found symptomatic expression in hysterical symptoms—and in which Freud apologized for writing something that read so much like a novel. In 1899 Freud published his massive *Die Traumdeutung,* or *The Interpretation of Dreams,* which, in explaining dreams as a coded expression of a desire, was probably most responsible for gaining international interest in his work, unless one gives that honor to the *Three Essays on Sexuality* that even today can seem revolutionary in their insistence on pansexuality and the normalcy of perversion. Freud continually revised his theories. After roughly 1907 he was doing so for a growing international movement that was already breaking up into factions and dissident movements, a tendency more characteristic of an artistic movement like surrealism than a scientific movement. Freud hardly limited himself to medical thought as he delved into theories of culture and anthropology as well as into increasingly speculative work about the nature of the instincts and the structure of the psyche. All of his theorizing was bound together by a fairly consistent theory that repression of pleasure and sexual desire is the basis for culture, as well as the view that the psyche manages badly at best to reconcile itself to the necessities of culture. *The Ego and the Id, Civilization and Its Discontents,* or *Beyond the Pleasure Principle,* with its hypothesis about the death instinct, are a few titles that come to mind in this respect.

Freud never lost sight of the biological basis of human behavior, but, as his early unpublished *Entwurf einer Psychologie* (translated as *Project for a Scientific Psychology*) of 1895 shows, he was not able to translate his interest in neurology or biology into concepts that could relate psychoanalysis to work in those fields. He seems to have retained as a bedrock of faith that the "biological factor" is the ultimate explanatory factor, although to many it seems that this belief remained an article of faith with no conceptual rigor. This is not to say that there is no truth-value to Freud's claims about instinct and drive; but these concepts are not part of any contemporary scientific discourse. Freud's concepts are taken from the language games of everyday language, as well as literature and philosophy, and indirectly from the German romantics. These concepts are then transposed in order to fit into Freud's allegorical framework. And if Freud's descriptions and theories often seem to have a kind of incontrovertible truth about them, perhaps it is in part because they often rely on everyday language games that in fact organize our understanding of the world. We would have trouble, in our ordinary language, not using allegories in which "drives" motivate people around us or in which the pleasure principle, by definition, seems to demand that we negotiate cleverly with reality in order finally to maximize our pleasure. These are all stock principles, or characters, in our allegories of everyday life that have more than once received new life from the philosophers and the poets.

Freud differentiated psychoanalysis from psychiatry through his literary mode of explanation. To demonstrate my claim, I turn, almost arbitrarily, to the *Introductory Lectures* Freud gave in 1916–17 in Vienna for a mixed audience of doctors and laymen. In these lectures Freud was seeking to convince a general public that psychoanalysis deserved credence, for he squarely faced the question as to what are the limits of psychiatry and psychoanalysis and what are the criteria by which to judge the use and truth of each doctrine. Freud's criteria for psychoanalysis do not include a clear empirical demonstration that explains a given phenomenon by accounting for a limited number of features. Rather, in lecture 16 he has a rather curious answer to the question as to why one should accept psychoanalysis. Conviction about psychoanalysis will come only as a process: "Sie sollen anhoren und auf sich wirken lassen, was ich Ihnen erzähle."[9] The audience must listen and allow Freud's thought to "work on them." Conviction can come only after longer experience, through a process of revelation in which insight suddenly appears.

Freud is arguing here for the truth of insight that is based on different criteria from those used for scientific proof. Criteria for scientific truth minimally demand that a theory give results that can be publicly repeated, and, according to most epistemologists, demand that one should also be able to give procedures for falsifying as well as verifying in some positive sense the theory that a scientist proposes. This type of proof cannot be given by psychoanalysis, since it must deal with unique exemplars in conditions that can never be repeated. Freud is quite aware of this difference and explicitly states in his lecture that psychoanalysis is a question of experience, of experience that can be *unsagbar*—ineffable or unsayable. In this lecture Freud also rejects the idea that he is proposing, in psychoanalysis, a speculative system. He reiterates that psychoanalysis is like experience: *Erfahrung*. Though I have argued elsewhere that Freud is more systematic than he admits here, I would also suggest that Freud is proposing essentially the same criteria for psychoanalysis and the experience it offers that we use for judging our unmediated response to a literary work.[10] Conviction comes through the experience of the individual work after time, through a process of revelation in which the literary work—or the psychoanalytical experience—reveals itself to be an essential structure of a unique experience. Or in other terms, this argument says that Freud is using the criteria for authenticity that underwrite modernist aesthetics: the goal of much modernist poetry is knowledge granted by the revelation of the essence of the unique particular. Therefore, it is not surprising that many modernists felt that Freud was on the side of the mad poets in their revolt against psychiatry.

Let us pursue the introductory lectures. In lecture 16 Freud challenges his audience to try to allow the psychoanalytical concepts to "grow up" next to psychiatric concepts until they reach the point where they can be judged in their influences on each other; and then they can reach a decision about "unifying" them ("Versuchen Sie also auch, die psychoanalytische Auffassung neben der popularen oder der psychiatrischen ruhig in sich aufwachsen zu lassen, bis sich die Gelegenheit ergeben, bei denen die beiden sich beeinflussen, sich messen und sich zu einer Entscheidung vereinigen können" (p. 250). To demonstrate what he means by this rather strange request, Freud gives a demonstration of how psychiatry and psychoanalysis can deal with the same singular case history.

He narrates the story of a happily married woman who receives one day an anonymous letter telling her that her husband is having an affair with a young woman employed in his factory. Though it subsequently turns out that this letter had been written by a jealous maid who wished to cause harm to the accused woman, the married woman cannot get rid of the obsessive jealousy that she now feels and that is destroying her happiness. What would a psychiatrist do with such a case, asks Freud: he answers that the medical doctor would search first for an essential trait that characterizes the symptom ("zunächst das Symptom durch eine wesentliche Eigenschaft zu Charackterisieren" [pp. 256–57]). Freud emphasizes that the psychiatrist faces the woman's anguish as a taxonomical operation in which he evaluates the inner experience or ideas of the woman: "Ideas of this sort that are inaccessible to logical arguments based on reality are commonly called insane ideas *[Wahnideen]*. The good woman is suffering from insane jealousy *[Eifersuchtswahn]*. That is indeed the essential characteristic of this case of sickness" (p. 257). Like a botanist, or so Freud suggests, the psychiatrist looks for the differentiating characteristic that will given him a clear "species" distinction.

The next question to be asked is etiological: if these insane ideas do not come from reality, where do they originate? Freud says the psychiatrist will do some research and then probably come forth with the following explanation: "Insane ideas occur in those people in whose families other comparable psychic disturbances have repeatedly occurred." These people are disposed to such illnesses "through hereditary transmission" (p. 257). And that, says Freud, is all that the psychiatrist can offer without, in his own terms, appearing to be a scoundrel. The psychiatrist must content himself, in spite of his "rich experience," with an uncertain prognosis about the future course of the disturbance.

What could psychoanalysis do in this case? Freud's demonstration that psychoanalytic theory can find meaning in mental disturbance is already under way in this tale, since Freud has embedded the case in an ongoing narration. He starts a story mentioning the detail that the woman's son-in-law brought her to Freud for help. And the narration continues with Freud's post facto reconstitution of a story line that pulls all the elements together with consummate narrative logic. Little wonder that Hollywood once loved psychoanalysis: analysis often relies on a cinematic flashback to get to the revelation of meaning. The woman was—and perhaps is—in love with the son-in-law and is projecting onto her husband a fictional desire for another woman in order to justify her own illicit desire. Moreover, it seems that she, perhaps intentionally if unconsciously, suggested the damning letter to the guilty maid. For she once said, in the maid's presence, that nothing would distress her more than to know that her husband was unfaithful. Freud's narration turns up other "causes." For it can be surmised that the woman, now in her fifties, has an increased sexual desire, while her husband's potency is perhaps decreasing. Or, suggesting a mythic analogue to the relations of Hippolytus and Phaedra, modernist mythologizer Freud recalls that the relation between a mother-in-law and a son-in-law has always been a delicate one, so that primitive peoples have powerful taboos interdicting the contact of the two (p. 261).

Freud's constant appeal to anthropology and myth is characteristic of the modernist literary mind: the narration of a unique case finds meaningful illumination in the way the case stands in a relation of analogy to universal myths. In his hermeneutics Freud contrasts the mythic and narrative understanding that analysis uncovers to the taxonomic or nosological understanding that psychiatry teaches in the medical arenas. Freud's narration is a form of understanding in that it organizes the experience of the unique case in terms that are amenable to public purview, even if the narrative does not succeed in answering all the questions that one could ask about this case. A unique case can produce an excess of meanings that no single narrative can organize. However, Freud's point of view is that narrative, enhanced by reference to universal mythic structures, can reveal the meaning of the absurd particular. This revelation constitutes the basic form of psychoanalytic understanding. It is not unlike the goal of the literary modernism one finds in Joyce and Proust: Stephen's dilemmas in *Ulysses* are illuminated by his relations to the Ulysses-Telemachus myth, and the narrator in Proust's *A la recherche* is acting out the drama of the universal Fall from paradise that leads to the cities in the plain. Specific dramas are enactments of great mythic structures. This literary approach to understanding the meaning of pathologies is the basis for Freud's hermeneutics. From this perspective we can understand Freud's doubts about psychiatry's belief that hereditary determinism underlies pathologies because this determinism deprives pathology of any meaning.

Another aspect of Freud's critique of psychiatry in this regard is spelled out in *Three Essays on Sexuality,* in the forward to the third edition of the work in 1914 (first published in 1905). Here Freud likens psychoanalytical understanding to a judicial procedure. Psychoanalysis is based on the constant observance of a process of appeals, such as is followed in judging a case. English translations have notorious difficulties with this kind of Freudian metaphor, but the argument depends upon building a web of metaphors. In the forward to the edition of 1914, for example, he refers to the *Instanzenzug,* or process of judicial appeals that metaphorically describes the elaboration of psychoanalytic understanding. In this process of understanding the mind, as in a hearing, the accidental or the chance moments in the case should be pushed forward, and the dispositional or hereditary factors should be left in the background. The latter do not account for the unique exemplar in the case that stands before the court of analysis. Compounding metaphors, Freud adds that the necessity of judging the individual case means that the analyst must consider the ontogenetic in preference to the phylogenetic—the biologically unique and not the species. Biology is analogous to the law to which one may make appeal; but the individual case is the grounds upon which the analyst must appeal to a general law. For the disposition to illness is manifested only in the accidental particular. And "the accidental plays the chief role in analysis, for it is accidental experience that must be mastered by analysis" [Das Akzidentelle spielt nämlich die Hauptrolle in der Analyse, es wird durch sie fast restlos bewältigt]. What emerges from these analogies is that Freud consciously marks off the field of psychoanalysis as a field of knowledge different from that of medicine. In the "Vorwort" he is, in fact, breaking with psychiatry by declaring that hereditary dispositions are outside the "field of work" of psychoanalysis.[11]

The basic "unit" of psychoanalytical explanation is the narrative telling the individual case that is then explained by a larger allegorical narrative. In these psychoanalytical narratives we consistently find the modernist impulse to discover therein the mythical allegory that offers the revelation of a universal structure. This impulse is clearly revealed in Freud's metapsychological works, to use the term designating Freud's theoretical works that explain the grounds for his interpretation of his narratives. The metapsychological works are far-reaching allegories that elucidate mythic structures. They present mythic constructs that offer keys for an allegorical interpretation of the absurd particular contained in the narrative. In these works Freud offers general allegories to explain the self and its functions, which allow him then to explain psychic disturbances and pathologies in agonistic terms. These agons, to use the term for conflict in Greek tragedy, are the conflicts acted out by allegorical actors on the stage of the psyche.

Most important is the allegory set forth by the three actors lodged in the Freudian topography of the self—the id, the ego, and the superego—which even in these absurd translations of *Es, Ich,* and *Uberich* retain their allegorical character in the battles that they wage among themselves. Or of equal interest is the drama of the Oedipal complex that Freud increasingly placed at the center of the development of personality, or the universal drama of our coming to grips with our particular neuroses. The Oedipal complex is a literary structure, a type of master narrative, endowed with mythical dimensions. Telling us that we can never overcome our desire for the paradise of childhood desire, the complex allows the translation in dramatic terms of the permanent alienation that Freud conceived to be the center of the self. We all desired our mother or our father; but every human being has his or her own special dynamics that give rise to a unique neurotic stance by which we adjust to the world and the denial of our desire. Each development remains a variant on the schema given by the master allegory of Oedipus. Every child passes through a tripartite drama in which the id, ego, and superego are developed through the conflicts created by impossible desires and forever delayed gratifications. Both German romanticism and classical philosophy seem united in this view that passion is the agent for all mental illness, and repression the only way of mastering desires that, if realized, would be madness; or, if they were not successfully repressed, would call upon fantasy to create a psychosis to compensate for our lack.

But there is also the postromantic context in which we should interpret the Oedipus complex and understand Freud's appeal for writers. In disclosing an essential alienation, I have suggested that Freud's allegory is like comparable visions that describe the impossibility of plenitude in writers like Kafka, Joyce, and Proust. Nearly every modernist sees the self as a product of loss, as a victim of what the poet Cocteau called, in his version of Oedipus, the infernal machine. It is pointless to speak of Freud's influence on these modernists, though many of them knew his work quite well. Their works all spring from a postromantic matrix in which conflict, loss, and alienation are the essential themes to characterize the self in its relation to a world that always deceives it. Kafka's work, for example, turns constantly on the quest for the revelation of the absent center wherein the Father's law would reveal meaning: Kafka's characters are forever questing for access to the Law that would make sense of the quest enjoined—to seek the Law. The Law remains, even after God, the father, or whoever, has disappeared that gave us the Command. This is not unlike the basic situation in Freud's allegory, according to which the Oedipal revelation is the disclosure of the absent father's perduring presence in the form of the superego and its impossible demands. Logos, the Word, and the Law point to mythical structures that underwrite both Freud and Kafka. Proust's novel *A la recherche du temps perdu* describes the same absence of a center of values that, present to the narrator through their absence, condemn the narrator to a meaningless life after he becomes an adult. With the same sense that Freud saw childhood as the locus of forever retrospective bliss, Proust's narrator falls from a paradise of childhood that can seemingly exist only once it is lost. And so one might say that Freud's unconscious is an alterity that is so alienated that it could never exist except by not being present. And that his superego is the center of a logos that exists only to show us that we are never present to it except through our inadequacy.

For modernists like these, to enter adult life is to enter a realm of loss and alienation from an essential center of meaning. Art, that product of the imagination, may compensate for this loss. Joyce's artist as a young man calls upon the myth of Daedalus to imagine some fullness that might compensate for his loss of childhood plenitude, though the reader knows that fallen Icarus is more likely to be the mythic character to whom the adult bears the closest relation. *Ulysses* bears this out. To recapitulate, then, the modernist lives his alienation as the specification of an invariant mythic narrative—the Fall, Oedipus, Icarus, Electra, Odysseus—that makes of alienation our normal condition. The normal state of being abnormal is the absurd condition of the alienated modern. Like Proust's narrator, every one of Freud's children sucked in, on the maternal breast, a dream of eternal fulfillment; but then found that identification with the father meant forever giving up that eternity of bliss. This renunciation is imposed not only because of the violence that fathers always threaten to work like so many Abrahams on so many Isaacs; it is also because resembling the father means being alienated from all the meaning that the father once promised, but never delivered. The father lives on, in his absence, through the tortured memory that the superego maintains, tortured by a law that it barely understands. The way into the Law, as one of Kafka's parables portrays it, is nonetheless meant for each unique individual, and each gate therein has its own gatekeeper to keep it closed. In both Freud and Kafka the unique subject can always be the grounds for a universal allegory about the absence of universal logos.

Freud and Madness

These paradoxical alienations are grounds for angst, neurosis, and Woody Allen movies, but are not necessarily sufficient for the psychoses that we put into our asylums when we do not condemn them to live on the streets. Freud did not care much for the mad, for those truly psychotic who need internment. He thought that psychotics were not amenable to transference and hence could not enter into the analytic transaction that would help them deal with their conflicts through cathartic recognition. In practical terms psychoanalysts have largely left treatment of the mad to their psychiatric brethren. Nonetheless, Freud's view of madness has been pervasively influential. The Freudian account of psychosis is not in fact greatly different from his theory of neurosis, though the psychotic's strategies of adaptation are radically different from those of the neurotics. Neurotics deal with unsuccessful repression of forbidden desires by denying a piece of reality, whereas psychotics handle their failure to repress successfully by re-creating reality. Their pathology is to be altogether more successful than neurotics in compensating for their failure to adjust to reality—whether it be the reality of our inner desires that repression cannot eliminate or the reality of the demands of the exterior world. Psychotics are the successful artists who use the imagination to re-create their world and then live in it. Novalis and Hoffmann live on in this account of the power of dream and the imagination.

From the Freudian perspective all adaptive behaviors are in a sense abnormal, hence normal, and so we are all on intimate grounds with mental pathology. For example, we all experience a nightly bout of psychosis in dream. Freud maintained throughout his life that dream is a form of wish fulfillment. Renewing the romantic notion that dream is a form of compensatory madness, in a relatively late work like the *New Introductory Lectures on Psychoanalysis* (first published in 1933) Freud proposes that dream is a normal pathological product that represents, like psychosis, a turning away from reality. Freud explored this topic on a number of occasions. In his lecture "Revision of Dream Theory," Freud gives two reasons why the psychotic or dreaming self flees reality: either the repressed unconscious is too strong and overwhelms the conscious self trying to cling to reality, or reality becomes so unbearably painful that the threatened ego throws itself into the arms of the unconscious impulses.[12] This analysis is couched in the language of allegory, though a medical theorist could say that Freud has transposed the psychiatric concepts of endogenous and exogenous etiology. And to which a deconstructive critique might add with malice that the metaphysics of inner and outer have had a long life. But neither metaphysics nor transposed psychiatric concepts explain why psychoanalysis has had such purchase on our imaginations in its explanation of mental pathology.

I would suggest that Freud's appeal lies in his dramatic models for madness, in which a cast of actors, drawn from a multiple dramatis personae, are engaged in frontal encounters of great violence. The Oedipal conflict with its agon between parent and child, played out on the child's imaginary stage, pits with biblical intensity the son against the father. When the son cannot deal with the castration that will end his desire, he must submit to the demands of culture or take refuge in madness. Or consider the Freudian drama used to explain depression and melancholy. Id, ego, and superego strive for supremacy in a struggle that has the reverberations of a Shakespearean tragedy, complete with conspiracies and absurd lust for power. For example, Freud invents the following scenario for enacting depression in *The Ego and the Id* of 1923:

> How is it that the super-ego manifests itself essentially as a sense of guilt (or rather as criticism—for the sense of guilt is the perception in the ego answering to this criticism) and moreover develops such extraordinary harshness and severity towards the ego? If we turn to melancholia first, we find that the

excessively strong super-ego which has obtained a hold upon consciousness rages against the ego with merciless violence, as if it had taken possession of the whole of the sadism available in the person concerned. Following our view of sadism, we should say that the destructive component had entrenched itself in the super-ego and turned against the ego. What is now holding sway in the super-ego is, as it were, a pure culture of the death instinct, and in fact it often enough succeeds in driving the ego into death, if the latter does not fend off its tyrant in time by the change round into mania.[13]

In his ironic commentary on this battle, Malcolm Bowie notes that "the super-ego here acts upon the ego as an Attila or a Tamburlaine."[14] These tyrants are the heroes of the Jacobean tragedies that madness produces for us in psychosis. Freud's gift is to describe those natural events of our everyday life—shameful desires, guilt, a will to power, sadism, the desire to die—with allegorical agents whose drama he creates with a tragic necessity we had not seen since Shakespeare.

Freud is a continuator of the romantics, but central to his dramas is the positivist principle that the pathological is part of the normal; it is a normal development of a continuum of deviance for which there are no clear criteria for deciding what is healthy or unhealthy. It is also true that the neurotic demands of society that inform the superego's sadistic judgments suggest that our cultural norms are also deviant, at least by some obscure rational standard that Freud evokes with hesitation. The empirical evidence dictates that our common drama is all to be condemned to be deviant, and that is the norm—whatever be the dreams of reason.

Superimposed on this positivist principle, however, is the romantic belief that madness can effect a revelation of truths hidden in the psyche's depths. Any number of Freudian texts can be cited to show that Freud subscribed to this proposition. In *An Autobiographical Study* Freud addressed, near the end of his life, the question of truth by asking what psychoanalysis could do for the insane. He felt that medical practice had been wrong to have separated neuroses from psychoses so as to treat them as nervous diseases. The study of neuroses is necessary, since the knowledge of neurosis is an introduction to the understanding of psychosis, whatever be the therapeutic results analysis may have in dealing with psychotics:

Mental patients are as a rule without the capacity for forming a positive transference, so that the principal instrument of analytical technique is inapplicable to them. There are nonetheless a number of methods of approach to be found. Transference is often not so completely absent but that it can be used to a certain extent; and analysis has achieved undoubted success with cyclical depressions, light paranoic modifications, and partial schizophrenias. It has at least been a benefit to science that in many cases the diagnosis can oscillate for quite a long time between assuming the presence of a psychoneurosis or of a dementia praecox; for therapeutic attempts initiated in such cases have resulted in valuable discoveries before they have had to be broken off. But the chief consideration in this connection is that so many things that in the neuroses have to be laboriously fetched up from the depths are found in the psychoses upon the surface, visible to every eye.[15]

Madness is, as Freud says in the *New Lectures,* a privileged path leading to "internal psychic reality" (p. 85). Freud's belief in revelation shows again that romantic psychiatrists developed the conceptual conditions of possibility for something like a Freudian discourse. Working out of that matrix, Freud, doctor turned literary thinker, inevitably found in madness a form of revelation akin to poetic truth, since, for both psychoanalysis and romantic psychiatry, poetry itself is a compensatory activity akin to dreaming and psychosis.

Literature and Madness in Freud

Freud's theory of literature is part and parcel of his analytical theory of madness, just as his analytical practice is, in the broadest sense, founded on the literary working of allegory and metaphor to explain experience. His theory of art and literature derives logically from his theory of how the psyche deals with the real—or rather cannot deal with the real. We have noted that at the heart of this theory is the romantic equation that identifies madness and dream, and dream and art, which adds up to the view that art shares common features with psychosis. Art brings to the surface, in the creation of a world, that which is normally repressed; or as Freud writes, with his peculiar irony, on Leonardo da Vinci, "Kindly nature has given the artist the ability to express his most secret mental impulses, which are hidden even from himself, by means of the works that he creates; and these works have a powerful effect on others who are strangers to the artist, and who are themselves unaware of the source of their emotion."[16] In the experience of art, one unconscious sends to another unconscious messages that none can dare behold. Psychosis and dreaming come from the same depths and communicate much the same coded message as art: they create a world whose meaning escapes the creator and whose revelation is only dimly understood by those who are privy to it—unless they be versed in the Freudian art of allegorical hermeneutics.

In the papers dealing with psychosis as well as art and literature Freud spells out that fantasy allows the insane to replace outer reality with a constructed reality that the self can live with. For instance, in "The Loss of Reality in Neurosis" he dramatically describes the capacity of the ego to tear itself away from reality and to create a new version thereof that the ego does not find objectionable. Psychosis is an art form, for it literally remodels reality by creating a new "outer world" that it attempts to set in place of "external reality."[17] Freud places art and pathology together as comparable strategies of adaptation, for artists and neurotics—and a fortiori psychotics—find common strategies for the impossibility of satisfactory repression by turning to the imagination. In *An Autobiographic Study* Freud offers a medical diagnosis of how the imagination allows the libido to get around the repressive demands of reality:

> The realm of the imagination was evidently a "sanctuary" made during the painful transition from the pleasure principle to the reality principle in order to provide a substitute for the gratification of instincts which had to be given up in real life. The artist, like the neurotic, had withdrawn from an unsatisfying reality into this world of imagination; but unlike the neurotic, he knew how to find a way back from it and once more to get a firm foothold in reality. (P. 118)

With the example of Goethe constantly before him, Freud pays homage to the notion of artistic triumph over adversity. And a cliché about artistic triumph becomes the etiology of the imagination in the allegorical drama Freud has constructed to explain the war within the psyche. Basic to the drama is the agon between the pleasure principle and the reality principle. These all-embracing a priori principles that Freud saw behind all the psyche's internecine wars—until he added a death instinct—are creators of secondary agencies that can negotiate the impossibility of finding psychic equilibrium. And, as Freud's French successor Lacan was to emphasize later, the imagination is born to compensate for an inherent lack in the subject, or, simply, to mitigate the pain of being.

The positivist side of Freud came to the fore when he ultimately, and perhaps contradictorily, propounded a harsh judgment about the value of the artistic triumph of the imagination: the artistic work is really too much like a pathological product. This may be the norm, but Freud was also disdainful of a norm that looks so much like impotence. And so in *An Autobiographical Study* Freud seems, in the same breath in which he expresses admiration, to dismiss the artist whom he praises: "His creations, works of art, were the imaginary gratifications of unconscious wishes, just as dreams are; and like them they are in the nature of compromises, since they too were forced to avoid any open conflict with the forces of repression" (p. 118). Dreams are the nightly psychosis that allow us all to know wish fulfillment, whereas art is a form of psychopathology reserved for the privileged few. But it is not clear that this privilege merits great respect. Therefore, we see that art, insanity, and essential revelation are bound up in Freud in ways that are at once positive and negative. On the one hand, if art is akin to madness, then like psychosis it can be a way into the inner truth. Psychosis, dream, and art can open up depths that are not directly accessible to critical reason—until reason has been schooled in analysis. On the other hand, the reverse side of this analytical coin is a rationalist contempt for art. As Freud's paper "Writers and Day-Dreaming" spells it out, poetry is a kind of child's play that apes a reality it cannot attain. Imitation and representation are mere surrogate compensations for frustrated desire and bespeak a weakness, a failing, endemic to the species, when, from Freud's perspective, art and mimesis are not a sign of an individual's weakness of character. Mimesis is the product of a sick animal, and it is appropriate to see a reflection of the Platonic tradition and its condemnation of art as mere imitation in Freud's ambiguous attitude toward the genesis and ontology of the artwork. Art is a substitute gratification for those who cannot deal with the real. Artists may be justified to feel themselves as much condemned by Freud as by Griesinger if they desire.

But artists rarely want to be rejected, and most practitioners of the mimetic arts have preferred to focus on the Freudian position that vouchsafes a positive equivalency to art and madness. This viewpoint allows the mad to look upon themselves as artists and, conversely, artists to look upon themselves as privileged madmen. This side of the Freudian legacy has been used as a defense of both art and madness. It seems to renew another Greek tradition, the portrayal of poets as melancholiacs, going back to Aristotle's *Thirtieth Problem*. Freud is thus not responsible for the belief in the aesthetics of madness or the madness of aesthetics. But he has granted a patina of scientific plausibility to this essentially romantic defense of poetry and madness. Therefore, if psychoanalysis had not arisen to contest medical psychiatry's refusal to give meaning to madness, and seemingly give the artist a right to use his or her madness, it is quite likely that the shape of twentieth-century art and literature would be different from what it is.

What modern literature might have been without Freud is a matter for speculation; and one can argue that Freud is as much a symptom as a cause of the fact that madness has been granted a preponderant voice in modern literature. But one cannot deny that madness has become a dominant voice in the modernist quest for essential revelation. This voice speaks a distrust of, or a revolt against, psychiatry, a willingness to welcome the irrational and the deviant, and finally an often suicidal desire to "believe" in madness in some positive sense. These are some of the leitmotifs to which we shall now turn in order to understand what mad discourse in poetry offered us in the now declining twentieth century. Most writers have embraced Freud's positive legacy, especially mad writers, perhaps largely in hopes of keeping the psychiatrists from sequestering them or forcing them to submit to therapeutic treatments that, it must be said, have been far more brutal than the psychoanalytic couch of remembered dreams. Lobotomies and electroshock treaties may have therapeutic effects, but artistic creation does not seem to be one of them.

Chapter 9

Modernist Poetic Discourses in Madness

An Approach to Modernist Writers

It has been very difficult to be pointlessly, outrageously insane in the twentieth century. When the mad have not found their discourse immediately used as so many symbols for the purposes of psychiatric or analytical discourse, they have been anthologized to offer discourses in madness that, called madness or poetry, the critics then interpret. It would seem that madness has become readable. The ironic-minded may think that this is indeed fortunate, since there have been an extraordinary number of writers who have been certifiably insane in our century. In addition, the multitude of certifiably insane writers finds numerous fellow travelers in the legions of writers who have mimicked being mad, or the often borderline insane, or those sane who sought revelation in alienated discourse. One thinks immediately of Céline and Pound, Breton and Artaud, Berryman and Plath. An accurate list of writers illustrating this point would undoubtedly be interminable.

To bring, hopefully, some understanding to this diversity, I offer the hypothesis that there exists a modernist experience of madness in literature. To demonstrate this thesis, I propose to study a few major writers, all poets, exemplifying three dominant modes of literary expression: German expressionism, French surrealism, and American confessional poetry. These three rubrics can serve to center our readings of mad discourses that are central to modernist poetic practices. These movements are of great intrinsic interest for understanding modern culture, and I have selected them because they allow us to situate, in terms of our modernity, a few writers and their representation of the mad self, as well as the role pathologies play in that revelation of self. Moreover, by looking at these different movements, we shall see that modern writers of quite diverse cultural backgrounds have all been obliged to use and reflect upon the psychiatric and psychoanalytic theories that relentlessly make sense, in negative and positive ways, of the madness that informs their discourse.

Much of modern literature is a response to madness. The encounter with madness can involve the writer's own insanity, or the madness that the writer perceives as revealing some insight into our usually fallen condition. The encounter with madness is usually mediated through the categories of psychiatry and psychoanalysis. Psychoanalysis is often used against psychiatry (the converse is rarely the case, *pace* Nabokov). For, by and large, modern writers have viewed psychiatry as an enemy, at once imperious in its claims to have the power to classify the deviant self and fraudulent in its reduction of madness to some hereditary or organic cause. Freud has often come to the rescue of the writer in search of a self that is not the product of a psychiatric tragedy, since Freud seems to explain to writers that their deviance is quite normal, especially in response to a culture that is crazy in itself. However, Freud's view that poetry is a surrogate gratification can also be taken as an indictment: the writer must also ponder the dilemma of being reduced to an infantile dreamer incapable of facing the demands of reality. Medical explanations of madness present a minefield of unpleasant possibilities that writers tread at the risk of losing their self.

In addition, the truly psychotic poet must also face society's institutionalized juridical power; and the psychiatrists of the world—Kraepelin and not Freud—legally define what madness is and what power society should use against it. Hence the rage of many a writer is directed against the psychiatrist, for mad writers find that they cannot articulate their own experience without finding the doctor there, ready to control the logos that a writer must live by. The doctor is ready, in short, to reduce writing to the categories of a taxonomy that determines what society will do with the body of the insane writer, with the asylum awaiting those who cannot control themselves. In this regard, the poet seems to have been especially vulnerable to disasters, though the following chapter could be written using only novelists or painters for examples—substituting, say, often suicidal abstract expressionists for poets who shared this bent for self-destruction.

German Expressionism and Hereditary Madness

In a broad sense, expressionism is the dominant aesthetics of our century, starting in Germany before World War I. The continuities of our cultural history are underscored in the self-conscious way the German expressionists enlarged upon the French poets of the preceding decades in making pathology, personal and cultural, central to their works. Coming from the same milieu, it is perhaps not surprising that psychoanalysis shares the expressionist axiom that pathologies characterize our daily being. In this regard, Walter Sokel sees an analogy between the Freudian view of the artist as a displaced psychotic and the expressionist view of the artist as an empty vessel needing art as a compensation for his constitutional inferiority.[1] In conformity with psychiatric views of madness, the expressionists saw themselves as victims of their constitution, of an *Anlage* that imposed hereditary determinism on them. Their rage against a condemnation to decadence and dissolution underlies the often apocalyptical views of the expressionist revolt. Hereditary determinism decrees that deviance and decline is a normal state of affairs. Expressionists found madness everywhere, with an overdeterminism that, through the rhetoric of expressionist hyperbole, transforms everything into a metaphor for insanity.

In expressionist art the mad are present everywhere: they are the ubiquitous psychic double of every writer, wandering in every expressionist landscape and city scene. Insanity reveals the violence at the heart of being. It offers an apocalyptic revelation that the psychiatrist's discourse cannot master, and so there is often something gleeful about the expressionist revelation of madness. There is rebellious delight found in showing that medical rationality has no purchase on the universal presence of insanity. This is what Georg Heym demonstrates in his much anthologized poem "Die Irren" (The mad) of 1910.[2] When confronting a psychiatrist, the mad can therapeutically chat with equanimity about Hume, the philosopher who symbolizes Enlightenment rationalism, before they suddenly give into madness and smash the doctor's head. This poem's irony, if that is the term, conveys a complicitous fascination with the power of the irrational. There is at once a pessimistic acceptance of the psychiatrist's judgment that the mad are condemned to remain in their folly and a joy in the affirmation that the outburst of the irrational is a natural occurrence. Insane violence is natural like a volcano exploding, or, in Heym's image, like spiders and mice scurrying about as they follow their natural instincts. There is a complicity with the mad in many of these texts, suggesting that the mad should have the upper hand over the doctors. Or perhaps that they would have the upper hand, if it were not for the whip that enforces the power of medical discourse over the mad, those mad who, like Heym's mice, run everywhere throughout our cityscapes.

For expressionists like Heym or the doctor Gottfried Benn, madness is a direct revelation of a cultural and physical decadence in which they revel with various degrees of romantic irony. Their general belief in constitutional decadence is summed up in their favored theme of the "twilight of the Gods," since the fall of the gods is in effect the fall of logos into morbid pathology. Sickness and pathology are thus conceived as a disclosure of the unsavory truth. This expressionist credo also leads to a contradictory stance: the poet views the mad at once as totally other, as alienated cripples deprived of logos, as it were; and as angels of revelation who offer knowledge that no other source can grant. In Ernst Stadler's poem "Irrenhaus" (Insane asylum) the mad inmates are first presented as mutes bereft of self-consciousness:

> Hier ist Leben, das nichts mehr von sich weiss—
> Bewusstsein tausand Klafter tief ins All gesunken.

> [Here is life that knows nothing more about itself—
> Consciousness sunk a thousand fathoms deep into the cosmos.]

But then, in syntax recalling Hölderlin, Stadler describes their sudden insane cries as breaches in the cosmic silence:

> Vielen aber ist Himmel aufgetan.
> Sie hören die toten Stimmen aller Dinge
> sie umkreisen
> Und die schwebende Musik des Alls.
> (*Expressionisme,* p. 147)

> [But to many heaven is opened.
> They hear the dead voices of all things go around them
> And the swaying music of the cosmos.]

This polarity of pathology and cosmic revelation reflects the oscillations of a culture that cannot decide where to relegate the mad, or if madness has a message. It reflects a fundamental indecision about the truth-value of madness that is mirrored in the positions of psychiatry and psychoanalysis. Is madness the mute spectacle of some decadent fall out of logos, or does it reveal the most intimate workings of mind?

And in the specific German context, we read in expressionism the irrational rationalities that became the monstrous political history we have not yet really understood. This is not to say that all expressionists were proto-Nazis in their exaltation of the fall into madness—though some, like the physician Benn or the philosopher Heidegger, turned from analyzing cultural pathology to embracing it by endorsing, for various periods of time, the insanities of National Socialism. This adherence to Nazi ideology was a move that, for many, was conceived of as therapeutic. In combatting madness with madness, expressionism set forth ideological contradictions that could, and did, lead to the self-fulfilling vision of cultural insanity of the Nazi movement.

There was of course another side to expressionism, one that harks back to the romantics and that we find rejuvenated in the surrealists and, later, on the American scene: that is, the desire to explore the inner self. Expressionism's goal was proclaimed to be self-expression; as Kasimir Edschmid wrote in a lecture in 1917, it was to get beyond the "mere facts" of experience and to show in a literary work "the hand of the artist who grasps them." But it seems inevitable that, for the expressionists, this desire for self-expression was tied up with a concept of pathology. Pathology is a mode of being and a form of revelation. And so, in the same lecture, Edschmid described how artists and poets can enter into the world of the sick through an identification with their disease.[3] The pathology to be explored could apparently be one within or one without. Expressionism thus came down at once on the side of doctors and against them, needing their clinical tableaux to understand their own decadence, and hating them for using their medical power to abuse the interned, those poets from the streets.

Trakl and Experience of Psychiatric Determinations of Madness

The poet who is most torn by these opposing impulses was Georg Trakl (1887–1914), the greatest expressionist and, after Hölderlin, perhaps the most powerful mad poet of all time. To show the hand of the artist, the poet turned to his own madness, but not with an innocent eye, for he brought to bear on his own experience the medical categories that, as a pharmacist, Trakl would have known well even if he had never been treated unto death by civilian and military psychiatrists. Through his own madness he spoke for the fall of all those anonymous mad he saw in the asylums. His encounter with his own madness was mediated by the psychiatric understanding that reigned victorious in prewar Austria, the same milieu in which Freud was first trained. Trakl faced his alienation with the anguish of the writer who finds that, in madness, his discourse is not really his own. Psychiatry had marked him with a hereditary curse. Facing psychiatry, it seems Trakl believed he could give meaning to his own experience of himself only by inventing a rhetoric, or perhaps a language, that would circumvent the psychiatric categories that, as a patient, he was obliged to accept.

Trakl's poetic exploration was motivated by this desire for an idiolect, for a self-created logos uncontaminated by medicine and reason. This also explains what many see as Trakl's hermeticism—or, for that matter, the hermeticism of many modern poets after Rimbaud. But Trakl is hermetic only to those who are unable to enter the concrete experience of alienation in a discourse that tries to redefine the inner world as an objective world. Drawing upon the French symbolist experience of poetic madness, Trakl's achievement is the creation of a rhetoric that can encompass experiences not encoded in ordinary language games, nor in the medical taxonomies. Lucia Getsi's translation of a late poem, "Klage" (Lament), a poem written during World War I while the poet was confined to a mental hospital in Kraków, gives immediate access to Trakl's world:

> Sleep and death, the dark eagles
> Sweep around this head all night long:
> The icy wave of eternity
> Would engulf the golden image of man.
> His purple body
> Shatters on terrible reefs,
> And the dark voice spreads lamentation
> Over the sea.
> Sister of stormy sorrow,
> Look, an anguished boat sinks
> Beneath the stars,
> The silent face of night.[4]

Trakl's expressionism conveys an experience of madness by drawing on images from the Western tradition: depicting the poet's inner experience of going under, he demonstrates his submission to the exterior disorder that his body cannot resist. Madness is the anguish experienced while the exterior world, the stars, remains indifferent to this wreck. Insanity is the extinguishing of light in the *Umnachtung,* the literal term for being lost in night as the light of reason is drenched in the waters of madness. The sister, the object undoubtedly of illicit incestuous desire, is called upon to witness this destruction in which she seems to be at once an innocent and guilty participant. In fine, "Lament" is, paradoxically, a quite unified experience of dissolution, moving from the presentation of the allegorical figures of death and sleep, to an image of the body's destruction, and finishing with an apostrophe to the personified image of melancholy, the sister, calling upon her to see the boat go under.

It is not the wrecked body that makes this description, but some observer who, in terms of the rhetorical axis of the poem, is outside the wreck. This observing presence that speaks for, but also at a distance from, the mad person is like a psychiatric observer set within the poem. The observer's distance sets off the fall that the self undergoes. Implicitly present is a viewer who sees the fall, but does not participate in the conflictive dynamics that make up the experience of madness. The observer can describe, judge, and on occasion condemn. These are the roles of a psychiatric observer who threatens to suppress the experiencing self with an objectivity that menaces the mad self. But this objectivity is nonetheless necessary to set off the poet's world in its alterity.

The polarities I describe here—the quest for the pure experience of madness and the rhetoric that demands an objective experience of madness—characterize the dilemma of the mad writer who wants to be mad on his or her own terms. For writers are obliged to mediate this madness through terms imposed by an exterior observer, be it the psychiatrist or the analyst, whose presence as logos establishes their rupture with logos. This polarity reflects the divided nature of the poetic self as it contemplates itself in its otherness. The cost of this experiencing one's own self as other is dramatized in Trakl's "Helian," a long poem in which the poet experiences himself as dead. Excluded from contact with the living word, he is decaying and rotting, or so he is described in the final five stanzas of the twenty-nine irregular stanzas, again in Getsi's version, in which the poet describes himself and his double Helian:

> Let the song also remember the body,
> His madness and white brows and his leavetaking,
> The decayed one, who bluely opens his eyes.
> O how sorrowful is this reunion.
>
> Stairs of madness in black rooms,
> Shadows of old men under the open door,
> Where Helian's soul sees itself in a rosy mirror
> And snow and leprosy fall from his forehead.
>
> On the walls the stars have died
> And the white shapes of the light.
>
> Bones of graves arise from the carpet
> Silence of rotted crosses on the hill,
> Sweetness of incense in the purple night wind.
>
> O you broken eyes in black mouths,
> When the grandson in the tender darkness of his mind
> Ponders alone the darker ending,
> The still god lowers his blue eyelids over him.

(P. 79)

The distance between observed and observer is expressed here in a poem that is almost pure self-reflexive commentary on the poetic capture of madness. The work ponders its own coming to be at the same time that the creating mind knows that it is headed toward madness. In *Helian* Trakl has set forth a multifaceted double: Helian is the sun god, the enshrined prophet, the poet in contact with the sun and thus logos; and in all these guises he observes himself as undergoing death, a metaphor for the body's going under in madness. Multiple oppositions undergird this. The poet is himself and another, he is torn between the purity of snow and the leprosy of inner experience, he experiences light and, finally, darkness. Darkness—madness as *Umnachtung*—means the loss of vision, hence the light of reason, and signifies the fall into the night beyond logos and the god's presence. And, without irony, the god represents those forces of reason that might make sense of this fall, and perhaps even the psychiatrists who thought Trakl suffered from dementia praecox.

The psychiatric determination of madness as a fall into dissolute inner states dominates Trakl's experience of his insanity, and this experience is buttressed by the psychiatric rationalization of madness as a hereditary curse. This psychiatric denial of meaning to madness coincides with the tragedy Trakl feels he lives in his rupture with logos, though his tragedy finds its determining fate in medical determinism. Psychiatric views of madness press themselves upon the poet and explain to him finally that his poems are predestined. "Helian" is again a key text for this experience of insanity as a form of "going under" that destroys a family, a generation, and perhaps even an entire race of those damned by their heredity, which Trakl portrays in the work's central stanzas:

> At vespers the stranger is lost in black November devastation,
> Under rotten branches, along leprous walls,
> Where earlier his holy brother walked,
> Drowned in the faint string music of his madness.
>
> O how lonely the evening wind ceases.
> Dying, the head bows in the darkness of olive trees.
>
> Awesome is the decline of this race.
> In this hour the gazing man's eyes fill
> With the gold of his stars.
>
> (P. 77)

"Erschütternd ist der Untergang des Geschlechts": a family, a generation goes under in madness. Like earlier expressionists, the poet reads this destiny in the stars that make of him, as representative of the race, a scapegoat in madness. And this insanity writ large becomes the expressionist version of the apocalypse: the twilight of all the gods.

In a late prose poem, "Dream and Derangement"—"Traum und Umnachtung"—Trakl describes the family at the origins of his madness with a kind of diagnostic savagery: "At night the father grew old; in dark rooms the mother's face turned to stone, and the curse of a debased race weighed upon the body" (p. 146). The curse of the "debased race"— "entarteten Geschlechts"—unwittingly echoes the future Nazi diagnosis of cultural pathology. In Trakl's case the race is Germanic, and the place of the curse can be located, as Herbert Lindenberger puts it, in "the Salzburg world of Trakl's childhood, a setting of old churches, uninhabited castles, cemeteries, winding rivers, and wooded mountains."[5] This "real" decor is essential in that it comes to symbolize the family and the race, it is the concrete place of the hereditary curse where the father reigns, the patriarch who is at once the transmitter of the curse and the source of the reason that purports to explain the curse. In revolting against the father-doctor, the poet enacts a revolt against the God who condemns the mad writer. As in Freud, God is the displaced father who controls language and reason. And he is interchangeable with the psychiatrist who judges the experience of madness as the victim of insanity falls from language. God, father, the deified shrink, all are the object of the poet's revolt at the same time that he is helpless not to accept their reason: "He sat upon the icy stair, feverish, raging against God in a wish for death. O the gray face of terror as he raised his round eyes over the mutilated throat of a dove" (p. 149). The death of the dove suggests the loss of any religious solace or salvation, for God himself is the source of the condemnation to madness that weighs upon the poet. He hears the condemnation in the father's voice:

> All night long he lived in a crystal cave and lepers' scabs grew silver upon his brow. A shadow, he moved down the mule-track under autumn stars. Snow fell, and blue gloom filled the house. A blind man's voice rang out, the harsh voice of the father, and confirmed the dread. (P. 151)

In images reminiscent of Lautréamont and Rimbaud, Trakl describes the body as the locus of a fall that derives from, and is paradoxically condemned, by the father. This is not cultivated madness, however. This madness is a lived contradiction for which there is no mediation or dialectical resolution except the suicide that did indeed put an end to it. After more than one attempt Trakl finally killed himself.

Surrealist Solutions to Expressionist Dilemmas

One solution to Trakl's double bind is to reject the very idea that the race is a locus for the hereditary decadence leading to madness. Another would be to reject the idea of decadence. After World War I the French surrealists took both tacks. Not only did they reject hereditary tragedies, but they also exulted in contradiction as they decreed madness to be superior to medicine. Two of the most important surrealists, Louis Aragon and André Breton, were trained as doctors; and in their work in military clinics during World War I they were trained in the same kind of psychiatry that treated Trakl at the outset of the War. The rejection of medicine is especially clear in the work of the chief theorist of surrealism, André Breton, who saw in psychiatry's collaboration with the war effort, the intellectual bankruptcy of European medicine. If Breton subsequently saluted Freud as a master, it was largely because, in rejecting bourgeois medicine, Breton could then project onto Freud his own utopian program for using the revelations of insanity to transform conscious life. Renewing the German romantics in his own way, Breton proposed that the unconscious and the pathologies associated with it are the key to all intellectual and creative activity. Not surprisingly, Breton and his followers willingly endorsed Freud's belief that dream offers access to the true self. Breton's valorization of dream, like Freud's, came as a response to the psychiatric rationalism that, for Breton as for Freud, had no purchase upon the most pressing psychic phenomena.

Unlike Freud, however, Breton and his followers were utopian revolutionaries who believed that psychiatry represented the very codification of the kind of insane rationality that had led to the massacres of four years of trench warfare. Their revolt against the war's rationalized insanity was unconditional. Logically—or illogically as one will—the surrealist hatred of psychiatry led Breton to call upon the mad to murder their psychiatrists. And psychiatrists as diverse as Janet and Clérambault, to name two famous examples, took Breton's histrionics seriously enough to demand that the police conduct an investigation.[6] This homicidal example shows at any rate that surrealism's revolt that was totally antithetical to Freud's conservative, pessimistic beliefs that culture is the result of necessary repression. From Freud's perspective, Breton's call for the liberation of instinct would result, if it were possible, in an orgy of instant gratification that would destroy everything civilization is founded on. It is impossible to imagine Freud entertaining the call for a surrogate deicide by killing the gods of medicine; nor can one seriously entertain an image of Freud calling for the destruction of repressive rationality so as to allow the unconscious to flower forth in a

Rimbaudesque revelation of perpetual Christmas. I stress this perhaps obvious point, since more than one revolutionary current in our recent past has wanted, with rather simplistic hopes, to annex Freud.

As opposed to the expressionist apocalypse, in his histrionics Breton called upon all to live insanity as revelation. From this utopian perspective, psychoanalysis was a doctrine that showed the necessity of liberating the unconscious and transforming pathology into poetry. Madness and art were never more closely linked, theoretically at least, than in this moment when Freud's doctrine for curing neuroses became a basis for an aesthetics that understood itself to be the pathway to permanent revolution. This was the message to be gleaned from the first *Manifesto of Surrealism* of 1924, according to which the goal of all surrealist activity was simply the revelation of the "actual functioning of thought."[7] By this Breton means all that has been repressed by the bourgeois superego. Breton's hyperevaluation of the revelations of the insane was part of a desire to devalue the ideology he detested.

Attacking ideology, Breton countered the belief in the hereditary determinism of insanity with the charge that social causes are primarily responsible for madness—and that psychiatrists are the first of these social causes. This accusation is voiced of Breton's quasi novel, *Nadja*. In this autobiographical narrative, Breton spends much time with a young woman, Nadja, who, struggling with incipient insanity, finally ends up in an asylum. Breton portrays his attempts to help her, but Nadja cannot cope with the exigencies of everyday life. In condemning a society that incarcerates those who cannot adjust to societal rules, Breton categorically declares, "You must have never entered an asylum not to know that the insane are produced there just as thieves are produced in jails."[8] The antipsychiatry movement of the 1960s is prefigured in Breton's indictment of the asylum as a producer of insanity:

> Is there anything more hateful than these institutions *[appareils]* supposedly for the conservation of society but which, for the least offense, for the slightest failure to observe decorum or common sense, hurl a poor subject into the company of other subjects whose company can only be harmful to him and, above all, systematically deprive him of relations with all those whose moral and practical sense has better foundations than his. (P. 161)

The asylum is the pivotal point for understanding how society exercises its power over the insane, which is to say, from Breton's perspective, all those who fail to subscribe to the dominant ideology of bourgeois rationality that it is psychiatry's task to enforce.

Madness is a fissure in ideology, and according to Breton this endows madness with its superiority over psychiatric medicine. It was not merely during the war that medicine had dishonored itself by forcing sane men to submit to institutionalized insanity; Breton later described nearly all psychiatric syndromes as codifications of moral prescriptions of some sort. Typical of this critique of nosology is an essay published, in 1930, in *Point du jour*. In it he attacked, for example, Bleuler for his notion of autism. Breton saw this clinical entity to be a deceptive way of turning egotism into a medical problem. Psychiatric clinical entities are merely, as Breton put it, a form of facile bourgeois denunciation "that allows one to consider as pathological everything that in humanity is not pure and simple adaptation to the exterior conditions of life, since it [this denunciation] aims secretly at exhausting all those cases of refusal, of rebellion, and of desertion that may or may not have appeared until now worthy of respect." By the latter Breton means such things as poetry, art, passion, or revolutionary action. In brief, doctors in the service of ideology are no longer doctors, they are jailers, or outfitters for prisons and scaffolds (pp. 91–92).

Polemics aside, surrealism did give the coup de grâce to the belief in norms in art. Surrealism accepted enthusiastically the Freudian version of the positivist axiom that, on the continuum from the normal to the abnormal, there is no break. Against the doctors, this axiom, according to surrealism, ultimately denies the existence of insanity and deviance: there are only repressions and denials. Demonstration of this axiom is another goal of *Nadja*. In demonstrating Nadja's incapacity to deal with reality—which means respecting a bourgeois sense of propriety—Breton declares, "The well-known absence of borderline between madness and nonmadness does not dispose me to grant a different value to the ideas and perceptions that are the affair of one state or the other" (p. 171). Madness disappears, and so does sanity, in this willingness to entertain the idea that all perceptions have equal interest. This is a curiously positivistic idea that underlines the power that positivism has had to shape our mental landscape. (I recall that the idea of pan-normality came into Freud through the work of nineteenth-century scientists like Claude Bernard for whom all that exists in nature is normal in the sense that it is the product of physiological processes that can be described by the always "normal" laws of chemistry and physics.) In praising folly Breton wants to abolish distinctions between the normal and the pathological by using the doctors' theory against them.

To this end he thus narrates the consequences of his dealings with Nadja.

This young woman, leading a marginal existence wandering on the streets, is not normal, and Breton knows that she is not normal, though it is not clear initially to what extent she is incapable of functioning in society. At the end of the book she apparently can no longer adapt herself to social demands and is placed in an institution. Breton is shaken, for it is at least arguable that his influence had been instrumental in her failure to adjust to social necessities. Can the unstable profit from surrealism? Breton admits that he had attempted to teach her the paramount surrealist lesson, that

> the freedom that one has acquired here at the price of a thousand of the most difficult renunciations demands that one enjoy it without restriction during the time in which this freedom is given, without any pragmatic consideration of any sort, and that because "human emancipation," conceived in definitive in the most simple revolutionary form, and which is nothing less than human emancipation in every respect, . . . remains the only cause that it is worthy to serve. (P. 168)

The contradictions involved in the utopian claim for absolute freedom are part of the surrealist stance in championing the rights of the insane to be insane. The right to be insane, totally insane, means the right to be a mass murderer like Charles Manson. Breton presumably knew full well that total freedom with no regard for others is not possible or desirable. But his poses sometimes suggest the contrary, and it does him little honor.

Breton wants the freedom to go mad to coincide with the liberation of the unconscious and all that is repressed. But when faced with real insanity and the social necessity of taking care of Nadja, he invokes a new principle that should somehow have intervened and protected her: the instinct of conservation must coexist with the desire for total freedom. Breton does not seem to me to be in good faith when he states in *Nadja* that he did not realize that Nadja could lose or perhaps had already lost that instinct for conservation that operates so that Breton and his surrealist friends all conduct themselves in conformity with the rules of bourgeois propriety (p. 169). The surrealists were willing to exploit the mad, but they were hardly willing to imitate them, at least not in the street.

Breton and his friends did imitate mad discourse, either explicitly, by imitating the discourses of the insane, or implicitly, by incorporating irrational associations into their work. What is of interest for my analysis of the modernist experience of madness is that Breton relied explicitly upon psychiatric classification when he supposedly wrote insane discourse. He did, or could, not propose some other way of dealing with madness. For example, to demonstrate the poetry of madness, Breton and Eluard published, in 1930, their collaborative work, *L'Immaculée Conception,* in which they simulated the discourse of severe mania, interpretive delirium, dementia praecox, general paralysis, and mental weakness—all this relying totally on psychiatric categories. This work wants to prove that, with proper poetic training, any normal person could produce madness: all of us can reach the poetry lying within, the poetry that rationality, from our earliest years, has repressed. Thus, from this democratic perspective, anyone can reach the utopian space of the marvelous or essential revelation. In simulating madness, in producing discourses that are the same as those produced by dementia praecox or severe mania, the first-person speaker of Breton and Eluard's text claims, in addition, to be destroying those "proud categories" used to pigeonhole the mad in the name of a rationality that "denies us every day the right to express ourselves by means that are instinctual in us":

> If I can, in succession, make speak through my own mouth the richest and the poorest being, the blind person and the hallucinating person, the most fearful and the most threatening being, how can I admit that this voice, which truly is just mine, comes to me from places that are even provisionally condemned, from places about which I must, with the common of mortals, despair of ever gaining access.[9]

With an irony that Hoffmann would have appreciated, Breton and Eluard declare that simulated madness may replace all other poetic genres. However, irony aside, it does not really seem that the homage paid psychiatric categories by imitating them would be the best way to destroy these categories.

In this work Eluard and Breton seem to believe that their delirious texts take the reader to a place that is normally beyond access. This place is variously the unconscious, the space of the repressed, or the locus of desire. Whatever be the formulation used to designate this essentially romantic space, it relies upon a metaphor that makes madness into a place, a space, a box, perhaps Pandora's box. This space is an enclosure into which one enters as into a room—though only surrealist activity offers a key to the door. In short, this spatializing of the unconscious transforms madness into a place. This is not a felicitous metaphor, neither in Freud nor in the surrealists. The idea that the unconscious is a type of space denies that madness is a series of disrupted relations that are often best characterized in terms of dynamics. When one gives up the notion that the self is a unified entity, characterized by an inner and outer dimension, it is quite difficult to conceive of any part of the self as some substantial place. This is a fundamental critique that one can make of the entire Freudian and subsequent surrealist topography of the self: it spatializes notions that should be looked upon simply as operative concepts, especially the notion of the unconscious. There is something remarkably simpleminded about the idea that one need merely gain access to a space in order to find the revelation of that true self—now expressed in madness—whose existence has been interdicted by social norms. This metaphor turns the self into a series of boxes. But this has been a powerful notion in the modernist experience of madness, of which surrealism can stand here as our most important exemplar. The power of misleading metaphors should never be underestimated.

With this metaphor in mind, the reader can plunge into a text of simulated madness and look for the "space" it opens. The last paragraph of an "Essai de simulation du délire d'interprétation"—or an attempt/test in simulating an interpretive delirium—gives a very lovely passage:

> Au commencement était le chant. Tout le monde aux fenêtres! On ne voit plus, d'un bord à l'autre, que Léda. Mes ailes tourbillonnantes sont les portes par lesquelles elle entre dans le cou du cygne, sur la grande place déserte qui est le coeur de l'oiseau de nuit. (P. 41)

> [In the beginning was the song. Everyone to the windows! Nothing can be seen, from one side to the other, except Leda. My swirling wings are the doors by which she enters into the neck of the swan, on the great deserted square that makes up the heart of the bird of night.]

There is really nothing in this text—a quite literary play with images taken from Greek myth—to differentiate it from many other surrealist texts. There is a series of irrational juxtapositions, obeying perfect grammar and syntax, that have a certain thematic coherence: they seem motivated by the revelation of night, which could characterize certain forms of insane discourse, especially if written by a gifted poet, whose self has lost its sense of the axis of discourse so that he or she cannot separate out the first and the third person. If this text is madness, then my very commentary shows to what extent madness has become readable by hermeneutic procedures that, at least since surrealism, are common property. Moreover, the aesthetics of surrealism allows the reader to recuperate the text's irrational disjunctions as surrealist poetry, and within the context of a book about insane texts, the poem is read as a text designed to illustrate the poetry of madness. This is a rather unsatisfactory way of explaining the modernist recourse to madness, but it must be said that readers of modern poetry must often use this hermeneutic axiom in order to find a way of entry into much modern literature.

Interpreting the Certifiably Insane Poetic Text:
Alexander and Artaud

In spite of its ambiguities and bad faith, surrealism is nonetheless largely responsible for the fact that we believe something can be found in insane discourse. After surrealism, it seems we are often drawn to poetry by the truly mad precisely for what we hope it may show about their capacity to plumb their own condition. Admittedly, what is usually revealed is that only a small percentage of the mad is gifted in the use of language. By making mad discourse a central issue for our modernity, surrealism brought about the necessity of sharpening our sense of contexts, of the necessity of rules for interpretation, as well as a belief in the aesthetic value of discourses that escape from those traditional language games that we call poetry, fiction, or simply literature.

To sharpen our discussion of what is at stake, then, in modernist incursions into madness, it seems imperative to read a poem by a certified schizophrenic, a "writer" who was incapable of functioning outside the asylum in which he was interned for life. Such a writer is Alexander. Alexander's poems have been collected by the psychiatrist Leo Navratil in his anthology of mad writings, *Schizophrenie und Sprache: Zur Psychologie der Dichtung.* Work like Alexander's brings up, most pointedly, questions as to whether the mad are surrealists, and, equally as important, what is the context for reading mad discourse? Has the modernist belief in madness made it possible to read what is written from within madness? Perhaps an answer can be given by a marvelous little text like Alexander's "Rot" (Red):

> Rot ist der Wein, rot sind die Nelken.
> Rot ist schön. Rote Blumen und rote.
> Farbe dazu ist schön.
> Die rote Farbe ist rot.
> Rot ist die Fahne, rot der Mohn.
> Rot sind die Lippen und der Mund.
> Rot ist die Wirklichkeit und der
> Herbst. Rot sind manche Blaue Blätter.[10]

> [Red is wine, red are the carnations.
> Red is beautiful. Red flowers and red.
> Color added to it is beautiful.
> The red color is red
> Red is the flag, red the poppy.

Red are the lips and the mouth.
Red is reality and the
autumn. Red are many blue leaves.]

This short poem immediately leaves the impression that one is confronting at once an automatism and a poetic sense that language can indeed color the world. Navratil, a psychiatrist with great sympathy for the needs of his patients, claims that such a text shows that the *Geist* within Alexander cannot be totally disturbed (p. 101). For the poem shows some inner dimension that has not been fully perturbed by madness. But the doctor also recognizes that schizophrenic discourse follows automatic patterns in its arbitrary associations and mannerisms; and, as he says, "In general these characteristics do not spring from the free will of the sick, but are underwritten by compulsions, automatic responses, and opposing impulses *[Gegenantriebe]*. What appears to us to be voluntary is experienced by the schizophrenic as unwilled, imposed, or even done by others" (p. 98). From this perspective, the poem is the product of uncontrolled forces that produce meaningless combinatory orders, meaningless because they do not correspond to any "will" to communicate. Yet, the aleatory associations do "reveal" an order of meaning that is independent of any intent that a schizophrenic may have had. The question is whether this order is imposed by language or, as the surrealists and Freudians hold, this order corresponds to something in Alexander's unconscious.

With this question the reader must face questions of context for the rules of interpretation. How does a "schizophrenic" line like "Red are many blue leaves" differ from a surrealist line, say, Eluard's "La terre est bleu comme une orange" [The earth is blue like an orange]? Formally, the two lines are the same: both are contradictory in terms of the logic of properties. Both are patent contradictions that flaunt our ordinary rules for usage.

But does an ambiguity remain after we contextualize these lines? Eluard's contradiction is part of a surrealist game in which we can look for associations that resolve the contradiction. Eluard's line presupposes that we will look to the earth to find properties of azure, of the ideal, and thus a sense of fullness that recalls the perfect roundness of the fruit; and both images are joined in a jubilatory celebration of the world. The surrealist context allows other rules of usage, including one that recognizes contradiction as a poetic way of getting around the restraints of logic.

When the context is the asylum, or when the text is granted to us as part of a therapy, this context hardly seems to allow the freedom of contextualization that aims at a celebration of the world. In Alexander's case we may ask instead if we are dealing with the attempt at the creation of an idiolect, a private language game—which flies in the face of what we recognize to be a property of linguistic usage. Having said all this, perhaps all we can affirm is that the rules of the schizophrenic's language game remain obscure, however much we feel that in this poem about red, there is a revelation of semantic combinations and associations that we had not perceived before. And that is a poetic act. But the rules of interpretation seem to be sui generis, specific to Alexander, whomever he may be. Of course, the mad text may also be contextualized by medical rules, as when Navratil speaks of the compulsions that produce it. This reductive reading hardly seems satisfactory for a poem like "Red"—for ultimately that reading means we are using psychiatric rationality to deny meaning to madness. The mad poem hovers on the borderline between a meaningless mechanism and an exploration of meaning that expands the possibilities of language.

Context is a constraint that madness renders problematic, for, if madness is a break with logos, then context is made impossible. However, interpretation of madness in literature has also been rendered problematic by the fact that, for various ideological reasons, modern literary theorists have often proposed models of interpretation that abolish context. Meaning is defined to be dependent only on the immediate context of rhetorical structures that the reader can supposedly perceive directly in the text. This belief in the immediate perception of meaning, promoted by doctrines as different as New Criticism or American deconstructionism, is part of the modernist belief in immediate revelation (or negative revelation in the case of deconstruction). Erroneously, this modernist hermeneutics dispenses with looking for a context, in which the rules for reading are established, in favor of an epiphanic revelation. However, a text by a surrealist poet, representing madness and thus undertaking a mimetic act, does not exist in the same context as a poem written by a schizophrenic writing when a doctor requests it. Surrealism denies the distinction, but this denial is born of a utopian desire for immediacy of meaning that transcends the limits of context. When pushed to the extreme, modernist hermeneutics reduces all texts to an eternal allegory, usually of desire, or lack, or some other eternal explanatory principle for which context is superfluous. Irony in New Criticism, desire in surrealism, self-representation in deconstruction are examples of this allegorical operation.

Expressionism and surrealism shared this belief in immediate meaning, however much some of their work problematizes it. Pathology was a universal allegory for the former, the expression of desire for the latter, and both are variants that make madness the ultimate referent of the modern text. It was, however, a former surrealist who most poignantly contested the possibility of the immediate revelation of meaning. The example of the truly insane Antonin Artaud (1896–1948) brings up the question of the hermeneutics of modern madness from a different perspective, for Artaud was a poet and he was mad. So he is another type of test case for whether madness can be an experience communicated by poetry. Artaud combines an Eluard and an Alexander, which decidedly complicates the rules for context. As a poet, actor, and theorist, in his madness Artaud wanted to express his authentic self. By this he meant revealing immediately, without language, some inner meaning of his self. To be "authentic," this revelation had to be unmediated by medical rationality, science, or universal logos. Thus Artaud believed that his true self was outside of any of the contexts that language needs for its operations. In short, it is impossible to name the self. Seeking immediate self-revelation in his madness, the poet had to contend with meanings that language automatically imposes upon the self. Artaud is emblematic of the modern poet who, struggling with recurrent insanity, believes that survival depends on making contact with his or her own self: the mad poet inevitably transforms this desire for authenticity into an existential odyssey that pursues a self that is beyond logos. Or, as Artaud wrote, with van Gogh's suicide in mind, "nobody ever wrote or painted, sculpted, or modeled, constructed or created, except to get in fact out of hell."[11]

Overcoming psychiatric determinations of madness is a matter of life and death, and more poets have died than survived in this struggle. In Artaud's archetypal struggle, the poet struggles with madness, not as some force within, but as an exteriority that besets the self, and psychiatry is part of that exteriority. Artaud reverses the dynamics of Freudian and surrealist spatial determinations for madness: insanity comes, not from within, but from without to besiege the self. Insanity is not a compensatory liberation, for Artaud's reversal portrays insanity as a place in discourse that is not spatially interiorized. Madness is lodged in the logos that invests and destroys the putative authentic self. It is hard to imagine a form of madness that is more perversely destructive for the poet, who has only language to work with.

Social repression is part of logos, and so the artist, like van Gogh, is "suicided" by society, and especially by doctors, who try to make him ingest language. In *Van Gogh le suicidé de la société* Artaud, like Breton, launches the attack on psychiatry for its role in creating the mad, though Artaud's attack is also part of a larger strategy by which he hopes to free himself from all the exterior forces—logos, God, society—that would determine his being as, he claims, they attempted to determine van Gogh's. This imposed exteriority is constitutive of his madness and van Gogh's:

> When I am sick, it's because I am enchanted, and I cannot believe that I am sick if I don't believe, on the other hand, that it is in someone's interest to take away my health and to profit from my health.
>
> Van Gogh also thought he was enchanted, and he said so. And I think quite pertinently that he was, too, and one day I'll tell how. (P. 34)

The paranoia of this text is obvious, and it is also obvious that paranoia says little about Artaud's madness. Artaud's madness is tied up with the very possibility—or impossibility—of creating a literature that would be more than literature: Artaud's project was to express his own being without using the common language—in short, God's logos. Language is the foundation of the self, and, if it cannot name itself, one can hardly "speak" of its existence. But anything that can be positively named is exterior to Artaud's being: hence his paradoxical sense of the total loss of any self, of any world, that might be his, precisely because language allows him to name an "I" that belongs not to him, but to language. Immediate expression is simply a deception worked by the wiles of God's logos.

For Artaud, the conflict with exteriority also characterizes being a body, a body that is at once the self and not the self, at once the source of being and of the pain and anguish that is inflicted upon the self by the body in its pathological alterity. The body is a contradictory presence that is lived as the excrescence that grants the poet an identity even as it ties him to the world as a pathological object. (Artaud often used drugs in an attempt to rid himself of the pain of having a body.) In his earliest texts of *Le pèse-neufs*—this "nerve balance"—that Louis Aragon published in 1925, Artaud began the search for a language that could correspond to physical states and thus "localize" the poet's being. Failing to find this language, he confronts his *impouvoir,* his lack of capacity, and experiences the loss of his own reality in each attempt: "Une espèce de déperdition constante du niveau normal de la réalité" [A constant wasting away of the normal level of reality].[12] This one-line text, simply naming the constant fading away of reality, could be the motto of the madness that haunts the modernist poet of loss. Even the body loses its cogency for the argument that, through a body, one belongs to the world.

Surrealist belief in immediate revelation seemed illusory to Artaud. At the beginning of *Le pèse-nerfs* Artaud made this clear in a critique of surrealism and its ambitions to find inner realms of plenitude:

I am still struck by this untiring, by this meteoric illusion that prompts us [souffle] with these limited, determined architectures, with thoughts, the segments of a crystallized soul, as if they were a great plastic page and were in osmosis with the rest of reality. And surreality is a shrinking of this osmosis, a sort of turned around communication. Rather than seeing in it a lessening of control, I see in it a greater control, but a control that, instead of acting, is distrustful, a control that stops encounters with the most ordinary reality and allows rarefied and subtle encounters, encounters that are worn down to the cord, and which catch fire and never break. (1:86)

Artaud still hoped for a means of discovering a plenitude of immediate presence in the form of an explosive reality: "I imagine a soul worked over and made into sulphur and phosphorous by these encounters, as the only acceptable state of reality." Anything less than a permanent incandescence is a wasting away, a loss of being, that Artaud could not tolerate. With this standard for existence, it is not difficult to see why Artaud never really believed in the immediacy of revelation that surrealism wanted to find in the self and its repressed world.

In spite of his desire to exist as a permanent incandescence, Artaud experienced his madness in infuriatingly traditional terms, for not even Artaud could escape culture. Artaud managed to overthrow psychiatry by destroying, symbolically, the body that would have made him a medical object. But at the same time he had to have recourse to traditional mediations to express himself. Consonant with all tradition, the myth of the fall is one of the central themes of his madness, as is the loss of paradise when the father threatens with the imagined castration that is also a saving crucifixion. In fact, Artaud often seems to have experienced his madness through myths that parallel the Freudian allegories of madness. The Oedipal myth in psychoanalysis transposes the Judeo-Christian myth of the Fall and the loss of paradise. After the fall, only through the fantasy of the castration-crucifixion can one reach the salvation of adulthood. Or, when this fails, one becomes a psychotic. Artaud lived his psychosis as a refusal to accept the crucifixion demanded by the father become superego, which is to say, the voice of divine logos that imposes laws as well as language.[13] The writer may revolt against the father, but this, too, can inflict destruction upon the rebel, for madness can result from the guilt the ambivalent son or daughter must feel about wanting to kill the parent. And with the parent's death every child feels an ambivalent loss, joyous over the death, and guilty about that joy, and even guilty about having, in fantasy terms, caused the death of the parental *Instanz* that judged the child. The complications of judgment and guilt are multiple and pervasive; and Artaud lived his madness as a dramatization of most of them. When not identifying with the Jesus whom God put on the cross, he was most resolutely determined to kill the original patriarch. Artaud did not commit suicide.

The Modern American Experience of Mad Discourse

In his madness Artaud nonetheless refused the Freudian romanticism of the quest for the revelation within. Artaud's example shows that a loss of the belief in inner revelation leaves intact the discourse on madness that takes madness to be a form of exteriority. This shift, from viewing insanity as inner revelation to seeing it as an exterior relation, centers madness on the body. It makes of insanity a relation to a world that is lived as intolerable loss. This description characterizes the way that, after Artaud, many modern poets have experienced madness in their poetry, especially a number of American confessional poets. After the demise of the surrealist utopian belief in inner madness, confessional poetry was written more in expressionist terms, again dictated by a vision of the pathology and dereliction of the body; and this is especially true of those American confessional poets who lived on the edge of sanity[14]—and who, unlike Artaud, often did not have a tenacious will to live and curse all those who robbed them of a self. With a sense of some mourning, both for American literature and for our culture, we can turn to two suicidal women for whom the experience of madness and poetry were much the same expressionist experience: Sylvia Plath and Anne Sexton. Their poetry shows these recurrent traits of the modernist experience of madness in a new guise, adjusted to a new context, in what we can see as the staging of the almost domestic confessional self.

Sylvia Plath (1932–1963) adopts in her poems a confessional stance that invites the reader at once into a world of madness while seemingly granting an ironic distance characteristic of romantic rhetoric. Once the reader realizes that this irony is part of the craft of madness, the poetic world Plath proposes is at times intolerable in its intensity. From her first encounter with madness, Plath wrote with what seems almost to be a premeditated savagery, preparing her second collection of poetry, *Ariel,* immediately before she killed herself (and which listeners can sense, I think, in her recorded reading of her poems). Her final poems read like a preparation for suicide, a kind of journal in which madness judges itself and justifies itself. As with Artaud, her madness is mediated at times by Freudian myth, at other times by the diagnosis of the white-coated doctors. The smell of electroshock treatment is never far way, and the doctor is at once friend and sadist. Tor-

tured and coy, such is the ambivalence of her poems as well as her autobiographical novel, *The Bell Jar* of 1960.

American confessional poets would like to believe in psychiatry, for faith
in doctors is part of the American credo. But much of their poetry documents, almost with pride, that medicine is not a match for madness. Plath
made that clear in a short story, "Johnny Panic and the Bible of Dreams,"
that can serve as an introduction to her poetry. Plath uses a nearly medieval
allegory to embody madness in a character called Johnny Panic. The story's
narrator knows that the doctors cannot rival with Panic. She knows much
about madness, because she works in an institution in which the mentally
disturbed are treated. Although she has yet to read all the dream records of
all the patients who have ever been to the clinic, she does type up the daily
records of the dreams of the unbalanced:

> [D]ay by day I see these psyche-doctors studying to win Johnny Panic's con-
> verts from him by hook, crook, and talk, talk, talk. Those deep-eyed, bush-
> bearded dream-collectors who precede me in history, and their contemporary
> inheritors with their white jackets and knotty-pine-paneled offices and
> leather couches, practised and still practise their dream-gathering for worldly
> ends: health and money, money and health. To be a true member of Johnny
> Panic's congregation one must forget the dreamer and remember the dream:
> the dreamer is merely a flimsy vehicle for the great Dream-Maker himself.
> This they will not do. Johnny Panic is gold in the bowels, and they try to root
> him out by spiritual stomach pumps.[15]

Doctors, with talk and stomach pumps, couches and dream collections, can
deal neither organically nor psychically with the allegorical figure who
invests the mad, the panic who uses the mad for his own expression.

Madness can be named only as something other than the "I," or perhaps
an "I" that is not really the self that the mad subject longs for. In this alienation, the self in distress can identify neither with its own madness nor with
the medical categories that the men in white jackets bandy about. Both
Trakl and Artaud show a comparable anguish about ever naming a self that
would be something other than a psychiatric category imposed by language.
Plath's confessional poetry engages in an equally hopeless struggle to end
the rupture that makes up the self's relation to the world. In despair her
work often takes the form of an apology for the necessity of death. Though
there are moments of revolt against the father, against the fascist patriarch
she erects as a kind of ideal psychotic superego, that revolt does not suffice.
She experiences the world as a total otherness to which death can be the
only satisfactory relation. Her well-known poem "Daddy" might at first
give the impression that, in violence or revolt, the poet can liberate herself

from the judgmental logos that condemns her to nonidentity. She apparently knows what liberation would entail, for like Artaud, she dreams a patricide:

> Daddy, I have had to kill you.
> You died before I had time—
> Marble-heavy, a bag full of God,
> Ghastly statue with one gray toe
> Big as a Frisco seal.[16]

In derision she notes that she has been to see the doctors and that they have used therapy on her:

> But they pulled me out of the sack,
> And they stuck me together with glue.
> And then I knew what to do.
> I made a model of you,
> A man in black with a Meinkampf look.
>
> And a love of the rack and the screw.
> And I said I do, I do.

In derision she shows that the sadism of the self-hatred she suffers is easily explained with Freudian allegories: she identifies with what persecutes her. The attempt to murder the father, to build for oneself an identity by destroying a "bag full of God," falls apart, however, when revolt fails to establish the relation of the self and a world. And every object in the world seems then to become an image of psychotic fantasies with which she identifies, since precisely that object isn't her. Paradoxically, objects are no identity, as one finds in her poem "Tulips."

Plath relies here as elsewhere upon Freudian categories to set up structures of intelligibility for what is essentially exterior to language: the utter dislocation of relationships that defies any discourse to account for them. In this regard "Tulips" is one of the most extraordinary texts presenting perception within madness and giving unique access to a psychotic state. The poem's speaker is in a hospital bed, the focal point for the disjuncture of self and world. She looks at the flowers in the room and finds that the "tulips are too excitable." In this opening line the dislocation of self and world is presented as a condition of things, for there is no self left to be a center to these relations:

> I am nobody; I have nothing to do with the explosions.
> I have given my name and my day-clothes up to the nurses

> And my history to the anaesthetist and my body to the surgeons.
>
> (P. 160)

Abandoning herself to the institution, to the others, to the ebb and flow of things, she compares herself to a nun: pure in some disconnected sense, approaching the purity of death and its lack of struggle. But the tulips remain, recalling the presence of the world that madness imposes upon her as a disruption:

> The tulips are too red in the first place, they hurt me.
> Even through the gift paper I could hear them breathe
> Lightly, through their white swaddlings, like an awful baby.
> Their redness talks to my wound, it corresponds.
>
> (P. 161)

In their expressionist alterity, things are present as a pathology that constitutes the narrator's world.

Paranoia can be easily invoked to characterize this experience of the world as a pathology in which things seem to watch the narrator, in which the "tulips eat up" her oxygen. But Plath's confessional image circumvents the category that would rob the poet of her madness by making it everyone's and anyone's ordinary madness. Hers is the madness of those moments in which a nobody—a void—is assaulted by the presence of things:

> The walls, also, seem to be warming themselves.
> The tulips should be behind bars like dangerous animals;
> They are opening like the mouth of some great African cat,
> And I am aware of my heart: it opens and closes
> Its bowl of red blooms out of sheer love of me.
> The water I taste is warm and salt, like the sea,
> And comes from a country far away as health.
>
> (P. 162)

With a distraught irony Plath closes this hallucination by making an implied comparison of tulips and heart, though the irony works to abolish any distinction between what would be inner and outer to the body, or an inner and outer self, leaving the poet a washed-over emptiness from which health is viewed as if on some distant shore.

The difficulty of being a voice belonging to no center of identity demands that the poet look constantly for doubles that "reflect" an identity that the poet does not really have. Identity can be had only by illogical assertion that identity is other than what the poetic persona is. In this way the poet is a mirror, something like an image or double of what she isn't. The second half of "Mirror" illustrates this well:

> Now I am a lake. A woman bends over me,
> Searching my reaches for what she really is.
> Then she turns to those liars, the candles or the moon.
> I see her back, and reflect it faithfully.
> She rewards me with tears and an agitation of hands.
> I am important to her. She comes and goes.
> Each morning it is her face that replaces the darkness.
> In me she has drowned a young girl, and in me an old woman
> Rises toward her day after day, like a terrible fish.
>
> (P. 174)

This poem presents a play of images recalling Kafka's expressionistic, psychotic gift for inverting logical relationships. The poet is the exterior image of herself, hence not herself, but an empty reflection of what she is, a double, but one without reality. She is at once other, and not anything, though, with the terrible destructive logic of the disintegrating mind, she can nonetheless become an image of the body's coming apart, its destruction leaping forward into consciousness with a flash of color "like a terrible fish."

Much of Plath's poetry, like much modernist experience of madness, explores its disintegration by finding images of exteriority that are doubles of itself—or nonself. These images are only indirectly presented as doubles, for the modernist mind, on the edge of chaos, refuses to suggest really solid links between the void that it takes for its identity and the image that it then offers of its nonbeing. Some images in Plath are, of course, expressionistic in their description of pathology, as when, in "Lady Lazarus," the poet's persona finds her "skin / bright as a Nazi lampshade" (p. 244), or, in "Elm," when the persona seemingly becomes a tree, inhabited by a cry, perhaps a nocturnal raptor, so that "Nightly it flaps out / Looking, with its hooks, for something to love" (p. 193). At other times there is a surrealist indirection to her presented disjunctions between the self and the exterior forces— father, logos, body—that besiege the not-real self. All of which comes madly together in *Ariel*'s "The Hanging Man":

> By the roots of my hair some god got hold of me.
> I sizzled in his blue volts like a desert prophet.
>
> The nights snapped out of sight like a lizard's eyelid:
> A world of bald white days in a shadeless socket.

> A vulturous boredom pinned me in this tree.
> If he were I, he would do what I did.

(Pp. 141–42)

The dialectic of self and exterior object finds a logical culmination in the image of Promethean emptiness that seems fated, without explanation, to endure an eternity of absurd torture to which the poet assents, perhaps as the only way to find some justification for being riveted to a mountain of psychosis.

It is with some relief that a reader leaves the tortured logic of the self-denying identities created by a poet like Plath and confronts the anguish of her contemporary, Anne Sexton (1928–1974). The relief is only temporary, for Sexton invites the reader to step into a lyrical realm of suicide. Sexton's domestic madness is our final exemplar, for she rounds out our view of the modernist experience of madness. Though both Plath and Sexton committed suicide, Sexton's itinerary through madness was the opposite of Plath's: Sexton was a poet who actively desired some exteriority that might allow her to mediate her madness. And she lived her madness largely through perception of it afforded by psychoanalysis. Plath's and Sexton's works thus offer complementarity in their exploring the opposing possibilities of modern madness. Plath's self-denying projections find an almost logical complement in Sexton's sweet madness that is all the more despairing in that it apparently seeks some mediating solace for the disjunctures that madness afflicts upon Sexton's fragile self. But, in despair, the only solution is again Death, at times an allegorical figure, but finally the real solution to which the poet had recourse after several unsuccessful attempts.

Suicide is the ultimate horizon of Sexton's world within which the confessional imagination tries to work through madness. Sexton calls upon some exterior figure—father, "father-doctor," some Oedipal deity, Jesus, God, or simply a family—that can anchor a world in which the nonreal self can find identity bestowed upon it from without.[17] It is in this sense that Sexton's work unfolds with reverse symmetry to Plath's work, or Artaud's, in the Freudian space that provided them with the arena for their revolt and rage. Unlike the Artaud who refused to Jesus the right to incarnate the logos that the poet wanted uniquely for himself, Sexton writes that "Mrs. Sexton went out looking for the gods," or so reads the first line of *The Death Notebooks* (p. 349). Her search presents another contradictory, modernist possibility in writing and living insanity: the impossible possibility that the poet, struggling with recurrent madness, might anchor the self in transcendence.

However, this is a disappointing transcendence that shows itself to be a projection of alienated need.

Like every child of Nietzsche, Freud, or Kafka, Sexton found that the gods had died, even if they live on in a memory that is sublimated into the present. The Hegelian notion of sublimation can be used to explain the modernist concept of time and history, or the sense of the fall that has been developing since the romantics. The concept of sublimation contains within it the idea that, though we have fallen into time, indeed we have lost the past, nonetheless the past lives on in the present sublimated as a form of reminiscence. The modernist lives nostalgically the present as a loss of the plenitude we believe to have once existed in the past—the past is lost but present as loss in the present. This view of sublimated loss is an essential feature of modernist consciousness, be it in Joyce, Proust, Kafka, or Freud. The fall into time is a destructive modernist possibility for living madness: madness also takes the form of nostalgia for the past as a present. It can take the form of death-oriented anguish about a continuity with the past after all relations to time have been severed. This theme of the past in the present is such a dominant modernist motif that it has led some theorists to consider the mad person's relation to time, in the form of regression, the key to all insanity. When the psychotic invents another world, his or her madness signifies a refusal of present reality: this refusal leads the mad to resurrect past infantile structures of consciousness that abolish the present and restore the past. In this vein, both the Freud of the unresolved Oedipal complex and the Foucault of *Mental Illness and Psychology* propose that the psychotic denial of reality is often, if not usually, an attempt to return to some past, to fix the past in the present as a recovered plenitude—which shows that the romantic belief in our fall into the finitude of time is an origin of much current theory about psychopathology.

Sexton's image for this nostalgia is that she was wedded to her teddy. In "Mothers" the regression from present emptiness is expressed with childlike simplicity that in itself is a refusal of the present:

> Oh mother,
> after this lap of childhood
> I will never go forth
> into the big people's world
> as an alien,
> a fabrication,
> or falter

> when someone else
> is as empty as a shoe.

(P. 465)

To justify this refusal to leave childhood, Sexton seizes upon motifs of the fall, for her present self is a void: the empty shoe that is at once self and other, present here and now, but longing for the past. To overcome this emptiness she constantly seeks, with childlike greediness, some exterior confirmation of her being that she knows will never really occur, since, Kafka-like, if it were to occur it would be insufficient.

The past thus becomes grist for the therapy session. In the posthumously published poems of *Words for Doctor Y.*, Sexton stages her needs in her therapeutic sessions with her psychiatrist. In these texts she confesses her evil nature, describes the voices that speak to her, and laments an exile from God that seems as much an exile from childhood. In her extreme need, even madness can be defended as a gift, desperately portrayed as an endowment from without:

> What about all the psychotics
> of the world?
> Why do they keep eating?
> Why do they keep making plans
> and meeting people at the appointed time?
> Don't they know there is nothing,
> a void, an eyeless socket,
> a grave with the corpse stolen?
> Don't they know that God gave them
> their miraculous sickness
> like a shield, like armor
> and if their eyes are in the wrong
> part of their heads, they shouldn't complain?
> What are they doing seeing their doctors
> when the world's up for grabs.

(P. 574)

Lamenting that even death can be stolen from the psychotic, this type of poem affirms and denies the value of madness in the same phrase. With ironic ambivalence, and a good bit of hubris, the poet demands as her own the very concept of "psychotic." If we grant her this rubric, she has a way of positioning herself between a world of loss, "a grave with the corpse stolen," and a world of miraculous being that, in spite of her childlike desire for faith, she does not really believe to exist.

In the same poems, a patriarchal doctor comes forward as the godlike figure who listens to her hallucinations and then breaks into her world, allowing her to resurrect some relationship with the past:

> My little illustrated armor,
> my hard, hard shell has cracked
> for Dr. Y. held my hand
> and with that touch
> my dead father rode on the Superchief
> back to me with dollar bills in his fist
> and my dead mother started to knit me a sweater
> and told me, as usual, to sit up straight,
> and my dead sister danced into the room
> to borrow something and I said
> yes, yes, yes

(P. 578)

Sexton longs to fuse with the past. But she is playing in despair with Freud and Joyce, whatever be the reality of the momentary solace she achieved in therapy. She throws herself into regression, but her madness is filtered through a series of intertextual reflections and mediations. In describing the magic of the doctor's holding her hand, Sexton alludes knowingly to the Freudian therapeutic transference. Transference should open up the resurrected past, the past a child remembers when the Superchief locomotive, associated with the dead father, was the image of what the recent past took for modernity. It is a past in which the mythical family of fragmented memory suddenly lives, affirmed in the final line by the repetition of the last lines of Molly Bloom's soliloquy in Joyce's *Ulysses*. Sexton's identification with Molly, also found in "The Dead Heart," is revealing. Joyce's heroine speaks these lines in a kind of cosmic affirmation of love, which is what the psychotic undoubtedly hopes to find in the therapeutic transaction.

Literature can be affirmation—what Kafka called prayer. Prayer articulates the hope allowing at least momentary escape from madness, as in Sexton's prayer called "For the Year of the Insane." She prays to the Virgin Mary to be intercessor, to be a therapeutic goddess. The poetess wants to see Mary point to a way that will lead out of the anguish of the ongoing dead past, and away from the pain of the body that is the concrete place for the anguish about the sublimation of the past. Sexton experiences anguish about losing the past in the body. Pain is there, and the body with its blood is a prison:

> O Mary, open your eyelids.
> I am in the domain of silence,

the kingdom of the crazy and the sleeper.
there is blood here
and I have eaten it.
O mother of the womb,
did I come for blood alone?
O little mother,
I am in my own mind.
I am locked in the wrong house.

(P. 133)

She is locked in a house in whose cellar one finds "Freud shoveling dirt" (p. 569). On the main floor struggles the ego convicted of narcissism. The struggle takes place in the physical house of the body wherein the dead father, the allegorical superego, continues to live, creating despair by his present absence, and pain by his sublimated dead presence. The contradictory logic of Freudian space was perhaps never better portrayed than in these intolerably painful poems. Locked in the haunted house of the self, the poet experiences the Freudian spatial topography as her body's way of being mad.

To say that madness is lived in terms of the dominant discourse of a period, of modernism in Sexton's case, is to say again that madness elects whatever discourse is available to it. Unfortunately, this is not to say that the dominant discourse allows the poet to triumph over madness. On the contrary, it seems that living out psychiatric categories or a Freudian allegory is more often a cause for despair. And Sexton found no more solace in the transcendental modern doctor than in the God of her childhood.

In their suicidal anguish, these examples of modernist discourses in madness—those of Trakl and Artaud, of Plath and Sexton—suggest a unified experience that characterized the writing and living out of madness by modern writers. These examples finally show that the extraordinary number of modernist poets for whom madness was the central issue of their work originates in a historical moment when madness became readable because we wanted to read the aberrations of our self and our culture. I hope to have shown that these poetic discourses share, even when they contest, the same axioms that modern medical discourses have used to describe insanity. In one sense this has meant that poets have lived their madness in terms of discourses that ask them to give credibility to madness at the same time these discourses denigrate or deny madness any meaning. This ambivalence, to use a good Freudian term, has not been eliminated by simply proposing that the poet must chose between Freud and Kraepelin, psychoanalysis or psychiatry, to explain madness. Our examples depict the suffering with which modern poets have been obliged to live their madness through both discourses, and neither have provided a mediation that allows madness to be lived as anything but anguish and despair. But perhaps there has been more triumph in these poets than I have suggested. Since antiquity it has been evident that an animal like *homo sapiens* is unique in the capacity to write poems and go insane. Modernism sharpens our understanding that the imaginative use of language often resembles going insane, for both can share the common project to create a world through language. In this creation poetry is sometimes successful, madness often is not. And perhaps there is a bitter success in the very fact that a Trakl or a Plath could use language to create the record of defeat by madness, or the defeat of medicine by insanity. For, to conclude and to recapitulate, during most of the twentieth century, the matrix allowing literature to speak madness has been fixed by those psychiatric and psychoanalytic discourses that have determined not only how we analyze the mad, but how the mad experience and write about their own fall from reason, into despair, melancholy, and hallucinatory worlds, which often results in suicide, but also sometimes in fragile triumphs called poetry.

Chapter 10

The Contemporary Scene's Affirmation of and Rebellion against Logos

Logos and Cybernetic and Linguistic Theories of the Psyche

Since roughly World War II cybernetics and linguistics have inspired new theories of madness. These new theories have not rejected psychiatry and psychoanalysis; rather, cybernetics and linguistics have tried to incorporate these medical discourses into their far-reaching theories of mind and madness. The new theories reflect a widely held belief that the human mind can be described by concepts of cybernetic governance and information flow or that the mind is (something like) a computer. A variant on this belief is that the mind is the locus of actualization of a linguistic system and its functioning. Even when recognizing neurological concepts, contemporary thought is fascinated by the idea that mind is more than a biological dependency: the postmodern mind is an agent of communication, information flow, or language processing. In this regard postmodern thought seems to have effected a return to Greek thought. For, today, mind is considered to be constituted by some milieu larger than itself, and it can be argued that this milieu seems quite analogous to what the Greeks meant by logos: the transindividual milieu of language, reason, mathematics, and harmonious relations.

The contemporary doctrine of logos proposes that a culture's language—or the cultural cybernetic system or ecosystem—makes of the individual mind itself a localized feedback system, a recursive function, or a second-order system, all of these ordered by the larger system conceived as the information system making up culture or language. These views propose a mind that is neither entirely metaphysical nor biological. Rather, postmodern thought theorizes that, in addition to or beyond metaphysics or physiology, mind is more like a software system programmed by culture, or a matrix informed by language and hence by cultural programs. Brain cells and neurological linkage are the hardware, to use a dubious metaphor; but mind itself is part of a larger informational system. The concept of logos in the Greek sense of language and relations can also describe this pancultural system, since the metaphor of hardware links up easily with the notion that language or culture is software that programs the individual mind.

Metaphors, however misleading, should not be hidden. When "software" is used as a metaphor to describe the contents of mind, the effect is to make of mind a position in a logos transcending the individual mind. Software is culture seen as a program. In brief, then, our postmodern metaphors compare the mind to a kind of program using a biological terminal plugged into a larger system. It is the larger system that grants mind its capacity to function sanely by its participation in culture, understood also as what is encoded or programmed in language.

Psychopathology, understood as a rupture in the program or logos, is defined cybernetically as some kind of disturbance in the system. This systemic view appears to rob madness of much of its poetical and mythical functions. Programmers are little inclined to believe that an entropic dysfunction can bring about a mystical revelation. And one would not expect to find a promise of revelation in the exemplary theory of madness proposed by psychiatrist Jurgen Ruesch and anthropologist Gregory Bateson when they adapt psychiatry to cybernetics (or vice versa?):

> Psychopathology is defined in terms of disturbances of communication. This statement may come as a surprise, but if the reader cares to open a textbook on psychiatry and to read about the manic-depressive or the schizophrenic psychosis, for example, he is likely to find terms such as "illusions," "delusions," "hallucinations," "flight of ideas," "disassociation," "mental retardation," "elation," "withdrawal," and many others, which refer specifically to disturbances of communication; they imply either that perception is distorted or that expression—that is, transmission—is unintelligible.[1]

Hallucinations or disassociation are here turned into a question of communication, since these perturbations can be described as breakdowns in circuitry, or, alternatively, as purposeful attempts at managing semantic networks that have gone astray. Subjective phenomena such as delusions are transformed, by the axioms of the methodology, into a public phenomenon: madness must be a question of public channels because communication can only be defined as a public area to which, by definition, we all have access.

There is necessarily a social dimension to madness if insanity reflects a distortion in communication, in systems, or language circuits. Whence comes much of the impetus for recent antipsychiatry with its insistence that madness reflects social pathologies that express themselves through the individual victim of madness. And whence derives the contemporary literary text that wants to make of madness a revelation of our social dysfunctions.

But we shall deal with literature only after we have staked out the territory in which madness is made into a cybernetic or a linguistic phenomenon.

Since World War II there have been so many schools, movements, factions, and counterfactions in abnormal psychology and therapy that it may seem almost absurd to privilege any one of them. But if we keep in mind the question of systemics and the correlated view that madness has a social matrix, we can make sense of most of these movements as so many variants on a theme—complicated by their use of traditional psychiatric and psychoanalytical models that are still quite dominant. To speak of postmodernity, therefore, I feel justified to select two influential thinkers who illustrate cybernetic and linguistic theories of madness that do break with traditional models. These thinkers are the English anthropologist Gregory Bateson and the French psychoanalyst Jacques Lacan. Both have had great influence in molding contemporary thought by propounding generalized theories about mind and logos. Bateson's influence in psychotherapy is perhaps waning, though it is not impossible that his thought on the relation of mind and ecology, on mental health and homeostasis, could in some form become the dominant view of madness in the future. Lacan's influence has been great among humanists, who have been attracted to his attempt to "rethink" Freud through structural linguistics. In Europe and Latin America Lacan has had a major influence on the practice of psychotherapy as well as on theory.

It is remarkable to what extent comparable axioms undergird the thought of these two thinkers from different disciplines. Though Lacan was a medical doctor trained in psychiatry, and Bateson began as an academic anthropologist, in their attempt to rethink madness they both enlarged their theory by borrowing from other disciplines. Structural linguistics and Lévi-Strauss's anthropology are dominant influences on Lacan's work, whereas the anthropologist Bateson worked in psychotherapy after being initiated into Norbert Wiener's cybernetics and Shannon's formalization of information theory. Their theories of madness presuppose theories about communication and information theory according to which language and communication are the key to social adaptation. Psychosis is primarily a question of not having access to the proper circuits, or of being excluded from a culture's symbolic system, since sanity demands that the self be integrated into an information-flow system. Like tragedians with computers, Bateson and Lacan have refurbished, then, a doctrine of logos for the information era.

The individual mind is a locus in communication circuits that are larger than the individual mind. From a biological viewpoint these circuits include the ecological system of which any mind is a realization. From an anthropological viewpoint, the system is identified with language itself and all the cultural codes that language embodies. This view of mind breaks with positivist medicine, for mind is coextensive with culture and the codes that make it up; or mind is viewed as an individual instance within the ecology of mind composed of all the interconnecting systems of culture and neurology. According to Bateson, mind is a false reification when considered apart from the "interlocking processes" of communication systems that make up our ecology.[2] Or, according to Lacan, the "subject" is always absent to itself since the subject is a position in the symbolic system of language. Both of these viewpoints appear to reject the traditional humanist claim that, in its autonomy, the self is a self-empowered agent. In their demystification of human autonomy, Bateson and Lacan join the hosts of other contemporary demystifiers, from Marxists to behaviorists, who reduce the self, if not to an illusion, at least to what Sartre called, speaking satirically about the Freudian self, the "dear absent one."[3] But Sartre was once a humanist.

Bateson, Schizophrenia, and the Theory of the Double Bind

The self is a process, not a substance; or it can be likened to a matrix for processing symbols encoding social values. When this matrix is perturbed, insanity results. Psychotherapy is possible if the therapist can find and correct the disruptions of the feedback procedures that normally allow for equilibrium and a healthy adaptation to the world (*Psychiatry,* p. 233). Or as Bateson and Ruesch succinctly state, with a terminology that wants to reconcile biology and cybernetics, the "organism" is a self-corrective entity that needs adequate data about its errors. Bateson's later papers in *Steps to an Ecology of Mind* (1972) evince less interest in biological concepts, for he is more interested in a theory of madness based on communication. Biology is integrated into a larger concept of ecology. In these papers he formulates the theory of the "double bind" as a way of describing a perturbation in communication. The double bind is a derangement of information flow, and it explains the etiology of schizophrenia strictly in communicational and hence social terms. The etiology of schizophrenia is not engendered by a single trauma. Rather schizophrenics are produced by "sequential patterns" in families in which children receive conflicting messages (*Steps,* p. 206). Parents sabotage their children by giving them contradictory information patterns; and finally the children are no longer capable of sorting out types of messages. This disorder in turn results in the disruption of normal corrective feedback procedures that allow children to understand messages, information, and the levels and types of statements they are receiving.

The contradiction at the heart of the double bind is simple enough. Parents communicate a contradictory message—or "two orders of message" (p. 213)—that is simultaneously decoded as containing contradictory imperatives: the parent says at once, "Love me or I'll kill you," and "If you love me, I'll kill you." The first might be communicated linguistically, the second with body language. Bateson proposes that there is in a real sense unconscious communication, especially dealing with "matters of relation" between human beings and with their environment, communication that can rapidly become pathogenic (p. 413). Psychotic behavior can be construed then to be a defense on the part of a victim who does not know, after confronting these patterns of contradictory messages, how to sort out and decipher messages in terms of content, levels, and types. As Bateson makes clear, this reaction is part of an information flow, since, if a person cannot decode in a proper fashion, then he or she "is like any self-correcting system which has lost its governor; it spirals into never-ending, but always systematic, distortions" (pp. 212–13).

The popularity of Bateson's views may be due in part to the clarity with which he expressed tragic pathos about a cybernetic system gone amuck. Bateson himself encouraged the application of his thought to a great variety of situations, wherever communication can be taken to be a key to the analysis of social or individual phenomena.[4] His success can also be explained by his appeal to Americans' optimistic enthusiasm for any broad-ranging theory that promises pragmatic results. Bateson's work says that therapy is possible, because even the past can be changed. Dealing with the regressive angst of modernist nostalgia, Bateson's therapist is capable of changing the way the schizophrenics deal with their past: "What exists today are only messages about the past which we call memories, and these messages can always be framed and modulated from moment to moment" (p. 233). Bateson's psychic cybernetician is able to reorder the past—and perhaps even abolish the tragic destiny that Freud deterministically ascribed to every unresolved Oedipal crisis. Moreover, Bateson's theories of memory are consonant with recent views that the past *is* a type of neurological circuit. For example, the neurologist Gerald Edelman says that memory is a process of continuous reordering of mappings of neuronal groups. Edelman seems remarkably close to the psychotherapist when he says that through new contextualizations and synaptic associations there is a continual alteration in global mappings that constitute the mind's view of its past.[5]

Bateson and other communication theorists use, however, little in the way of direct neurological investigation to argue the a priori necessity with which communication theory can describe all levels of biological organization as forms of messages. Bateson is clear on this point:

> A priori it can be argued that all perception and all response, all behavior and all classes of behavior, all learning and all genetics, all neurophysiology and endocrinology, all organization and all evolution—one entire subject matter—must be regarded as communicational in nature, and therefore subject to the great generalizations or "laws" which apply to communicative phenomena. (*Steps*, pp. 282–83)

Without disputing Bateson's claims that logos in the form of codes, messages, and information flow is at work in all biological organization, including mind, the historical reader inevitably recalls that Bateson's claims are reminiscent of the all-encompassing theories of, say, mechanics in the eighteenth century. In the eighteenth century it was impossible to think beyond the models provided by mechanics. Is this the case today with regard to models of mind provided by computers and information theory? And with regard to schizophrenia, Bateson's claims about the double bind may seem to do little more than demonstrate how a single-variable all-encompassing model—if not metaphor—can always be applied to every type of inquiry. Families produce schizophrenics, says this model, and the producer of madness is the absence of the homeostatic circuit of communication that every family ought to have in place. The proof is found in the dissolute mind of the schizophrenic that perforce must have some kind of family. This may seem circular; but proof is always difficult in matters of mind, since whatever the mind can imagine about itself often becomes the case.

Lacanian Tragedies in Logos

Jacques Lacan brought a different emphasis to the understanding madness, one allowing for the work of the imagination. Wanting to "rethink" psychoanalysis, he transformed psychoanalysis into a theory of communication, or of the failure of communication. Taking structural linguistics and anthropology as his guide, Lacan conceived the human subject not as a presence, but rather as an absence. The subject is never present to itself, Lacan claims, because it is an effect of language: the subject is the subject of language and, as such, is always elsewhere, immanent to the linguistic system that unconsciously forms the subject. Consciousness is not the primary place to look for the self, for the total mind is larger than the conscious self—which is often informed by the imaginary. The self or ego is not conscious of the totality of mind.

The view that the human self is larger than the individual conscious ego is of course Freudian. But, different from Freud, Lacan shares with Bateson the belief that mind is not immanent to the circuitry contained within a single "brain and body," but, as Bateson says, that "mind is immanent in the larger system—man *plus* environment" (*Steps,* p. 317). Lacan shares the view that mind is essentially programmed by culture, through the larger environment of language. For his specific concepts, however, Lacan turns to structural linguistics and its description of language as a system made up of signs. Signs are constituted by signifieds (concepts) and signifiers, or the material embodiment of the signifieds, that can only be identified by their difference from each other. Lacan argues that meaning is produced by the differing play of signifiers that refer to something other than themselves. This differential flow of signifiers means that the self is decentered by the signifiers that institute it. The self is not present to itself, a paradoxical view that Bateson also defended. In his terms Bateson argues that, if consciousness has feedback upon mind and if consciousness deals with only a skewed sample of the events of the total mind, then "there must exist a *systematic* (i. e. nonrandom) difference between the conscious views of self and the world, and the true nature of self and the world" (p. 444). The alienation of the knowing self from itself characterizes both Lacan and Bateson's supposedly normal subject as it processes the information flow and signifiers that constitute it.

Once their axioms are in place, Lacan and Bateson both develop a powerful model for explaining the perpetual miscommunication that is central to the subject. Lacan's subject is in this regard a tragic self forever dispossessed of the world it desires; and Lacan's type of analysis can be called literary if we mean by literary a tragic view based on the way language shapes the self—or subject, as Lacanians prefer, reserving the notion of ego for that deceptive image that imagination grants to consciousness. The tragic subject is unconsciously tragic, however, since Lacan theorizes language as the medium in which the subject, unknown to itself, is constituted by the unconscious messages that logos codifies, seemingly, for itself.

The elaboration of this doctrine is found in Lacan's *Ecrits* (1966), the volume containing his principal texts written for publication. In them Lacan betrays a high priest's desire to use an oracular style that must be mastered before the neophyte can be initiated into the master's world of metapsychological reflection. His seminars are different. Full of an arrogant pedagogue's sarcasm and sometimes affectionate scorn for his benighted pupils, these transcriptions reveal the tragic thinker, masquerading at times as a clown, who doubts that communication can ever take place, least of all in a seminar. In these essays and seminars Lacan asks us to entertain something like the following question: if we are born into a culture that is coextensive with language, what are the requirements for a psychiatry consonant with the hypothesis that there is no human self without language? If this hypothesis is accepted as incontrovertible—and it probably isn't—then a structuralist theory can presuppose acceptance of the axioms declaring that language is an autonomous system and that the linguistic system is dominant in defining the cultural matrix that constitutes the subject. Language transcends any individual speaker so that, again from the structuralist viewpoint, language must inform the individual subject. This interesting, if dubious, axiom leads to the view that the subject is a position within a linguistic matrix. The subject exists as a realization of the combinatory possibilities of language, so that each subject is a repository for the cultural possibilities encoded in the language that speaks through the individual.

For a neo-Freudian confronting cybernetics, the structuralist paradigm has the attraction that it allows the theorist to situate the unconscious in a nonspatial way somewhere in the unfolding of logos. The unconscious is defined as a "space" in language, not as some physical locus, like Anne Sexton's metaphysical cellar in which the id is lodged like a raging captive. The unconscious is a necessary operational hypothesis to account for certain effects of psychic life as informed by language. So, Lacan adds, the unconscious is structured like a language, if it is not language. The unconscious is that place where language unfolds, the locus of the symbolic system by which we are formed but to which we are never completely consciously present. Paradoxically enough, for contemporary theory the conscious mind is more of a problem than the unconscious one. In considering Freud's achievement, for example, Bateson after Lacan finds himself obliged to resolve the great problem of consciousness:

> We presume that consciousness is not entirely without effect—that it is not a mere collateral resonance without feedback into the system, an observer behind a one-way mirror, a TV monitor which does not itself affect the program. We believe that consciousness has feedback into the remainder of mind and so an effect upon action. (P. 444)

But these "effects" are unknown to the information theorist.

According to Lacan, in a state of consciousness we are present to ourselves as the ego or *moi* that is a creation of the imaginary. The imaginary is the second coordinate, after the symbolic, in Lacan's psychoanalytic description of the self. In early work Lacan described the formation of the ego as a product of images, and he formulated the idea that we all pass through a mirror stage in our assuming an ego that we usually believe to have some substantial reality. Or to offer a sample of Lacanese from "Le Stade du mirroir" of 1949:

> L'assomption jubilatoire de son image spéculaire par l'être encore plongé dans l'impuissance motrice et la dépendance du nourrissage qu'est le petit homme à ce stade *infans,* nous paraîtra dès lors manifester en une situation exemplaire la matrice symbolique où le *je* se précipite en une forme primordiale, avant qu'il ne s'objective dans la dialectique de l'identification à l'autre et que le langage ne lui restitue dans l'universel sa fonction de sujet.[6]

This remarkable sentence about the mirror stage recapitulates what I have said, I hope, up to this point; in a paraphrase translation, the child assumes in jubilation his specular image, at a time when he is undeveloped in terms of motor functions and still dependent on nursing; and this assumption of his image by the little man in the infantile stage causes to appear, in an exemplary situation, the symbolic matrix into which the "I" is, in a nascent form, plunged, before this "I" enters into the dialectic of identity with the other and before language confers upon him his function as a subject existing in the sphere of symbolic universality. So the infant first acquires the imaginary function through vision, then enters into symbolic relations through language, relations that are perforce mediated by others, or by the Other as Lacan says.

The mirror stage is an update of the speculum of romantic psychiatry. It remains fundamental throughout Lacan's thought, for it is the experience of an initial alienation that sets the stage for all the other alienations he describes. In the later essay "La chose freudienne" (1955) he ties ego development more closely to the development of desire and narcissism. In addition to the romantic ironist there lurks in Lacan an old-fashioned Ciceronian *moraliste* ready to berate the passions, for he discovers that the imaginary functions through passion to form the "I." "I" am formed when passion brings to every relation with the image "that is constantly represented" a meaning that "makes me exist as this image, in such a dependency, that this image ties to the desire of the other all the objects of my desires, in the most intimate way to the desire that they arouse in me" (1:238). Desire is mediated by the other both in the sense that one desires what the other desires because the other desires it, and in the sense that one desires something other than oneself—for desire is always desire beyond a lack in the self.

Psychic life is tied, through the imagination, to an image of self that depends on others; and through the symbolic order to a reign of linguistically encoded messages that are forever absent from consciousness. The self is a product of a double alienation. The subject only exists as the other, or through the symbolic order represented in Western culture ultimately by the "name of the father," the guarantor of the "phallic signifier" that grounds all other signifiers in culture and language. Lacan is quite clear: it is the paternal imago that offers access to the symbolic order. And psychosis can be avoided only if the subject is integrated into the order of signifiers identified with the father and the phallus. Logos is identified with the patriarch—a question to which we shall return at the end of this chapter in our considerations of the feminist way of contesting logos.

The third coordinate that constitutes psychic life for Lacan is the "real." The real is what exists for the subject outside of the realm of language; perhaps it is best looked upon as the realm of trauma and, finally, death. The real cannot be said; but it is ready to tear asunder the realm of language, the symbolic, which is the ground of the self. Mental illness hovers over Lacan's vision of the subject, since the ego exists for us only in illusory identifications of the imaginary, and our "authentic being" is in the absent world of signifiers over which we have no control. Or perhaps one should speak of a perpetual split, in which the unstable ego floats in intersection with the alienated subject. In an early seminar on the ego in Freud's work, Lacan seems to regard insanity as an intrinsic part of the relations of the ego and the subject since, to paraphrase the untranslatable, the ego is a point of attachment between common discourse in which the subject is caught and alienated, and the subject's own psychological reality. Moreover, the imaginary relation (involving both images and that which is phantasmic) is deviant in human beings insofar as here is where is found the opening or gap through which death acquires presence. The symbolic world, whose very foundation is based on the phenomenon of insistent repetition (since signs acquire identity through repetition), is alienating for the subject, or more exactly, this world is the cause of the fact that the subject's truth is always hidden from him somewhere. The ego exists at the point of intersection of one and of the other—which I would gloss as the point where the subject carves out a space in the flow of information, communication, and signifiers that actualize a subject.[7]

Lacan's point is that this flow of signifiers is alienating by its very nature. It is always somewhere other than where we think it is, so communication seems impossible in any real sense. From his tragic perspective, Lacan uses a communication model to describe madness, madness that may appear to be our daily lot. Psychosis occurs when there is a *béance*—a break or gap—

in the chain of signifiers that constitute the subject. The causes for this break, the etiology of psychosis, are as varied as the patients who find themselves unable to engage in the normal repression that characterizes the relatively sane subject. The mad find themselves overwhelmed by the flow of signifiers that make up the unconscious. Language is no longer organized, since the "name of the father," the phallic signifier, has been "foreclosed." This is the term Lacan uses to say that the central paternal signifier has lost its position as the foundation of discourse. In psychosis the subject is inundated by a flow of linguistic signifiers, which enacts the refusal to accept the symbolic order. Lacan's tragedy plays out its final act when the psychotic falls from logos, floundering in the real, or the awareness of death outside of language.

Lacan's theory also says that madness is somewhat akin to a cybernetic system that has lost its feedback mechanism. In his seminar on psychoses, Lacan entertains this idea, one entailed by his view of the "primacy of the signifier." Who controls the material signifier of language, if, in its autonomy, language is not subject to feedback control mechanisms? In the seminar Lacan is not comfortable with the idea that he has reduced the subject to a dysfunctional cybernetics machine. To distinguish a subject from a computer he needs to differentiate the mechanical act of sending and receiving a message from an act of signification involving the symbolic order. (This is another way of formulating the problem of meaning in Alexander and schizophrenic poetry, discussed in the preceding chapter.) If the self is a cybernetics system, it seems pertinent to ask if a computer could go insane. According to Lacan this would make sense only if one could say that the messages received by a mechanical system were in some sense subjectively received, "qu'au point d'arrivée du message, on prend acte du message" [that at the arrival point of the message someone takes note of it].[8] Lacan would not admit that this distinction reintroduces classical subjectivity into his psychic system. But either he must introduce some notion of subjectivity, or, it seems to me, he transforms the subject into a type of communication system not essentially different from any other Turing machine or cybernetic system. The human world in which madness can occur, as he puts it, includes not only significations, but also the order of the signifier. But this ponderous distinction, meaning that language is reserved for human beings, and that animals have instincts, merely renews the classical idea that animals do not share logos; and it hardly differentiates a human being from a troubled computer.

To offer a perhaps helpful recapitulation at this point, Lacan was an antihumanist humanist who did not want to see natural science and especially biology explain the human subject by reducing behavior to questions of physiology and neurology. To this end he adapted a structuralism that makes of the subject a tragic being who is never really subjectively present to itself, except through the delusions of the imaginary expressed through the ego. Like a dysfunctional cybernetic system, the subject goes mad when the program fails to include the signified that orders the system, when the name-of-the-father fails to occupy the place of the Other, as Lacanians say in describing the dysfunction in the programming of the subject. Or, as feminists in revolt have said, when the subject is not adapted to patriarchal ideology, the subject is declared mad because of its refusal of logos. With that thought, it is appropriate now to turn to a new issue in this study: gender.

Gender and Madness

Both Lacan's psychosis and Bateson's schizophrenia send us looking for the social site of madness. Social ties are first made through information circulated in the closed circuitry of the family, the first level of organization in the social network or the ecosystem. Lacan and Bateson both introduce questions of gender into the etiology of madness because they both place heavy responsibility on the mother for producing psychotics. Bateson's double bind is clearly mother-centered; and Lacan's teachings attribute to the "phallic mother" the responsibility for the child's failure to integrate the name-of-the-father, and hence be programmed properly by the signifying chain in which phallic values organize the world. It is true that Lacan's thought has actually enjoyed a great vogue among feminists, though I personally find it difficult to reconcile feminism with the idea that psychotics are produced when the mother's discourse displaces the signifier that Lacan calls the name of the father. The mother's role is central in the family drama, and so the Lacanian Joël Dor explains psychosis by saying, quite literally, that the circulation of the phallus in the maternal genealogy leaves no place for the symbolic father and hence no place for the symbolizing of the law of the father through the institution of a symbolic castration.[9] There is something quite disturbing about the way Bateson and Lacan find the causes of madness in women's role as mother. However, we shall presently consider some women writers for whom the rupture with logos is a positive or necessary task, and in their desire for madness, they curiously affirm Bateson and especially Lacan's theory.

The role assigned the mother in recent theories of madness brings up the question if there is a gender determinant of madness. To put it mildly, gender has become a key in the contemporary understanding of self, personal identity, and madness. It is true that the idea that there are male and female modes of madness is as old as Greek medicine. And it is also true that many historians and feminist revisionists argue that women have always lived madness in ways that are different from men. In *Woman and Madness* Phyllis Chesler states the thesis most baldly: "Madness and asylums generally function as mirror images of the female experience, and as penalties for *being* 'female,' as well as for desiring or daring *not* to be."[10] Feminist revisionists have argued this point of view with cogency, though this cogency springs from an a priori identification of femininity with insanity, or with whatever is other than reason—reason being identified with the masculine. However, I do not think that it is true that these a priori identifications reflect the complexities of historical reality, however much medicine may have contributed to the patriarchal ideology that, with reason, feminists wish to attack. Some women have experienced their madness as an intrinsic part of being woman—some but hardly all—just as some, but hardly all, doctors thought women were intrinsically insane.

I would argue that in the history of understanding the discourses of madness, gender distinction really plays an active role for the first time in contemporary writing. Before the contemporary period mad women have written works of literature and have been portrayed in literature. And gender has played a supporting role in the allegorical explanations of madness that have characterized much discourse on madness. However, only in contemporary texts have women asserted that madness is a product of woman's condition—and have made this assertion in order to express a revolt that refuses sanity, or at least the sanity that requires integration into the patriarchal cybernetic system called culture. For this reason contemporary culture demands that one contrast male and female understandings of madness in literary texts. Madness in writing has become a part of sexual politics. In attacking the tyranny of male logos, women are obliged of course to use logos to defend the right to go mad, since they must use language to explore in writing their rupture with logos. This development of a woman's literature that wants to use madness against culture and its codifications prompts me, therefore, to discuss recent literature depicting madness, first as written by men, then by women. I make this separation to facilitate the exposition of the following thesis: both men's and women's works often contest the systemic characterization of the self we find in theorists like Bateson and Lacan. But, in this contestation, both men and women are obliged to entertain the idea that madness is a systemic dysfunction in communication, or, alternatively, that insanity results from being excluded from language and the culture that exists through language. Dialectically, revolt often begins by an affirmation of what one wants to contest.

Male Postmodern Madness

Historical accuracy demands that we note that, in advance on our psychiatric theorists, Franz Kafka (1883–1924) was the real precursor in presenting madness as a psychotic dysfunction in semiotic functions. His novels and stories are well described as feedback systems that, in their loopings, only succeed in designating their failure to have meaning. The postmodern text, after Kafka, is often a self-referential circuit. It threatens to tumble over into psychotic disassociation, paranoid reasoning, and hallucinatory states, but maintains an appearance of functioning only by representing its own dysfunction. Moreover, Kafka described the original double bind of literary psychosis when he disallowed that we would ever understand the message that enjoins us to understand the message declaring itself incomprehensible. He portrays Lacan's desire for the signifier—the absent signifier promised by the absent father—that remains a paradoxical present absence, even if the law, or the castle, or some other distant source of logos promises redemption for our lack. In this regard *The Trial* and *The Castle,* and many of Kafka's short stories and parables, prefigure not only Lacan and Bateson, but the postmodern belief that the function of literature is to explore the function of literature—to suggest a certain crazy circularity about this belief that all communication works as a feedback system.

Kafka opens the literary space of postmodern explorations of madness. Is this madness marked by gender? One could argue that madness unmarked by gender considerations is precisely the masculine form and that, at least in much contemporary literature, feminine madness is experienced as marked by gender. Certainly there seems to be little concern with gender in the case of the two exemplary male writers I select to illustrate how the linguistic and cybernetic understanding of madness have come to dominate the works of the European and American postmodernists: the Irishman Samuel Beckett and the American Thomas Pynchon. After Kafka, the most important writer for a schizoid experience of the contradictions of textual feedback is Beckett (1906–1989). With regard to gender perhaps Beckett's work can be aptly called androgynous. The narrative self often seems male, but in its madness the self, like the female self described by feminists, is never empowered to speak truly itself. Rather, the self must pass through signifiers, through his culture's linguistic system. And so, by using language, Beckett's narrators lament that they must use what is exterior to themselves to express their self. In a sense they must use what they are not to be what they are. Every self-reflexive statement proclaims itself a contradiction through which an unnameable names itself. The view that language is alterity, that it is other than the self, makes of insanity the normal condition of any self that reflects on itself, perforce through language, and finds that it is always alienated in language. Or, in Beckett's schizoid terms, Beckett's narrators must say "I" when the word "I" clearly is not "me." "I" is simply a token in the linguistic system that, the narrator says, the tribe crams down your throat from the moment of birth. "I" cannot therefore be an expression of "my" self.

In Beckett's narrated madness, we find nameless narrators, or a narrator with no fixed name, listening to the flow of messages that are sent, do not arrive, or, if they arrive, are not understood, for the self is forever beyond language, or alienated in a language that is not the subject's. Language is perhaps an autonomous system, and the power of the system is seductively to foster the belief that communication is possible. Accordingly, Beckett's characters spend much time entertaining the hypothesis that a message with meaning might arrive—in dramatized form this lasts the two acts during which Didi and Gogo wait for a message from Godot. Or in narrative it can last the time Moran spends in *Molloy* trying to catch up with Molloy, to bring this cripple a message before their bodies undergo total entropic disintegration. But messages all go astray, information is forever lost, and the self undergoes the dissolution that entropy promises all, body and mind. Madness is constitutive of being in the world. The consequence of thermodynamics, for beings such as ourselves, is the entropic madness deriving from the dissolution of organization, and thus of communication and meaning. Or, as information theory postulates in its version of entropy, the most probable event in the universe is chaos; to which Beckett adds that madness is more probable than sanity.

Beckett's fascination with entropy and madness—his own and that of others—is evident in his early novel, *Murphy,* published in 1938 about the time Lacan was developing his theory of the mirror stage and when Turing was working out his theory of mechanical thinking machines. Beckett's later texts, increasingly written from within madness, are, so to speak, preceded by a work of reflection on madness, in that in *Murphy* Beckett has his hero Murphy escape from the world by hiding him in MMM, a madhouse. As an attendant and thus an observer in the asylum, Murphy can enjoy the delectation of all the interned varieties of madness that he once contemplated on the outside:

Melancholics, motionless and brooding, holding their heads or bellies according to type. Paranoids, feverishly covering sheets of paper with complaints against their treatment or verbatim reports of their inner voices. A hebephrenic playing the piano intently. A hypomanic teaching slosh to a Korsakow's syndrome. An emaciated schizoid, petrified in a toppling attitude as though condemned to an eternal *tableau vivant,* his left hand rhetorically extended holding a cigarette half smoked and out.[11]

The psychiatric manual is a repertory of types that the narrator evaluates with affection. For the mad have withdrawn from the flow of messages, information, and language that plagues Beckett's narrators throughout his work. For this, Murphy admires the insane and finds in them a philosophical model: "Except for the manic, who was like an epitome of all the self-made plutolaters who ever triumphed over empty pockets and clean hands, the impression he [Murphy] received was of that self-immersed indifference to the contingencies of the contingent world which he had chosen for himself as the only felicity and achieved so seldom" (p. 168). Murphy's is not a romantic admiration of insanity as an oracular state. The mad offer no revelations of meaning. On the contrary, in their "self-immersed indifference" they contest any science of self by refusing insertion into a network of meaning. They want to live outside the symbolic system that plagues them with messages.

In *Murphy* Beckett's challenge to our view that sanity means living successfully in an informational matrix is first articulated through Murphy's emphatic rejection of psychiatry. The mad get along quite well without language, they have no desire to be inserted into an informational circuit or a classificatory system. Murphy's favorite patient is Mr. Endon, a chess-playing schizophrenic whose case presents, as A. Alvarez notes, great analogies with Beckett's narrators in later works, from Watt and Molloy through Winnie, Joe, and the narrator of *How It Is.*[12] Mr. Endon is continuously visited by inner voices, though there is one "inner voice" that "did not harangue him, it was unobtrusive and melodious, gentle continuo in the whole consort of his hallucinations" (p. 186). In his relationship to language, Beckett's first schizophrenic provides a model for successful adaptation. His is a typical relation to language that obtains among Beckett's later narrators, language, and the world. Fiction is a voice, originating somewhere, listened to somewhere, a product of autonomous language floating among other hallucinations called the world. There is a split between listener, or narrator, and language. Language is alterity, though it invests the narrator like a flowing force, a logos from some unknown god; and, with other imperatives, it often enjoins the narrator to speak.

The imperative of language imposes the double-bind situation in which Beckett's narrators are all enjoined to speak in order to say that they can't; hence Beckett's frequently quoted contradictions about the necessity to speak when one has nothing to say and nothing to say it with. Or to quote the schizoid narrator of *The Unnameable* and his sense of obligation expressed in the language that is not his:

> It's of me now I must speak, even if I have to do it with their language, it will be a start, a step toward silence and the end of madness, the madness of having to speak and not being able to, except of things that don't concern me, that don't count, that I don't believe, that they have crammed me full of to prevent me from saying who I am, where I am, and from doing what I have to do in the only way that can put an end to it, from doing what I have to do. How they must hate me![13]

The locus of this double bind is a social space, a place where the "they" imposes its injunctions on the alienated unnameable:

> Not to be able to open my mouth without proclaiming them, and our fellowship, that's what they imagine they'll have reduced me to. It's a poor trick that consists in ramming a set of words down your gullet on the principle that you can't bring them up without being branded as belonging to their breed. (P. 324)

In this demented lamentation the psychiatrist may see schizophrenia, and the linguist may find, somewhat metaphorically, a description of the linguistic contract that one must accept by being born into a linguistic community. Both are right. For Beckett this contract is a pact with alienation, since this pact makes the self a product of language that is exterior to the self. Or, according to Lacan, the signifier is always the Other's—which shows perhaps that Lacan was quite as mad as any of Beckett's narrators.

Beckett, writing in English and French, can stand as the exemplar of European postmodernity, with a tradition of philosophy, science, and linguistics that comes to an entropic end in the dementia of his fumbling characters. American postmodernity, infatuated with the technologies of communication that often seem to usurp interest in all other sciences today, can be well illustrated by Thomas Pynchon and, more generally, by what has been called cybernetic fiction.[14] Pynchon, a reclusive, but still active, American writer who, for all we know, is quite sane, narrates insanity in novels in which madness can be defined as the overflowing of messages through circuitry in which everything connects with everything else. Cybernetic flow generates overloads that are experienced as paranoia. Like one of Beckett's heroes, Pynchon seems to believe that the only way to escape this madness is to disconnect, which is what happens to Pynchon's character, the protean Puritan Slopthroth. In *Gravity's Rainbow* (1973) he enters an antiparanoid state in which nothing connects to nothing. Sanity is a communicational void.

Most of the time, however, Pynchon's characters are caught up in an overload of messages so that the world signifies far too much. His most accessible character in this respect is the archetypical quester, Oedipa Maas, of *The Crying of Lot 49* (1967). Her name suggests an excess of Oedipal desire, or perhaps the source of the psychic energy fueling her quest to find out if there is an alternative communication system lurking somewhere in California. Years of seeing a shrink have not, however, set her internal circuitry flow in equilibrium; and her ventures into the hyperreality of southern California demonstrate that no informational equilibrium between inner desire and outer world is possible. To live in this hyperreality is indeed the same as living within a gigantic cybernetic system. And it appears meaningless for her to ask if she might find something outside this system. The circuits of signification are a form of closure for thought. The attempt to create new forms of signification, to get outside the system, can only be madness even if, in this paranoid form of closure, to remain within the system is also to experience insane overload.

To the chagrin of Pynchon's characters, signs and communication systems are programmed forms of insanity that someone, somewhere, has stuck into the hardware we once called the world. In contemporary American literature disbelief in this system and its codes is usually, contradictorily, juxtaposed with an affirmation that reality is accessed through constructs such as codes and linguistic systems. We are dramatically reductionist today in believing that the real is instituted by a program that can generate reality on the basis of a few combinatory rules. Schizo-texts engage us in the double bind of accepting these views even as these texts contest them. One form of contestation is to show that madness derives from a systematic elaboration of demented combinatory schemes, since, if imposed on the human sphere, computer language generates madness. Yet sanity also relies upon the computer's binary logic, for one cannot think without the law of the excluded middle, declaring that either a thing is or it isn't. What, Oedipa Maas wonders, does logic have to do with understanding the proliferation of signs that make up the reality encountered, say, on a California freeway?

Pynchon shows that, defined as a computer program, communication is deadly in its rigidity, for the rigidity of the logical binary oppositions that make up the code are not capable of explaining the contradictory possibilities that the world offers. Thus it is not inapposite to see the double bind again at work in a world of signs in which one is enjoined to understand at the same time that there is far too much information, far too many signs, for one mind ever to decode. In Beckett as in Pynchon, the schizo-text trades, too, on ethical contradiction, for we postmoderns are under the obligation to decipher communications that, on the metalinguistic level, declare that they are indecipherable madness. (Or as one inadequate, but popular interpretation of Gödel's theorem goes, self-reflective logos can never point to anything but its own failure to account for itself.) From this perspective reality is a cybernetic condition in which feedback processes produce only greater and greater loopings proclaiming insane loopings.

The grandest enactment of this programmed madness is Pynchon's novel *Gravity's Rainbow*. This work takes as its basic axiom that in the total cybernetic system, once called reality, everything is connected to everything—all messages interrelate, everything is interfaced. This means that every message and its contradiction can reach the receiver. And in this state of hypercommunication everything signifies everything. Interestingly, this is a condition of hyperinterpretation that seems to work out the implications of the madness we first saw in the poet Nerval. However, the cybernetic world of hypercommunication came into existence about the time of World War II, or at least this is the time Pynchon chooses for his cosmic conspiracy in which world history itself seems manipulated. History is the result of all the interconnecting relations put together by the System. The System exists as the total ecology of all events that, like a cybernetic system that has lost its governor, is out of control. History ends, entropically, as a form of insanity—history understood both as events and as the information system that gives access to those events. The end state of history seems to be the contrary of the advent of Hegelian reason, since in Pynchon's novel it is the demented Zone produced by the System.

The linear programming of the Zone results, for example, in the industrial wasteland of Germany at the end of World War II. An alternative to this system is found only in dream, such as might be found if we were able to dream of a world development based on cycles; or something that avoids the linear logic of the System that governs industrial society. The novel recalls that Friedrich August Kekulé (1829–1896) had such a dream. Supposedly in a dream Kekulé saw the circular shape of the benzene molecule, and his discovery gave organic chemistry to the System. But here Kekulé also dreams of the Great Serpent holding its tale in its mouth, and this dreaming Serpent in turn surrounds the world, or as the ever-harried voice of the narrator describes the dream and its opposite:

The Serpent that announces, "The World is a closed thing, cyclical, resonant, eternally-returning," is to be delivered into a system whose only aim is to *violate* the Cycle. Taking and not giving back, demanding that "productivity" and "earnings" keep on increasing with time, the System removing from the rest of the World these vast quantities of energy to keep its own tiny desperate fraction showing a profit: and not only most of humanity—most of the World, animal, vegetable and mineral, is laid waste in the process. The System may or may not understand that it's only buying time. And that time is an artificial resource to begin with, of no value to anyone or anything but the System, which sooner or later must crash to its death, when its addiction to energy has become more than the rest of the World can supply, dragging with it innocent souls all along the chain of life. Living inside the System is like riding across the country in a bus driven by a maniac bent on suicide.[15]

Pynchon's narrator faces the double bind imposed by the obligation to conceive a rational ecology of mind when the system informing the thinking mind is itself berserk. Since most of *Gravity's Rainbow* unfolds within circuits of the System, his novel gives indeed the impression that a maniac bent on suicide is the narrator. But, for a moment in *Gravity's Rainbow,* a dream affords an escape from the overloading connections, a dream of a rationality that escapes the linear program. The reversal of romantic motifs is important: dream is *not* the locus of madness. Dream allows escape from the information systems that, if not merely alienating, are savagely pathological in their construction of the real. The problem is to find a point outside the System that constitutes mind, so that one can judge the pathology of the System itself. But in the name of what criteria can one judge pathology when the System establishes the categories of reality? Or, to anticipate the feminist dilemma, what higher reason can judge reason in the service of destructive norms?

For Pynchon, the true disorder of hypercommunication, simulating order, leads to apocalyptic madness. The threat is to be taken seriously, since, at the end of *Gravity's Rainbow,* the communication system exists ready to send off the rocket that is, in the novel, already launched and poised to annihilate us all in the cinema where we are watching . . . the rocket. The rocket would be the System's ultimate product, the logical outgrowth of technology looping out of control, justifying itself because it is. The looping is mimicked by the novel's final recursive loop that marks closure by blowing us up. But the apocalypse is "always already" there—to use the terms of deconstructive hyperinterpretation and its heady paranoia—since the program contains its self-destructive end as one of its encoded logical possibilities: logically destruction is present from the beginning.

Feminist Visions of Rupture with (Male) Logos

Ecology is the study of how, within a system, all entities connect and corre-late. For the contemporary mind, it is one way to study sanity or to under-stand the lack thereof. Both Beckett and Pynchon illustrate the ruptures and overdeterminations that make of linguistic systems and cybernetic circuits producers of madness, or a dysfunctional ecology. And to return to the ques-tion of gender marking, these insane systems are not marked by male writers, though they may be considered as masculine by female writers who see in them products of patriarchal reason and logos. Feminists may then proclaim their right to alternative forms of madness—madness when judged by the logic of the insane (male) system. Yet male writers, like Pynchon and Beckett, have been rather much in agreement with many feminists about the ecologi-cal dysfunction of the cultural system. There is a symmetry here that points to a consensus about the way contemporary society produces madness.

But before considering this symmetry, we should again consider the claim, advanced by some feminists, that would annex all madness in order to make of it a characteristic of the feminine condition. To generalize this viewpoint, they contend that the mad man has assumed an essentially femi-nine position, and that madness is always the feminine pole opposed to male rationality, whatever be the biological gender of the mad person involved. (And so Kafka's or Beckett's texts might seem to have a feminine gender inscribed in them.) Therefore, or so it is argued, women have no choice but to contend for their identity in and through madness, and forge or claim an identity larger than the privative identity of being the irrational opposite of the supposedly rational male. This can mean that feminists in revolt want to blow apart the male logos that excludes the truly feminine voice from the information system that determines what counts as culture and rationality.

In variants on this argument—or political strategy—many women writ-ers want to affirm their madness to escape from the double bind that enjoins them to be rational, which is to say male, while contradictorily telling them to remain their feminine self, or irrational. This is the classic double bind imposed on women, and one can look back to earlier times, to, say, George Eliot's *Mill on the Floss* to find it at work in the determination of then nor-mal femininity. Today, by contrast with Eliot's social satire and irony, some women writers feel they must struggle with language itself, conceived of as a masculine logos that forms the system that destroys woman's identity. In their revolt against this belief, these women have chosen to affirm that their writing in madness is affirmative of a self beyond sanity determined by mas-culine rationality. These discourses affirming madness merit our attention for the contestation they direct against language conceived as a system, or a systematic codification that defines woman as mad. For purposes of exposition I shall limit myself to considering a few recent French women writers, primarily because it is especially in France that this revolt against the codifications of (male) reason has resulted in some of the most powerful writing of the past twenty years or so.

However, for purposes of clarity about the issues involved, I should like to examine the following argument about the revolt against reason. To wit, it has always been easy to argue that every rebel against social norms has always been judged mad, since by definition social norms exist to exclude dangerous alterity (as perceived of course by the norms). In the nineteenth century Emily Dickinson exposes the dilemma posed by the danger of her difference in terms of norms:

> Much madness is divinest sense
> To a discerning eye;
> Much sense the starkest madness.
> 'Tis the majority
> In this, as all prevail
> Assent, and you are sane;
> Demur,—you're straightway dangerous,
> And handled with a chain.[16]

In this dialectic, claims to reason are at stake, and the right to madness is vindicated by a reason superior to social norms. The norm has little to do with reason, for it is a matter of assent. Higher, or true, reason may perceive the failures of the norm, but at the risk of being judged insane. This dialectic between higher and lower, or false, reason is probably inevitable in historical change, and points to the fact that the claims of reason have little to do with gender—even if women have been and are still the victims of irrational oppression. In this dialectic the claims of reason remain the claims of reason, and declare that Emily Dickinson is sane. Such is the circle of rationality that Emily Dickinson illustrates with her usual concision.

Contemporary French women writers claiming the right to madness are not directly interested in the dialectic of higher and false reason. Though it is difficult, perhaps impossible, not to resort to this dialectic to vindicate oneself, many women seek to circumvent this dialectic by proclaiming the otherness of woman. Claims to alterity in essays by feminist theorists such as Cixous and Irigaray have become standards in feminist polemic. Our interest here, however, is not in theory, but in several texts in which madness is written to show or defend a female way of being in the world that avoids the dialectic of superior and inferior reason. They want to do so by portraying the otherness of madness. Woman's madness is outside of the (male) systems of communication and cannot be integrated into the social circuits of normal social ecology. As such, these texts in and around madness may not always make directly feminist claims. Rather, they present woman's madness as simply other, beyond rationalization perhaps, and clearly beyond the rationality of medical reason. By claiming, implicitly and explicitly, the desire and the right to be mad, writers such as Marguerite Duras, Emma Santos, and Jeanne Hyvrard have attempted to open up a space for women that is not regulated by the binary oppositions of cybernetic reason or the constraints of (masculine) logos and reason. Pursuing a desire to blow open from within the realm of codified signifiers, or the cybernetic system of male logos, these writers attempt to write from within madness, largely in refusal of language and communication systems as they now exist.

Marguerite Duras and the Silence of Madness

Marguerite Duras, who until her death in 1997 was perhaps the most influential female writer in the world, compels attention for her creations that escape the double bind entailed in using reason to decry reason as irrational. It is noteworthy that Lacan said that she is one of the few to see the truth of the subject as he taught it, but it is perhaps more relevant that Duras has dismissed the "male" concern with theory as a matter for imbeciles.[17] Theory is an attempt at dominance, a masculine concern with mastery through logos; and Duras's novels, plays, and films are aggressive in their refusal to set forth a theoretical framework for understanding the psyche. Many of her characters are mad, or in borderline states, if judged by common categories of understanding. Unconcerned with these categories, Duras allows in her work women—and men—their madness as a right needing no justification. Viewed usually from the exterior, in films, novels, and plays, these characters exist in a state of rupture with the communicational system that would pin them down and force them to signify. Duras refuses theory, but one can understand why Lacan praised her work: the mad in Duras's work are not situated in the "symbolic order," or the signifying matrix of culture. They exist as presences, disruptions, caught up in a world of erotic viewing and passionate seeing; they are pure projections, from the Lacanian perspective, of the imaginary, the realm of passion. And once this disjuncture takes place, logos is powerless to patch over the gap and explain the rupture that has occurred.

Madness exists in Duras beyond conceptualization, for mad characters are not integrated in the circuits of language. They speak, but they do not speak texts that can be grasped by some hermeneutics that will reinsert their deviance into a symbolic system. The heroine of *Le Ravissement de Lol V. Stein* (1964) goes mad in a traumatic moment when her fiancé abandons her at a ball; he walks out on her with another woman. One can—and many critics have—speculate about the etiology of Lol's insanity, but finally her madness is simply a brute fact. It defies any category that can reduce it to a case study. Knowledge can only be negative, as is suggested when Lol's best friend says about her that "not to know anything about Lol was to know her already."[18] Moreover, there is no truth-value to madness—or as viewers of Duras's cinematic works recall, the truth of madness is the cry, the direct scream of madness, a smashing of the order of signifiers. There is only the raw truth of madness as presence, or as Lol says about the truth-value of her madness, she wasn't lying when she cried.

In Duras's world passion is generating by viewing, often by the triangular viewing in which one desires what the other desires. Language is devalued, almost in direct proportion to the inflation of desire. Detached from the world, language often seems, to use a linguistic notion, to have no transitive function. Names do not name (p. 113). Or language even appears to empty the world. It is guilty of some ontological fault, and the male narrator of *Lol V. Stein* can speculate that perhaps Lol's madness came about because of some lack in language—the original sin flawing Lacanian logos. Imagining the ball at which she was abandoned, the narrator asks what might have happened:

> Lol cannot go far into the unknown upon which this moment opens. She has no memory, not even imaginary, she hasn't a single idea about this unknown. But what she believes is that she was to enter into it, that that's what she had to do, that it would have been forever, for her head and for her body, their greater pain and their greater joy confounded and joined in their definition that had become totally singular, but unnameable for lack of a word. . . . if Lol is silent in life it's because she believed, for the briefest moment, that that word could exist. For lack of its existence, she remains quiet. It would have been a word of absence, a word in the form of a hole, dug out in the center of a hole, of this hole where all the other words would have been buried. (P. 48)

So, he speculates, Lol needed a word beyond language, unsayable, but whose presence would have transformed the world. That word may not have been Lacan's "name of the father," but, whatever it be, there must be a founding concept that has to give a center to meaning if sanity can exist. But if the system has no center, then sanity is an illusion, an illusion usually entertained by men.

Biological gender thus plays at most a secondary role in the genesis of madness in Duras's work. Madness is a question of a position in culture and language: to be outside, in silence, is to be a feminine position, and mad. Duras's world is fissured between the poles of masculine reason and feminine desire and madness—but male and female characters can be attracted to either pole, and most go to the feminine pole, the pole of lack and void when compared with the illusory masculine world of ready-made systems. For instance, in her *Les Yeux bleus, cheveux noirs* (1986) Duras presents a probably insane female protagonist who goes to live in a solitary room with a probably homosexual male protagonist. The male is also a character of loss and madness and is described, by the female, as existing in a feminine void:

> She looks at him. This is how she sees him in his absence, such as he is there. Full of silent images, drunk with diverse suffering, with the desire to find again a lost object as well as to buy one that he doesn't have yet and which suddenly becomes the justification of his existence, a suit, a watch, a lover, a car. Wherever he may be, whatever he may do, always a complete disaster, all by himself.[19]

Madness is the state of absence in which a male longs for something other than what is—and wants to possess something beyond possession. Desire cannot be described, only shown to be a disaster, and so drama is the most fitting rhetorical mode for madness—which seems to explain the rather enigmatic way Duras places, in *Les Yeux bleus, cheveux noirs,* recurrent stage directions for how actors might handle the novel as a play. It also explains why Duras makes little distinction among her plays, narrations, and films based thereon. Madness can be staged as emptiness in all genres.

The male pole, with its perennial illusions, is hardly staged as triumphant logos in Duras's novels, films, and plays. Male reason often takes the form of the fear that a usually male character experiences when he confronts the "unintelligibility of truth," as a male conversational partner says in *Emily L.* (1987). He makes this statement once he has heard his female partner tell him the tale of a distraught English woman, a poet, whose husband is frightened by the texts she writes, and by one poem in particular. In this poem the English poet writes that on certain afternoons of winter the rays of the sun that filter into the naves of cathedrals oppressed you in the same way as the falling sonorities of the great organs. . . . that the wounds made by these same swords of the sun were inflicted by the heavens. That they left neither trace nor visible scar, neither in our body's flesh nor in our thoughts. That they neither wounded us nor gave us comfort. That it was something else. That it was elsewhere. Elsewhere and far from where you might think. That these wounds announced nothing, confirmed nothing that could have taught something or have been the object of provocation in the heart of God's kingdom. No, it was a question of the perception of the last difference: that one, interior, at the center of meanings.[20]

In this passage Duras has linked her fictional poetess with Emily Dickinson through allusions in which Duras's poet declares her difference, and in this difference, finds the wounds that lie at the heart of her near-madness. As Emily Dickinson said of "a certain Slant of light," it gives "Heavenly Hurt" there where "We can find no scar, / but internal difference, / Where the Meanings, are" (*Complete Works,* no. 258). A postmodern reading might also see this difference as the difference that grounds language and, I think, consciousness. In the same differentiating play that allows meanings to exist is found the "sovereign despair" of the human creature that comes to consciousness—and is capable of madness in reflecting upon difference, upon a torn consciousness that is at one with the world and severed from it, different and alone in the void. Duras's allusion to Dickinson makes, finally, reference to a tradition of women's writing in which the self is defined as separated from logos, defined through injury and lack.

This is not logical, from the codified (male) point of view, though this viewpoint is remarkably close to Lacanian formulations. The male character who lives with the fictional poetess is incapable of understanding his wife's poem with its "aerial voyage" leading to "the summits, the cold night of summer, the appearance of death" (p. 85). The poetic use of language brings the consciousness of death; and the void that death reveals in language shatters man's mastery over the world. Duras seems to want to show that the binary oppositions that many structuralists take to be the essence of reason cannot encode death's presence as absence. To conjure this threat of death, and the concomitant threat of madness arising from indifferentiation, the male character burns the poem. He cannot abide the poem's madness that denies mastery, denies power, denies language's purchase upon the world. In Duras's work, madness is a feminine privilege: in madness the fullness of our arbitrary being in the world is lived in a kind of tragic splendor. And to return to Lacan, her work communicates the tragic sense of non-communication that underwrites Lacan's description of our alienation in the symbolic system as well as the tragedy of the psychotic's unmediated confrontation with death. But against Lacan, her work shows the redundancy of illusory theory in this tragic world.

Two Psychotic Defenses of Madness

To continue this argument with, or against, theory, I now engage two women writers who, in defense of their psychosis, turn against the system of language itself and against the codes of narration contained therein. Like all writers, mad writers, narrating from within madness, must have recourse to language and to the system of narration codified in language. Confronting narrative structures, the mad must obey the synchronic rules, or the currently codified constraints, that dictate what counts as valid use. In this sense one can call narrative structure a system within the general system of language. The "system" of narrative has been well described by structuralists, semioticians, communication theorists, and other workers in the field of discourse analysis, or what one might call "applied logos." The mad writer wishing to find another model for communication can try to subvert the codified rules for communication. There is some hope of success, for history shows that the narrative system does not exist entirely because the rules for narration are "rational," have a "logic," or belong to eternal logos. Narration, like any aspect of the linguistic system, also has a diachronic side: it has evolved in history. The experimental writer—and in writing against the grain mad writers conduct experiments in communication—may feel warranted to invent new rules for what constitutes meaningful communication. The history of literature is in many respects a history of the successful recodifications of successive systems of communication; but it is also the history of the perduring constraints that have changed but little.

The contemporary mind has frequently considered narrative forms to be ideological constraints that limit the possibilities of communication. This belief has been held by both the mad and the relatively sane. To mad women writers, the system of narration appears to limit them specifically as women; or, in virtue of narration's codified restraints, to deny them the possibility of communicating their full experience of madness. This belief is a consequence of another of the beliefs at the heart of what is called the postmodern: there is a nearly axiomatic belief that holds that experience is what is communicated; reality is what can be codified by the linguistic system or encoded into the cybernetic network; or, in short, the real is what can be said. This may be a reductive axiom, and it may result in absurdities when it grants more reality to cyberspace than to our bodies—but it is a prevalent belief that reflects a new variant on the ancient logocentric doctrine that Reality is the Word. Pursuing a revolt against these beliefs—and, dialectically, embracing these beliefs to express their revolt—the final two contemporary women writers considered here, Emma Santos and Jeanne Hyvrard, are both experimental and both insane. They work against the communication system, the first by attempting to change the axis of communication that underwrites narration, the second by a poetic attempt at enlarging the experience that language, in the service of madness, might communicate. In their work being psychotic and being a woman are coexisting conditions, and in this regard they illustrate the most radical development of madness in its relation to gender. As women, they demand the right to be mad. This demand entails significant contradictions. It means using the (masculine) linguistic system to reject the system. It means using logos to break with (male) logos. And, most painfully, it seems to mean that they must desire the psychosis that destroys them.

Of the several narrative works written by Emma Santos, most of them usually available from the feminist publisher Editions des Femmes, I have selected for our purposes *La Loméchuse* (1978). Named after a species of beetle to whose body fluids some ants become addicted, this work narrates, in the third person, the tale of madness of a character—perhaps the author, perhaps her double—named Emma. It narrates her experience with a woman doctor with whom she tries to live, briefly, in a self-consciously "fusional" state; and then, after her rejection by the doctor, her near internment. At the novel's end, an insane Emma knows that she will soon be taken in charge by the authorities. This knowledge has seemingly allowed her to write.

Throughout the book flashbacks suggest numerous reasons for her insanity: childhood trauma, a thyroid operation that caused her to abort a child, or some congenital disposition to psychotic fantasy, expressed in her recurrent images of a shattered body. But etiology is an effect of the narration that organizes the symptoms in view of a psychiatric category. Emma refuses to allow her narration to be used by the psychiatric system that sees every narration concluding with a label for a résumé: schizophrenic, paranoid, or whatever is demanded by the system to effect closure. The narrator claims to live outside of words, the words that her doctor-lover Elisabeth knew, though she must of course have recourse to words to send, for example, her farewell to Elisabeth in the book's final chapter:

> Adieu, Elisabeth, she understands crime criminals and she's afraid in her turn. She forgives. She forgives the mad and the assassins. She'll become mad when the surroundings have judged her mad then criminal. The decor is for crime. They *[on]* impose upon her the role of assassin, they impose upon her the place of a mental defective capable of murder. She'll go take that place, that little place for adjusting her words to your doctor's language, for communicating finally with you and your kind.[21]

The strange distortion one feels on reading this passage is not just due to the pathos of an insane writer claiming that she is insane only according to some future judgment, or that she must adjust to the community's language if she is to communicate. It is also due to the systematic way Emma Santos writes in the first person using the third-person pronoun.

The normal axis of discourse, as linguistics or information theory describes it, is the axis established by the pronouns *I* and *you/thou.* The axis of the first and second person forms the syntagmatic axis of the linguistic system. This is the communicational axis that we all must use, but throughout most of the novel Santos replaces *I* with *she (elle),* until at the end of the novel, "she" makes the following assertion:

> An adult woman obliged to say I in place of THEY *[on]*, SHE ELISABE-MMA, she plunged into quicksand. Careful danger, it is written on the beach. She walks toward the water. She goes into a dime store. She selects a straw hat made in Java and an English style umbrella.
>
> Adieu Elisabeth, madness gets one by. She/it *[elle]* has a bird's head and a cat's smile. Adieu Elisabeth.
>
> Friday 5 May 1972. The narrative stops. The author is finally taken into custody by psychiatric care. The writing I becomes the written SHE. Privileged moment in which writing and life are melded in silence. (Pp. 154–55)

In *La Loméchuse* the first person has recognized her alienation written into the third person, the pronoun used as the object of reference in the linguistic system. Beckett's unnameable would feel a perfect schizoid affinity with this alienation; and he would endorse Santos's dreams of new pronouns and nouns that would express different relations from those codified by the linguistic system and its obligatory axis of communication. Their common break with logos is made in revolt against the destruction language works upon their identity, though for Santos this is a question of defending a gendered identity.

The mad reject language when they discover language cannot found the world of their desire. In Santos this discovery is tied up with doctors. For example, Emma desires maternity, but she lives in a world in which the doctors, who are portrayed as being in charge of language, prevent children from being born:

> She couldn't invent words, she listened to the child in silence. She doesn't know how to write. She writes with the emptiness of her womb. When she tried to speak, to explain her throat, to ovulate, they tore out her thyroid from all the way inside. It is reassuring to know that there is no longer anything, no longer a child, the infinite regenerates. The objects-mirrors frost over in the room without a roof and disappear. . . . One doesn't commit suicide, one is killed by the others. (P. 122)

It is nearly impossible to evaluate this outcry against doctors. They are, to be sure, emblematic of the patriarchy and the masculine double bind that enjoins Emma to use language to decry her lack of language. Suicide would be a response to this double bind. The double bind is also framed by a double system of language and madness, since Emma declares madness to be a system, too. Madness is perhaps the antisystem she opposes to language and the double bind formulated therein. Thus, she finds that one can be programmed by the circuitry of insanity, much as one can be by the communicational systems of language and information theory. It would seem plausible that Emma hits upon the notion of system because, precisely, in contesting the masculine domain, she is obliged to adopt a revolt that point by point is a negative version of what she rejects. And so finally, as the doctor Elizabeth says, in notes inserted into the middle of the novel, Emma's only recourse is to speak silence (p. 97). In silence, she speaks no negative affirmations. The double bind takes the form here, then, of the impossibility of speaking one's self in either sanity or madness. Yet Emma speaks, and perhaps we must interpret the transformation of the "I" into the "She" to be a strategy of her residual sanity, of the sanity residing somewhere within each psychosis. The transformation shows an intelligence that judges her alienation, and so sanity resides in the self-affirmation of an identity that, despite contradiction, resists the encroachment of doctors and perhaps the body's disease that doctors attempt to treat.

My second example of revolt in psychosis is Jeanne Hyvrard, a writer who has recently begun to receive critical attention. Her work can complete this discussion of gender determinations of madness, since, in it, Hyvrard carries the affirmation of her madness to a logical conclusion by affirming that men are right to lock her up. If not put in asylums, she says, the mad women of the world are capable of an uprising that will overthrow men and bring about a new ecology. Hyvrard is not vindictive, for the integration of all beings in a new relation to nature would include men. Her madness is utopian, and, I admit that, in the climate of cynicism of the late twentieth century, the reasonableness of utopian madness is tonic. In *Mère la mort* (1976) utopian madness chants a dirge to mother death, to the center of nature outside the codifications of the language and the logic that condemns Hyvrard to an asylum. Hyvrard's work claims there is a fullness beyond language, reached in madness, that (male) symbolic systems cannot encode. Addressing death—in which the Lacanian might see the real—the text's speaker is unnameable, outside of normal language, but somehow in contact with the elemental forces of nature, with the rocks and hills of the *causse* or plateau of southern France. The female narrator also appears to be writing from within the confines of a mental hospital. In *Mère la mort* the axis of discourse is respected, since in its dialogue the speaker addresses a second-person interlocutor, Mother Death, the feminine principle, the void, and perhaps the nocturnal abyss. But the discourse does exclude the ubiquitous third-person plural male pronoun—*ils*—from direct address: a constant object of reference, "they" in the masculine gender are excluded from real communication. Dialogue is a condition of femininity.

Hyvrard's narrator wants to overcome words and dictionary definitions; she desires to found a language adequate to new categories of being. In her madness Hyvrard wants to provide rules for yet-to-be-invented language games for which she can give no exemplars except a few powerful neologisms: notably, women driven mad are named *enfollées*. Hyvrard also wants to invent a new language system having three modes: the real, the imaginary, and the "fusional."[22] These modes correspond to the Lacanian coordinates of the self, but with a difference. Lacan's symbolic, founded on the phallus, is abolished for a feminine fusional mode of language in which symbolic difference would be replaced by identity. And with fusional identity, language, I think, would be plenitude, not lack.

Hyvrard claims that men will not allow new language games, for, judging with the categories of their truncated language, they declare her mad:

> They say that I invent words. They say that it is a sign of my sickness. They even give it a name. What already? They say that I am mad because I invent words. They oblige us to conjugate verbs in order to put chains on our sunrises *[Ils nous obligent à conjuguer les verbes pour enchaîner nos aurores]*. (P. 67)

Identifying dawn and liberation with surrealist gusto, Hyvrard presses into service a third rhetorical mode by which a woman can explore her madness, a poetical mode that overcomes male language by proposing a countermyth to the myth of male superiority. This is Hyvrard's way of circumventing the dialectic of superior and false reason. Myth, instead of superior reason, contains the counterargument that the mad poetess propounds in order to undo the destructive systems of masculine categories. She wants to embody the myth of a nature goddess that men cannot seize or possess. She would be a Daphne, illusive and beyond the power of Apollo, the male god of language and reason:

> A woman daughter of a river. A man pursues a woman. But when he seizes her, she becomes a laurel. They cut into our sentences and sign with our names. But it is their name that the crack in my forehead pronounces. For I have disappeared. They are alone. They think they appropriate me. But all they have in their hands is the crack that grows larger. I become the unnameable. (P. 65)

The myth of the unnameable may reach back to archaic sources, but, as we have amply seen, it is also a primary postmodern myth attached to madness in the era of hypercommunication and scientific determinations of information flow. The unnameable defies all systems that purport to order a, or the, world. But, unlike Duras's silent creatures of desire or Beckett's voluble schizo-narrators, Hyvrard wants to transcend the myth of the unnameable and create a myth of language beyond language, an order of communication that can only be hinted at by poetic or mythic indirection.

And so a second myth that animates Hyvrard's madness is the myth of a communication beyond communication, a fuller communication perhaps of an animistic nature, respecting the natural differences and identities of being. She dreams in madness of the total ecology of which mind is part and from which language alienates her. In her work madness reflects upon itself, upon its dysfunctional relation to the system that excludes her, but it does so without the usual contradictions of self-reference. Myth is successful in this regard, and in her litany of poetic incriminations quoted above, Hyvrard renews the myth of a logos that would respect the specific difference of things, all things, women and trees, living with their positive identities integrated into an ecology that respects the system of differences:

> I survive in the stones of the river. I survive in the laurel sheltering their horses.
>
> They need our strength in order to exist. But they cannot admit our difference. We have no need of them. But they can't accept it. I sit looking at the wall. They say I am mad. I am only looking for the piece that is lacking. The piece that would allow one to answer them. The piece that is lacking between power and identity. The piece that is lacking between the asylums where they lock us up and the power that they appropriate to themselves. (Pp. 65–66)

What the missing piece is, is unnameable. It would bridge the masculine realm of symbolic difference, the grounds of power, and the feminine domain of identity and specific difference. Hyvrard is still in the realm of myth, where the psychotic poetess can only designate by implication that which cannot be named. And perhaps Hyvrard's madness is to believe in or actually experience identity outside our circuits of communication—with all the passion of love and desire.

For Hyvrard is an angry poet of love. Her vision of her cosmic body, what she calls her insatiable body, does not exclude men from, one day, participating in her fuller ecology that men disrupt today. This is utopian madness and is a product of ideology, an ideology that her madness learned in order to speak its lack of discourse. The difficulty we have speaking this utopian ideology today, at the turn of the millennium, is perhaps more our loss than Hyvrard's, the woman who loves her *enfollées* "driven mad" by the masculine logos that refuses them their difference (p. 95). In aspiring to cause the limited "I" of discourse to explode and thus to open to all orders of difference, in wanting to give her *enfollées* a space of their own, Hyvrard proclaims the necessity of an ecology we have only dreamed of. Her utopian madness displaces the question of higher and lower reason and rephrases it as a question of freedom and enslavement that respects the various differences of natural orders. Freedom in Hyvrard's ecology would be granted to all to be what they are, from the so-called highest to the lowest order of creatures. For by what right, she asks, does the symbolic order grant the right to enslave or imprison or finally destroy what is different?

And we may ask, whence this freedom? Freedom arises in the moment of accepting death, mother death, and running with the tumor-ridden body into the streams of nature, for Daphne is a daughter of the rivers. There is a strong naturalism in Hyvrard's utopian acceptance of the body, its relation to nature, to births and bleeding. In many respects this is the freedom to overcome the double bind that enjoins us, on the theoretical level, to live with respect of nature and then, on the level of praxis, orders us to destroy our natural relationships to the earth. Hyvrard's madness is the experience of a total condemnation of the disequilibrium we have created in the "system" of postmodern industrial society—of which Pynchon's Zone is a variant vision.

To conclude, I note that Hyvrard brings madness back to a body, a sick and suffering body. Hyvrard seems to claim that her madness is due, in part, to a tumor. Then it is the case that this tumor drives her to seek a utopian language to express her desire to overcome her disequilibrium. Pathologies of the body can open the mind to mad discourse, but, as Santos and

Hyvrard show, there is no rigorous determination as to what discourse a mad person may speak. If the woman's ravaged body is another determinant of madness, then perhaps it is also true that disease can bring about a revelation of poetic truth. Clearly, disease can cause the mad woman to focus upon her condition as woman. And if the body can determine madness, and, by this, I mean madness that exists as a projection of personality in language and desire, then the Hyvrard of *Mère la mort* gives us a remarkable poetic meditation suggesting how we must make our thinking about madness multidimensional. The rage that crippled cells or pathological neurons may encode has a life unto itself that derives from cultural forms, and that in turn can inform culture. The affirmation of what woman's madness can reveal, in the name of freedom, has undoubtedly been one of the most important cultural events of our time—along with such events as the rapid evolution of cybernetics and the slow advent of ecological consciousness. Woman's madness suggests in fact that the restricted logic of contemporary cybernetic thinking may lead to the destruction of our basic ecology. The question now is to find higher reason in the midst of these contradictions.

Postscript: Madness between History and Neurology

As the twenty-first century begins, can we point to a model for understanding madness, say, one proposed by biology or biological psychiatry that is close to illuminating the obscurity of madness? Can we simply hope soon to see a demonstration of the causal relation between organic dysfunction and madness? My admiration for the many recent successes in neurology, molecular biology, and biological psychiatry does not lead, for the moment, to much optimism about understanding the relation between human biology and madness. Basically, I do not think that the questions have yet been framed in the proper terms. The simple accumulation of more and more neurological data will not automatically eventuate in any hypotheses or theories relating madness and organic pathological processes. I may of course be wrong—I hope that I am—but it seems to me that much medical research is directed by the belief in an "ever more facts" model. This belief supposes, with undue optimism, that ever greater descriptive accuracy of neurological functions will automatically generate a model for usefully describing the relation between organic and mental events. Or, as Gerald D. Fischbach succinctly puts it, in an introduction to a special issue of the *Scientific American* on mind and brain, more facts are all that is needed:

> [B]iological explanations of mental events may become evident once the component neural functions are more clearly defined. We will then have a more appropriate vocabulary for describing the emergent mind.[1]

Perhaps, but the past twenty or thirty years of redefined functions have not led to any theoretical model that can really describe the relation between neurological functions and mental events.

At most much research has accumulated data suggesting correlations between pathological anatomy and madness, but correlations are not causality. In the seventies we could read, for example, that research had shown that a drug whose mechanism of action has been linked to the dopamine system is d-amphetamine and that, as described by B. B. Bunney and G. K. Aghajanian, the drug "produces a paranoid psychosis that many feel is indistinguishable from paranoid schizophrenia and that is rapidly reversed by the antipsychotic agents used in the treatment of schizophrenia."[2] Suggestive claims of this type of research have been tantalizing since the development of neuroleptics in the 1950s, but they are hardly of the theoretical import that the popular press usually tries to make of them. Inducing madness with drugs is hardly a new phenomenon. This research does not mean that madness is something like a self-induced drug affliction (as Kraepelin thought). This type of research has been useful in finding, through empirical testing, that drug therapy can be efficacious in treating various syndromes. We know that the use of neuroleptics can block receptors of the neurotransmitter dopamine, for example, and we can be thankful for the empirical research that keeps leading to new discoveries in this area, such as the discovery of a third dopamine receptor, announced in *Nature* a few years ago, that seems to promise hope for new neuroleptics.[3] However, the implicit or explicit causal claim equating a hormone or a chemical agent with some mental syndrome is simplistic and fails to reckon with the levels of organizational complexity that biological explanations usually demand. Simplistic correlation fails to take into account the number of overdeterminations that seem to be at work in the neurological determinants of mental life.

Most biological paradigms are guided by a vertical sense of organization, and hence analysis, that allows the multiplicity of models that can have equal warrant in explaining whatever the scientific gaze is turned upon. For a simple thought experiment, I open a biology textbook used by my own university, and there I discover that the contemporary biological paradigm tells entering freshmen and departing seniors that no less than thirteen levels of analysis must be grasped in order to deal adequately with any living organism: beginning with the subatomic particle, analysis goes step by step "upward" through the atom, the molecule, the organelle (or structure within the cell), the cell, the tissues, the organs, the organ systems, the multicellular organism, and then makes an organizational leap to aggregates of individuals organized vertically upward as populations, communities (two or more populations), ecosystems, and the biosphere. In all good logic, then, medical models should be conceived in terms of multiple explanations, involving the biologist's sense of multiple levels of organization, that would demand, when viewed in terms of only thirteen levels of organization, the minimal computation of the linear permutations that these levels allow (or at least 13! combinations—i.e., 13 × 12 × 11 × 10 . . .). This is only a thought experiment, but it suggests the inadequacy of the simplistic causality that culminates in periodic press releases to the effect that science now understands the hormone imbalance that causes depression or schizophrenia (or sexual preferences or pair bonding or whatever). Hormonal imbalance may well be present in depression, schizophrenia, or my craving for chocolates: that fact in itself is neither a cause nor least of all a theory.

A sophisticated sense of scientific epistemology recognizes that the choice of model for explanation is as important as the data that one has to fit into the model. This recognition gives new importance to the so-called Mach-Duhem-Poincaré hypothesis according to which empirical reality, in its underdetermination, can be explained by an indefinite number of models. So, when asking if the brain is a neurological system that functions as a computer, we should first recognize that our cybernetic model is only one of many possible ways of viewing the mind. Or as Ervin Laszlo phrases it about "cybernetic modeling,"

> The choice of a specifically cybernetic model is not dictated by the nature of the phenomenon: as we know all empirical phenomena are under-determined by the data and permit the construction of an indefinite number of theories. . . . We would look in vain for data which would automatically select toward a cybernetic model; the very data we consider already implies a selection, and such selection in turn implies a theory.[4]

Is the mad mind a product of dysfunctional hormones, neurological circuitry, or, at another level, of perturbations of cultural software, historical patterns, or the fiction-making capacity of the cells that constitute the brain? The answer could be yes—since my thought experiment allows for mind to be a product of at least 13! combinations of development from subatomic particles to the largest cultural patterns that inform what we take to be our human ecology or biosphere. Some models obviously work better than others; they take more into account; and these models are to be preferred—though one must reject the model that, in taking everything into account, is vacuous in its empty totalization. (Literary scholars should warn their scientific colleagues that such theories are pandemic in historical and literary studies.)

My feeling is that, to understand mind and madness, it is time to overcome the "two cultures," the separation of humanities and science—or the separation of history and neurology. And if, as the mathematical physicist

Roger Penrose argues in *The Emperor's New Mind* (1989), many aspects of mind cannot be explained as algorithms—such as the mind's capacity to produce Gödel's theorem—then perhaps this is because beyond cybernetics lies a mind that must be understood as a model maker and a shaper of fictions. Some model is needed that explains how mind, constrained by and deriving from neurological circuits, comes to theorize itself and to entertain that it is constrained by neurological circuits. Mere self-reflexivity is not enough: a video camera, as Penrose points out, can take its own image. A video camera is not a mind, as even Lacan had to admit. In this model-making capacity lies the mind's capacity to understand and perhaps to be understood, for the model or models we are speaking of center upon the mind's capacity to theorize itself.

Arguing against Penrose, the philosopher Daniel C. Dennett proposes that the unified mind is a myth and that an understanding of the multiple selves within the mind means understanding that there is not simply one program for self. The philosophical interpretation of consciousness demands that one use a phenomenology that interprets the subject's behavior much as a reader must interpret works of fiction. In *Consciousness Explained* (1991) Dennett also introduces, albeit sotto voce, the necessity of history into his work of interpretation of consciousness, since the very notion of mind depends upon its concept—mind—in order to exist. Or, in Dennett's analogy, consciousness, like love or money, would not exist if the concept had not developed in the course of human history. Love has a biological base, money a cultural base, and both, I add, have unfolded in history so that we can see, or surmise, that there were moments in time when love, money, and consciousness did not exist as we know them today—or did not exist at all.[5]

My intent is not to take sides in the quarrel that pits a mathematical Platonist Penrose against Dennett, a philosopher of cognitive science. Rather, I want to suggest that the history of mind sets forth one indispensable base for finding models for mind, its function and its dysfunctions. Functions and dysfunctions are rooted in the history of the concepts that define what they are. And once a model for mind exists, the model becomes a plausible function of mind, even if the model is in some sense an invention or fiction. Fictions can and often do invest reality. Consider how cybernetics, in making of mind a form of *mathos*, is a renewal of Platonism. And we can see in this renewal of Platonism the possibility that the metaphysical construct known as mind is a plausible function of mind, a construct that depends on even as it defines the functioning of neurons. And, conversely, mapping neurological circuits may offer a concept of mind that will allow us to understand the multiple selves we all contain under the general rubric of mind or personality. Our selves may be plotted on multiple meandering neurological circuits that are beginning to suggest a new model of mind—once we find a model to relate neurons to history.

A new concept of self and mind is perhaps evolving that is more fluid than any we have seen in history before. Undoubtedly we shall find that it yields new ways of describing how madness perturbs the multiple relations of the self to its world. Clearly some new model, or models, are needed that go beyond the simplistic causality to which I have alluded in order to describe the multiple possibilities for pathological derangements of the interrelations of neurons and experience, biology and history; and undoubtedly these dichotomies need to be superseded, since the old opposition of nature and culture continues to make itself felt in them. These are, as we might say in borrowing from Kant, antinomies that are based on an older metaphysics, one that is probably not consonant with science or experience. However, my point here and throughout this study is that the historical determinations of madness seem to be part of the experience of madness: the conditions of possibility of certain types of madness are in part historical. The history of insanity has led to the elimination of clearly organic syndromes or ahistorical forms of dementia and neurological dysfunction from the province of madness, leaving classified as madness only those clinical entities that resist being described entirely as a form of organic pathology. One could trace out this history of elimination beginning roughly with general paralysis and going through epilepsy to Alzheimer's syndrome. Other syndromes may be removed from the province of madness, but there are probably limits to this process.

It is an article of faith in most medical research that there is no madness without some kind of organic transformation of the brain, usually some neurological or hormonal pathology. Recent work in molecular biology reinforces the belief that genetic determinants for madness, especially schizophrenia, will be found. As Beckett would have appreciated, recent work with Irish families, for example, proposes chromosome 6 as the susceptibility locus for schizophrenia.[6] This may well be the case—though it has not been conclusively demonstrated. Let us assume that all madness is accompanied by some kind of neurological or hormonal dysfunction, whether genetic in origin or not. If organizational complexity of madness always includes some organic anomaly, this will probably mean that an explanatory model of many forms of madness will have to be described by neurology and history in conjoined determinations. For the evidence already suggests that some basically ahistorical organic pathologies have taken demonstrably different forms in the history of madness.

For example, medical researchers need to ask why the mad no longer become witches or sleep with the devil, or at least rarely when compared with the sixteenth and seventeenth centuries. The specific content of madness is often an imaginative form of fictional construct, pathological to be sure, determined by a cultural matrix that informs the specific context within which neurons or hormones are programmed or that elicits whatever be the genetic determinants of madness. Systematic investigation of the history of melancholy or of the manic-depressive syndrome will probably reveal even greater cultural varieties than we realize today. Melancholy appears to have an invariant organic base and an equally variable cultural and historical component that has generated the variety of melancholias and depressions that have populated our literary and social history. Erotic madness seems to arise during the Renaissance: is this tied up with new types of sublimation? or desublimation? Is it accurate to say that it reaches it zenith in the Freudian concepts of pan-libidinal or erotic motivation and that it is disappearing in our postmodern era in which desire can be conceived as an effect of language? Was hysteria in the nineteenth century, as often argued, a culturally determined form of madness that disappeared when the cultural matrix changed? Empirical proof for answers to these types of questions is singularly difficult, but the questions and the theoretical understanding they may produce are necessary before we can know really what empirical proof might be. And all this must be conceived in the self-examining spirit that recognizes that the history of madness is a history of the understanding of the flexibility of our understanding of madness. This has contemporary implications. For example, the *Diagnostic and Statistical Manual (DSM)* of the American Psychiatric Association has more or less classified Charcot's hysteria out of existence, but recent Lacanian thought has tried to argue hysteria back into the clinic. Historical understanding is clearly at issue here.

The history of the relations between madness and literature is an important part of this historical understanding, for literature gives access to madness. Not only is madness a theme, in the traditional sense of "motif," in literary works; and not only is madness a producer of literature in the sense that the sane and the mad have exploited madness to produce literary texts. Madness and literature also overlap in many ways as projects of the multiple selves in a mind creating a relationship with the world, or in creating a world itself. Both madness and literature can be understood, historically, as ways of producing a world—the trinity of madmen, poets, and lovers in *A Midsummer Night's Dream* are all fiction makers. Madness and literature can be viewed as adaptive strategies, which have evolved in history, as the self has come to exist with a world, or, more aptly, the historical self became able to entertain the possibility of multiple worlds. In literature this capacity is a highly desirable state of affairs, in madness it is not. Madness is a pathology that derives, in part at least, from the capacity for literature. Some future model of brain and mind should account for this relationship; for the fact that the mind, through literature, can entertain multiple possible worlds is as astounding a fact as the fact that drugs can induce hallucinations or that hormonal changes may accompany the mad person's creation of nonexistent voices.

To conclude I should like to quote a passage from Monique Plaza's *Ecriture et folie,* a book on "writing and madness"; and then a passage from a fairly recent overview article about physiological research on "working memory" by Patricia S. Goldman-Rakic. The formulations by these two scholars—a literary critic and a neurobiologist—point to a future discursive possibility that posits literature and science as complementary discourses in explorations of mind and madness. We need to consider culture in terms of its multiple centers of historically unfolding signification. And we need to bring this understanding to bear on the mappings of neurological circuits, the mobile shiftings of alternative circuits that, in coordinating neurological functions, suggest the prodigious malleability of the brain in the production of that historical locus called mind. This is a suggestion, hardly a theory, though my two scholars suggest how historical understanding and science are ready to encounter each other. Plaza's understanding of Artaud's madness describes a historical way that madness existed in the poet's mind:

> Meaning coming from somewhere else imposes upon the writer an identity and a status that are totally antinomic with his current reality, and thus it menaces that reality with a danger that is social in origin.
>
> This meaning is a parasite on the writer's thought. Imported from various sources that the writer tries sometimes to name in order better to objectify them—or expel them from himself, to set himself free from them, or perhaps even to grant them existence—this meaning imposes laws that direct the writer's thought, thought that this exterior signification "tantalizes," to use Artaud's so accurate expression. [These painful intrusions] . . . are heterogeneous to the familiar functioning of psychic life; they have the strength of a devastating cry, a cry all the more painful in that, like a true ultrasound

image of the mind, it can neither be heard nor warded off. This cry destroys the obvious truths that life needs, and all the fragile constructions that are the basis for our mental life: questions such as who am I and who is the Other.[7]

This phenomenological description of madness is oriented by a historical understanding of being in the world that a mad writer proposes and that a literary scholar can articulate.

The neurobiologist, describing schizophrenic disruptions of memory, works at another level of analysis. But in her "Working Memory and the Mind" we recognize a commonality when Goldman-Rakic gropes for a general model for understanding schizophrenia:

> Perhaps researchers should begin to think of schizophrenia as a breakdown in the processes by which representational knowledge governs behavior. In my view, neural pathways in the prefrontal cortex update inner models of reality to reflect changing environmental demands and incoming information. Those pathways guide short-term memory and moment-to-moment behavior. If they fail, the brain views the world as series of disconnected events, like a slide-show, rather than as a continuous sequence, like a movie. The result is schizophrenic behavior, excessively dominated by immediate stimulation rather than by a balance of current, internal and past information.[8]

Her description is based on sketchy knowledge, but it suggests a theory that is complementary to the phenomenological portrayal of madness as a disruptive form of possession. The physiological description is in a sense verified by a description of the poet's own experience.

Disruption of short term memory is also complementary in some sense to the disruption of the long-term memory that we call history. We have some, though hardly complete, ideas about how culture is itself a memory system that imposes continuity upon those individuals who are born into it. A full explanation of madness will put together those various levels of explanation that link individuals, with their sometimes deviant hormonal and neural systems, to the cultural system that, in its own way, can induce pathology—or become pathological itself. This is a subject that opens onto another type of speculation at another level of analysis: when the ecology or the cultural matrix is mad itself. Analysis of modern history leads to the conclusion that madness is often encoded in culture itself. Any reading of German, Russian, or some aspects of modern American history is convincing in this regard. With what sweet simplicity might one wish that genes or hormones were the only factors needed to account for forms of homicidal deviance that so often seem the norm, we sometimes forget that they are insanity.

For this understanding of history, let me conclude by quoting again Emily Dickinson's lines that should be repeated like a mantra of rationality:

> Much madness is divinest sense
> To a discerning eye;
> Much sense the starkest madness.
> 'Tis the majority
> In this, as all prevail
> Assent, and you are sane;
> Demur,—you're straightway dangerous,
> And handled with a chain.

Notes

Part 1

1. Cf. Dieter Jetter, *Geschichte der Medizin* (Stuttgart: George Thieme, 1952), pp. 20–23.

2. I refer especially to Gerald M. Edelman, *The Remembered Present* (New York: Basic Books, 1989).

3. Throughout this book my references to Michel Foucault are to the full French text of *Histoire de la folie à l'âge classique* (and specifically to the 1972 edition by Gallimard also containing *Mon corps, ce papier, ce feu et La folie, l'absence d'oeuvre*) and not to the English translation that, somewhat scandalously, reproduces only part of the total book. I have developed at some length a critique of Foucault in a chapter on historicism in *The Power of Tautology: The Roots of Literary Theory* (Cranbury, N.J.: Associated University Presses, 1997).

4. Thomas Kuhn's argument is developed in *The Structure of Scientific Revolutions*, 2d ed. (Chicago: University of Chicago Press, 1970). Kuhn is a brilliant thinker, but his historical relativism, like Foucault's, has had undue influence, especially among humanists who, for their initiation into the history or philosophy of science, rely exclusively on these two "children of Bachelard"—as Kuhn called himself and Foucault at a lecture in response to a question I asked him about his views of Foucault.

Chapter 1

1. Who was Hippocrates? Undoubtedly a real doctor, though in this chapter and throughout I use the name to designate a group of writings, the "Hippocratic corpus," that has come down to us, from ancient editors, bearing Hippocrates' name. Scholars continue to debate which texts might have been written by the real Hippocrates, and which should be attributed to anonymous followers. There is a consensus that most of them were not written by Hippocrates himself, and some may have been written before Hippocrates lived. The flesh-and-blood Hippocrates was perhaps born at Cos in 460 B.C., perhaps died around 380. My favorite anecdote about the historical Hippocrates concerns his capacity to recognize reason in madness. Called upon to examine Democritus for his insanity, Hippocrates pronounced him to be the most powerful mind in Greece.

2. For Anaxagoras, see G. S. Kirk and J. E. Raven, *The Presocratic Philosophers* (Cambridge: Cambridge University Press, 1957), p. 372. See also Emile Bréhier, *The Hellenic Age,* trans. Joseph Thomas (Chicago: University of Chicago Press, 1963), p. 65.

3. I note here that, because of the peripatetic nature of scholarly life, I have used sources for this work found in libraries in the United States, France, and Germany, which explains the range of editions and translations for classical sources I have used here. For example, the remarkable holding of Renaissance and Enlightenment medical books at the Bibliothèque Méjane in Aix-en-Provence allowed me to look at translations of Hippocrates from several centuries, which suggest that a history of scientific translation would be a noteworthy introduction into the intellectual life of any given era. A 1697 French translation, *Les Oeuvres d'Hippocrates,* makes the psyche into a very Christian soul or *âme,* while the choice of intelligence, as proposed by the Budé edition, secularized Hippocrates for today.

4. *Hippocratic Writings,* trans. J. Chadwick and W. N. Mann (New York: Penguin Books, 1978), p. 248.

5. *Oeuvres anatomiques, physiologiques et médicales de Galien* (Paris: J. B. Baillière, 1854), 1:59, 67.

6. Stanley Jackson, *Melancholia and Depression: From Hippocratic Times to Modern Times* (New Haven: Yale University Press, 1990), p. 30.

7. Critical studies from Ainsworth O'Brien-Moore's early thesis *Madness in Ancient Literature* (Weimar: R. Wagner, 1924) to Lilliane Feder's *Madness in Literature* (Princeton: Princeton University Press, 1980) have been rather unified in attributing to Sophocles the first development of a self that defines itself in opposition to forces that besiege it.

8. *Ajax,* in *Sophocles II,* ed. David Grene and Richard Lattimore (New York: Washington Square Press, 1967), p. 39, ll. 776–77.

9. *Heracles,* in *Euripides I,* ed. David Grene and Richard Lattimore (New York: Modern Library, n.d.), p. 359, ll. 1311–15.

10. *The Bacchae,* trans. Minos Volanakis, in *Euripides,* ed. Robert W. Corrigan (New York: Dell, 1965), p. 168, ll. 31–36.

11. Some of these notions can be found in Fridolf Kudlien, *Der Beginn des Medizinischen Denkens bei den Griechen* (Zurich: Artemis, 1967), p. 56; also Giusseppe Roccatagliata, *A History of Ancient Psychiatry* (New York: Greenwood Press, 1987).

12. Cedric Whitman, *Aristophanes and the Comic Hero* (Cambridge: Harvard University Press, 1964), p. 10.

13. *Five Comedies of Aristophanes* ed. Andrew Chiappe (Garden City, N.Y.: Doubleday Anchor Books).

14. Cf. Bennett Simon, *Mind and Madness in Ancient Greece* (Ithaca, N.Y.: Cornell University Press, 1978), pp. 161–62.

15. *Plato's Cosmology: The Timaeus of Plato,* trans. Donald Cornford (Indianapolis: Bobbs-Merrill, n.d.), 86e.

16. Ernst Robert Curtius, *European Literature and Latin Middle Ages,* 2d ed., trans. Willard R. Trask (Princeton: Princeton University Press, 1967), pp. 49–50.

17. Cicéron [Cicero], *Oeuvres philosophiques, Tusculanes,* book 3, trans. Jules Humbert (Paris: Ed. Les Belles Lettres; Association G. Budé, 1931), p. 7.

18. I draw here largely upon St. Thomas Aquinas, *Philosophical Texts,* trans. Thomas Gilby (London: Oxford University Press, 1962).

19. Jackson, *Melancholia and Depression,* p. 42.

20. Jean Starobinski, *Histoire du traitement de la mélancholie des origines à 1900* (Basel: Acta Psychosomatica, 1960), p. 26.

Chapter 2

1. Marie-José-Imbault-Huart, *La Médicine au Moyen Age* (Paris: Edition de la Porte Verte, Bibliothèque Nationale, 1983).

2. Robert Burton, *The Anatomy of Melancholy,* ed. Joan K. Peters (New York: Frederick Ungar, 1979), p. 16.

3. Thomas Hoccleve, *Selected Poems,* ed. Bernard O'Donoghue (Manchester: Carcanet, 1982), p. 26. Here I leave out of consideration a number of visionary writers, usually having religious visions, especially in the fourteenth century. In England Julian of Norwich or a Margery Kempe had visions and heard voices. If they were insane—and one is inclined to think so today—they illustrate my thesis here that one goes mad within the cultural paradigms that allow the expression of madness.

4. *Dante's Purgatorio,* trans. John D. Sinclair (New York: Oxford University Press, 1968), p. 213.

5. See Jean Delumeau, *La Peur en Occident* (Paris: Hachette-Pluriel, 1980).

6. Erasmus, *The Praise of Folly,* trans. John Wilson (New York: John Simon, 1979), p. 23. This is a new edition of a 1668 translation.

7. Though my comments on Ficino are not flattering, this is largely because I am considering only his role in medicine and medical psychology. A fuller assessment of his historical importance would recognize the role Ficino played, through his Platonism, in bringing about the understanding that, to paraphrase Galileo, nature is written in mathematics. Americo Castro, for instance, has advanced this argument in his pages on Ficino in *El pensamiento de Cervantes* (1925; Barcelona: Editorial Crítica, 1987).

8. Paul Oskar Kristeller, *The Philosophy of Marsilio Ficino,* trans. Virginia Conant (Gloucester, Mass.: Peter Smith, 1964), p. 259.

9. A. Koyré, *Mystiques, spirituels, alchimistes du XVIe siècle allemand* (Paris: Gallimard, Collection Idées, 1972), p. 94.

10. Walter Pagel, *Paracelsus: An Introduction to Philosophical Medicine in the Era of the Renaissance* (Basel: Karger, 1958), p. 150.

11. Cf. Koyré, *Mystiques, spirituels, alchimistes,* p. 82.

12. Paracelsus, *Werke,* ed. Will-Erich Peuchert (Stuttgart: Schwabe, 1965), 2:449. All translations not otherwise attributed are my own.

328 • Notes to Pages 61–106

13. Paracelsus, *Vom Licht der Natur und des Geistes* (Stuttgart: Philippe Reclam, 1960), p. 45.

14. Here I quote from a Renaissance translation found in the Bibliothèque Méjane (Aix-en-Provence), *Les XIV Livres de Paragraphes de Ph. Theoph. Paracelse,* trans. C. de Sarcilly (Paris, 1631), p. 27.

15. I have yet to find a copy of the English translation, though the work was sufficiently popular in France to exist in French translation and Italian original in several of the French research libraries I have used for this work. Garzoni was obviously better known at the end of the Renaissance than he is today.

16. Garzoni, *Il Theatro de' varii e diverse cervelli mondani,* p. 12.

17. For these considerations of Duns Scotus I draw largely upon Emile Bréhier, "Moyen Age et Renaissance," in *Histoire de la philosophie,* ed. Maurice de Gandillac (Paris: Presses Universitaires de France, 1967), vol. 1, pt. 3, pp. 630–35.

18. Tasso, *Aminta* (Milan: Biblioteca Universale Rizzoli, 1987), p. 73, ll. 359–63.

19. Tasso, *Jerusalem Delivered,* trans. Ralph Nash (Detroit: Wayne State University Press, 1987), p. 470.

Chapter 3

1. I am translating here from *Discours de la conservation de la veue: Des maladies melancholiques: des catarrhes: & de la vieillesse,* 1597 ed., p. 110.

2. Or the "calor humida y sequedad," of the fifth chapter. I refer to the critical edition of Juan Huartes's *Examen de ingenios para las ciencias,* 1574 edition, edited by Esteban Torre (Madrid: Editorial Nacionale, 1976), p. 117.

3. *The Adventures of Don Quixote,* trans. J. M. Cohen (Baltimore: Penguin Books, 1970), pp. 31–32.

4. *Don Quijote de la Mancha,* ed. Martin de Riquer (Barcelona: Editorial Juventud, 1958), p. 390.

5. But only in the full French text: I recall that the English translation of Michel Foucault's *Histoire de la folie* is the translation of a truncated French version that does not contain Foucault's discussion of Descartes.

6. *Philosophical Works of Descartes,* trans. Elizabeth S. Haldane and G. R. T. Ross (New York: Dover Publications, 1955), 1:145. My addition of Latin terms.

Chapter 4

1. Emile Guyénot, *Les Sciences de vie aux XVIIe et XVIIIe siècles* (Paris: Albin Michel, 1941), p. 151.

2. *Les Oeuvres de Jean Baptiste Van Helmont, traitant des principes de*

Medecine et de Physique pour la guérison des maladies, trans. Jean Le Conte (Lyon, 1671), p. 232.

3. My discussion of Hoffmann is largely based on his *La Politique du Medecin,* trans. Jacques-Jean Brulier (Paris: Briasson, 1751), as well as *La Medecine raisonnée de Mr. Fr Hoffmann,* trans. Jacques-Jean Brulier, 2 vols. (Paris: Briasson, 1739).

4. Boerhaave, *Aphorismes,* 5th ed., no trans. given (Paris, 1745), p. 205.

5. Gaston Bachelard elaborates the idea that the "prescientific mind" is essentially characterized by the search for unity of thought, as in the case of Paracelsus. For the epistemologist this desire for unity is the major block to real research in prescientific cultures. Cf. *La Formation de l'esprit scientifique,* 4th ed. (Paris: Vrin, 1965), p. 88 and passim.

6. This is Diderot's answer to the mathematician D'Alembert in his *Entretiens entre D'Alembert et Diderot* of 1769. All the following quotations are from *Le Neveu de Rameau, suivi de six oeuvres philosophiques* (Paris: Livre de Poche, 1966), here p. 223.

7. La Mettrie, *Oeuvres de Médecine* (Berlin: Fromery, 1755), p. 112.

8. La Mettrie, *Oeuvres philosophiques, nouvelle edition corrigée et augmentée à Berlin* (1774), p. 316.

9. Jonathan Swift, *Gulliver's Travels and Other Writings,* ed. Ricardo Quintana (New York: Modern Library, 1958), p. 402.

10. Alexander Pope, *Poetical Works,* ed. Herbert Davis (New York: Oxford University Press, 1978), p. 239.

11. Max Byrd has written well on the Augustan hatred of the poor. Cf. the chapter on Pope, for example, in *Visit to Bedlam* (Columbia: University of South Carolina Press, 1974).

12. Diderot, *Lettre sur les aveugles* in *Le Neveu de Rameau,* p. 356.

13. Alphonse de Sade, *Juliette* (Paris: Editions Jean-Claude Lattès, 1979), pp. 246–47.

14. Quoted in Gilbert Lely, *Sade* (Paris: Gallimard, Collection Idées, 1967), p. 278.

Chapter 5

1. George Canguilhem, *Etudes d'histoire et de philosophie des sciences,* 5th ed. (Paris: Vrin, 1983), p. 228. And with further reference to von Haller, I think one can see in him the forerunner of medical positivism. In the *Elementa physiologicae* (Elements of physiology) Haller said that in his experience with autopsies of the mad he usually found abnormal brains and that the pathological alterations frequently extended to the spinal chord and the nerves. He asserted that "if nothing abnormal could be detected in these parts in rare cases, it should not be concluded that they were normal but that the disease process was located in the 'finest organization' of

these parts or that the examination had not been exact or careful." Trans. taken from John C. Hemmeter, *Master Minds in Medicine* (New York: Life Press, 1927), p. 205. The a priori assertion of the existence of fibers is implicit in this statement. However, Canguilhem also argues in his work that the mechanical paradigm came to an end with Haller's work. To which I would reply that Haller represents a different way of using the mechanical model. He introduced the notions of the irritability and sensibility of the muscles and the nerves. But he integrated his new ideas into the fibers physiology of the time: he began his work of physiology by declaring that the smallest fibers must exist if we are then to understand motion. Canguilhem's argument is persuasive, but Haller's contemporary Diderot endorsed Haller and even translated him because he was developing the mechanical paradigm.

2. Chant 2 of *Les Jardins* (1782), quoted in John Porter Houston, *The Demonic Imagination* (Baton Rouge: Louisiana State University Press, 1969), p. 10. This work also has a good chapter on the waning of literary neoclassicism.

3. Goethe, *The Sufferings of Young Werther,* trans. Harry Stein (New York: Bantam Dual Language Book, 1967), pp. 111, 113.

4. Jean Starobinski, "The Illness of Rousseau," *Yale French Studies* 28 (fall–winter, 1961–62): 69. Actually I find a fairly convincing case made for Rousseau's paranoid delusions, described as the classic syndrome of *délire d'interprétion,* made by Dr. Jacques Borel in his *Génie et folie de Jean-Jacques Rousseau* (Paris: José Corti, 1966).

5. *Hölderlin: Selected Verse,* trans. Michael Hamburger (Baltimore: Penguin, 1961), p. 75.

6. Jean-Jacques Rousseau, *Oeuvres complètes,* ed. Bernard Gagnebion and Marcel Raymond (Paris: Ed. de la Pléïade, 1959), 1:669.

7. *The Confessions of Jean Jacques Rousseau,* no trans. given (New York: Modern Library, n.d., p. 2.

8. Charles Singer and E. Ashworth Underwood, *A Short History of Medicine,* 2d ed. (New York: Oxford University Press, 1962), p. 281.

9. This is my translation from the first edition of 1800, available as a reprint edition of the copy in the Bibliothèque Nationale through Sladkine (Geneva, 1980), p. ix. The second edition of 1809 is also available in a reprint edition of the original in the series "Classics in Psychiatry" published by Arno Press (New York, 1976).

10. The works I refer to are P. A. Prost, *Coup d'oeil physiologique sur la folie* (Lyon, 1807) and Joseph Daquin, *Philosophie de la folie,* first published in 1791, then again, dedicated to Pinel, in 1804. The edition I have seen of Daquin's book was published in 1807 in Lyon, in the same volume containing Prost's book. The same volume, I note, contained a *Traité analytique de la folie* by a Dr. L. V. F. Amard, who, in praising Pinel, takes a view contrary to both Prost and Daquin. Asserting that the ancients expected too much from mere men—so much for Cicero—he affirms that mania finds its seat in the viscera; and goes on to expound the classic nosology of idiocy, dementia, mania with delirium, mania without delirium, the latter being either continuous or cyclical. This was a bargain volume.

11. Georget, *De la folie,* ed. J. Postal (Toulouse: Privat, 1972), p. 35.

Chapter 6

1. J. C. Reil, *Von der Lebenskraft,* first reprint by Karl Sudhoff (Leipzig, 1910); reprinted and ed. Karl Sudhoff (Leipzig: Klassiker der Medizin, 1968), p. 91.

2. Philippe Lersch, *Der Traum in der Deutschen Romantik* (Munich: Max Hueber, 1923); see p. 12 for Schubert, p. 34 for "dream as science."

3. So say Franz G. Alexander and Sheldon T. Selesnick in their very Freudian *History of Psychiatry* (New York: Harper and Row, 1966), p. 141.

4. Cf. Klaus Doerner, *Madmen and the Bourgeoisie: A Social History of Insanity and Psychiatry,* trans. Joachim Neugroschel and Jean Steinberg (Oxford: Basil Blackwell, 1981), pp. 238–45.

5. Emil Kraepelin, *One Hundred Years of Psychiatry,* trans. Wade Baskin (New York: Citadel Press, 1962), p. 79.

6. I draw upon Manfred Frank's discussion of Schlegel in Frank and Gianfranco Soldati, *Wittgenstein, Literat und Philosoph* (Pfullingen: Günther Neske, 1989), p. 28.

7. In *Deutsche Romantische Prosa,* ed. Eberhard Reichman (New York: Holt, Rinehart, and Winston, 1965), p. 38.

8. Unless otherwise noted, quotations from Hoffmann are from E. T. A. Hoffmann, *Werke in vier Bänden* (Salzburg: Berland Buch, 1985), here 1:45.

9. For English titles of Hoffmann's works I have used the useful bibliography of Leonard J. Kent and Elizabeth C. Knight, *Selected Writings of Hoffmann* (Chicago: University of Chicago Press, 1969), 2:348–52.

Chapter 7

1. There were of course precursory discoveries pointing to correlations between pathological phenomena and anatomy. For example, in the seventeenth century Willis and Morgani had demonstrated that a correlation often holds between hemiplegia and a lesion on the brain's corpus striatum. This type of localization suggested future research, once machine man died. For a history of neurological discoveries, see John D. Spillane, *The Doctrine of the Nerves* (New York: Oxford University Press, 1981).

2. E. H. Ackerknecht, *A Short History of Medicine,* rev. ed. (New York: Ronald Press, 1968), p. 149.

3. I paraphrase here Roger Bouissou's witty discussion of his compatriot in his *Histoire de la médecine* (Paris: Larousse, 1967), pp. 252–54.

4. For example, see John E. Lesch, *The Emergence of Experimental Medicine* (Cambridge: Harvard University Press, 1984). I have also drawn upon the French translation of Charles Lichtenthael's very useful *Geschichte der Medizin: Histoire de la médecine* (Paris: Fayard, 1978).

5. E. H. Ackerknecht, *A Short History of Psychiatry,* trans. Skulammith Wolff (New York: Hafner, 1959), p. 54.

6. See George Canguilhem, *Le Normal et le pathologique* (Paris: Presses Uni-

versitaires de France, 1961), especially his studies of Claude Bernard and experimental medicine.

7. Moreau de Tours, as he is usually called in French, published *Du haschich et de l'aliénation mental* in 1845. Quotation from Jacques Joseph Moreau, *Hashish and Mental Illness,* ed. Helene Peters and Gabriel G. Nahas, trans. Gordon J. Barnett (New York: Raven Press, 1973), p. 17.

8. Maurice Blanchot, *Entretiens infinis* (Paris: Gallimard, 1969), p. 298. Blanchot is interpreting Foucault's work.

9. Quoted by Albert Béguin in *Esprit,* December 1972, p. 779.

10. Nerval, *Aurélia* (Paris: Livre de Poche, 1972), p. 4.

11. Ross Chambers, "Récit d'aliénés, récits aliénés," *Poétique* 12, no. 53 (1983): 74.

12. Baudelaire, *Oeuvres complètes,* ed. Claude Pichois and Y.-G. Le Dantec (Paris: Ed. de la Pléïade, 1961), p. 1265.

13. The translation is Anthony Harley's prose version in *The Penguin Book of French Verse,* ed. Brian Woledge, Geoffrey Brereton, and Anthony Harley (New York: Penguin, 1977), pp. 406–7.

14. Lautréamont, *Les Chants de Maldoror* (Paris: Garnier-Flammarion, 1969), p. 205.

15. Renan, *Avenir de la science* (Paris: Classiques Larousse, n.d.), p. 22.

16. Rimbaud, *Poésies* (Paris: Gallimard, Collection Poésie, 1973), p. 126.

17. Jacqueline Biard, *Lectures de Rimbaud* (Paris: André Gugeau, 1962), p. 114.

Chapter 8

1. Bruno Latour, *Les Microbes, guerre et paix, suivi de irréductions* (Paris: Editions A. M. Métailié, 1984).

2. See, for example, the forward to the third edition of *Drei Abhandlungen zur Sexualtheorie* (Frankfurt: Fischer, 1984), p. 9.

3. Emil Kraepelin, *La Psychose irréversible,* trans. Odile Jeanteau, presented by Paul Bercherie (Paris: Navarin, 1987), p. 9.

4. Emil Kraepelin, *Clinical Psychiatry: A Facsimile Reproduction,* intro. Eric T. Carlson (New York: Scholars' Facsimiles and Reprints, Delmar, 1981), p. 219.

5. Emil Kraepelin, *Lectures on Clinical Psychiatry,* trans. Thomas Johnston, facsimile of the 1904 edition, intro. Oskar Diethelm (New York: Hafner, 1968) p. 155.

6. Michel Foucault, *Mental Illness and Psychology,* trans. Alan Sheridan (Berkeley and Los Angeles: University of California Press, 1987), p. 6.

7. Eugen Bleuler, *Dementia Praecox, or the Group of Schizophrenias,* trans. Joseph Zinkin (New York: International Universities Press, 1950), p. 7.

8. Peter Amarcher, *Freud's Neurological Education and Its Influence on Psychoanalytic Theory,* in *Psychological Issues,* vol. 4, no. 4, monograph 16 (New York: International Universities Press, 1965), pp. 40–41.

9. Freud, *Gesammelte Werke* (London: Imago, 1948), 11:250.

10. Cf. my "Freud, Lacan, and Structuralist Discourse," in the special issue "Structuralism and Poststructuralism," *Language Forum* 16, nos. 1–2 (1990): 69–92.

11. Freud, *Drei Abhandlungen zur Sexualtheorie,* p. 9.

12. Freud, *New Introductory Lectures on Psychoanalysis,* trans. James Strachey (New York: W. W. Norton, 1965), p. 16.

13. Freud, *The Ego and the Id,* trans. Joan Riviere, ed. James Strachey (New York: W. W. Norton, 1962), p. 43.

14. Malcolm Bowie, *Lacan* (Cambridge: Harvard University Press, 1991), p. 91. I read this work after I had finished my first draft of this chapter; however, I call attention to Bowie, especially since in his work he points out the transition from Freudian allegory to Lacanian allegory, which stresses, I think, that allegory is a central feature of all forms of psychoanalysis.

15. Freud, *An Autobiographical Study,* trans. James Strachey (London: Hogarth Press, 1950), pp. 110–11.

16. Freud, *Leonardo Da Vinci and a Memory of His Childhood,* trans. James Strachey, *Standard Edition* (London: Hogarth Press, 1953), p. 107.

17. Freud, *Collected Papers,* trans. supervised by Joan Riviere, vol. 2 (London: Hogarth Press, 1933). It is with great historical interest that I note that this volume was edited by Virginia and Leonard Woolf. Virginia Woolf's editing Freud suggests an essential dimension of what is meant by "modernism."

Chapter 9

1. Walter Sokel, *Der literarische Expressionismus* (Munich: Langen, Müller, 1970), p. 91.

2. Georg Heym, "Die Irren," in *Expressionnistes allemands,* ed. Lionel Richard (Paris: François Maspéro, 1974), pp. 138–39.

3. Kasimir Edschmid, *Uber den Expressionismus in der Literatur und die neue Dichtung,* 8th ed. (Berlin: Erich Reiss, 1921), p. 55.

4. In the interest of space I omit the German and quote only the excellent translations of Lucia Getsi, here "Klage," in Georg Trakl, *Poems* (Athens, Ohio: Artus Mundium, 1973), p. 166.

5. Herbert Lindenberger, *Georg Trakl* (New York: Twayne, 1972) p. 112.

6. At least Breton wanted his readers to think so: see Breton, *Point du jour* (Paris: Gallimard, Collection Idées, 1970), p. 89.

7. Breton, *Manifestoes of Surrealism,* trans. Richard Seaver and Helen R. Lane (Ann Arbor: University of Michigan Press, 1969), p. 26.

8. Breton, *Nadja* (Paris: Gallimard, Collection Folio, 1964), p. 161.

9. Breton and Paul Eluard, *L'Immaculée Conception* (Paris: Seghers, 1961), p. 24.

10. Leo Navratil, *Schizophrenie und Sprache: Zur Psychologie der Dichtung* (Munich: DTV, 1966), p. 105.

11. Artaud, *Van Gogh le suicidé de la société,* in *Oeuvres complètes* (Paris: Gallimard, 1974), 13:38.

12. Artaud, *Oeuvres complètes* (Paris: Gallimard, 1956), 1:89.

13. Cf. Jacques Derrida, "La parole soufflée," in *L'Ecriture et la différence* (Paris: Editions du Seuil, 1967).

14. As a matter of historical record I would suggest that the first confessional poem was written by ex-surrealist Raymond Queneau in *Chêne et chien* (Paris: Gallimard, Collection Poésies, 1969), first published in 1937. An autobiographical poem, Queneau narrates his depression and psychoanalysis.

15. Sylvia Plath, *Johnny Panic and the Bible of Dreams and Other Prose Writings* (London: Faber and Faber, 1977), p. 32.

16. Sylvia Plath, *Collected Poems,* ed. Ted Hughes (London: Faber and Faber, 1981), p. 243; all quotations are from this edition. Originally in *Ariel.*

17. The expression "father-doctor" is Sexton's in "Cripples and Other Stories," in *The Complete Poems* (Boston: Houghton Mifflin, 1981), p. 160. All quotations from this edition.

Chapter 10

1. Jurgen Ruesch and Gregory Bateson, *Communication: The Social Matrix of Psychiatry* (1951; New York: W. W. Norton, 1968), pp. 79–80.

2. Gregory Bateson, *Steps to an Ecology of Mind* (1972; New York: Ballantine Books, 1989), p. 331.

3. Jean-Paul Sartre, "L'Enfance d'un chef," in *Le Mur* (Paris: Gallimard Folio, 1972), p. 183. The context is a story in which the protagonist, upon being initiated into Freud, discovers he has complexes and that his real self is forever absent to himself. Needless to say, this parody is undertaken in defense of Sartre's belief in the primacy of consciousness. It is with regret that I have not included a section here on Sartre's rich phenomenology of psychopathology.

4. In later writings Bateson projected these ideas back onto the social systems he had studied earlier as an anthropologist. See his *Mind and Nature: A Necessary Unity* (New York: Bantam Books, 1980), where he develops the idea that social systems can go out of control and, losing cybernetic governance, break down. He invented the term *schismogenesis* to describe a runaway social system, which I think emphasizes the homology between individual self-corrective systems and collective ones. Societies can exhibit characteristics that we may call mad.

5. Edelman, *The Remembered Present,* p. 56.

6. Lacan, *Ecrits* (Paris: Editions du Seuil, Collection Points, 1971), 1:90.

7. Lacan, *Le Moi dans la théorie de Freud et dans la technique de la psychanalyse,* ed. Jacques-Alain Miller (Paris: Editions du Seuil, 1978), p. 245.

8. Lacan, *Les Psychoses,* ed. Jacques-Alain Miller (Paris: Editions du Seuil, 1981), p. 213.

9. Joël Dor, *Introduction à la lecture de Lacan* (Paris: Denoël, 1985), p. 126.

10. Phyllis Chesler, *Women and Madness* (New York: Avon, 1972), p. 16.

11. Beckett, *Murphy* (New York: Grove Press, 1957), pp. 167–68.

12. A. Alvarez, *Samuel Beckett* (New York: Viking Press, 1973), p. 33.

13. Beckett, *Three Novels* (New York: Grove Press, 1965), p. 294.

14. I refer in particular to David Porush, *The Soft Machine, Cybernetic Fiction* (New York: Methuen, 1985).

15. Thomas Pynchon, *Gravity's Rainbow* (New York: Viking, 1973), p. 412.

16. *The Complete Poems of Emily Dickinson*, ed. Thomas H. Johnson (Boston: Little, Brown, 1960), no. 435. Johnson's omission of the dashes.

17. Marguerite Duras and Xavière Gautier, *Les Parleuses* (Paris: Editions de Minuit, 1974), p. 36; cf. p. 48.

18. Marguerite Duras, *Le Ravissement de Lol V. Stein* (Paris: Gallimard Folio, 1976), p. 81.

19. Marguerite Duras, *Les Yeux bleus, cheveux noirs* (Paris: Gallimard, 1986), p. 65.

20. Marguerite Duras, *Emily L.* (Paris: Editions de Minuit, 1987), pp. 84–85.

21. Emma Santos, *La Lomécheuse* (Paris: Edition des Femmes, 1978), p. 152.

22. Jeanne Hyvrard, *Mère la mort* (Paris: Editions de Minuit, 1976), p. 60.

Postscript

1. Gerald D. Fischbach, "Mind and Brain," *Scientific American*, September 1992, p. 57. This is a special issue on mind and brain.

2. Benjamin S. Bunney and George K. Aghajanian, "Central Dopaminergic Neurons: A Model for Predicting the Efficacy of Putative Antipsychotic Drugs?" in *Model Systems in Biological Psychiatry*, ed. David J. Ingle and Harvey M. Shein (Cambridge: MIT Press, 1975), p. 105.

3. Solomon H. Snyder, "The Dopamine Connection," *Nature*, September 13, 1990, pp. 121–22. Presentation of research by Sokoloff, Giros, Martres, Bouthenet, and Schwartz, "Molecular Cloning and Characterization of a Novel Dopamine Receptor (D_3) as a Target for Neuroleptics," same issue, pp. 146–51.

4. Ervin Laszlo, "Uses and Limitations of the Cybernetic Modeling of Social Systems," in *Communication and Control*, ed. Klaus Krippendorff (New York: Gordon and Breach, 1979), p. 249.

5. Daniel C. Dennett, *Consciousness Explained* (Boston: Little, Brown, 1991), p. 24.

6. Eliot Marshall, "Dispute Splits Schizophrenia Study," *Science*, May 12, 1995, pp. 792–94.

7. Monique Plaza, *Ecriture et folie* (Paris: Presses Universitaires de France, 1986), p. 77.

8. Patricia S. Goldman-Rakic, "Working Memory and the Mind," *Scientific American*, September 1992, p. 117.

Index

Acharnians, The (Aristophanes), 36
Ackerknecht, E. H., 195, 197
Aeschylus, 14–15, 22
Agave, 27–28
Aghajanian, G. K., 317
Agrippa von Nettesheim, 54, 55,
  57–59, 61, 63, 73, 85, 94
Ajax, 22–24, 25, 26, 36, 156, 157
Ajax (Sophocles), 22–24
A la recherche du temps perdu (Proust),
  240, 242
alchemy, 55, 58–62, 104
"Alchemy of the Verb" (Rimbaud), 220
Alcina the Fairy, 65
Alcmene, 25
Alcmeon, 29
Alexander, 265–67
allegory: breakdown of Christian master
  allegory, 49–50, 51; in Du Laurens,
  75; Freud's use of, 241–42, 243, 244;
  and Galenic orthodoxy, 73; German
  Romantics' text as allegory for psy-
  che, 182–85; and Heinroth, 176–77;
  Ideler's drives and instincts as,
  177–82; madness stripped of allegori-
  cal dimensions in Shakespeare, 76,
  77, 79; in Paracelsus, 60–62; in psy-
  choanalysis, 194, 224, 333n. 14; and
  self, 72; in Tasso, 69, 70
All's Well That Ends Well (Shakespeare), 78–80
Alphonso II of Este, 69
Alvarez, A., 297
Alzheimer's syndrome, 225, 320
Amacher, Peter, 235
Amard, L. V. F., 330n. 10
amathia (stupidity), 39
Ambrose, 40

amentia, 235
American confessional poetry, 271–81
American Psychiatric Association, 321
Aminta (Tasso), 69
*Amore, Commentarium in Convivium
  Platonis, De* (Ficino), 55–56
Amphitryon, 25
analogy principle, 208–11
anatomy, 64. *See also* pathological
  anatomy
Anatomy of Melancholy (Burton),
  45–46
Anaxagoras, 16–17
anima, 3, 39–40, 42
animality. *See* bestiality
animal magnetism, 146
anthropology, 239–40, 284–85
Aphorisms (Boerhaave), 108
Aphrodite, 25
Apollo, 313
Aquinas, Thomas, 40–41, 48
Aragon, Louis, 259, 269
Arcanum, 61
Archeus faber ("generative spirit"),
  104, 106
Ariel (Plath), 271, 275–76
Ariosto, Ludovico, 51, 65, 68, 92
Aristophanes, 31, 32, 33, 34–36, 51, 118
Aristotle and Aristotelianism: on
  causality, 17, 46; and Christianity,
  40–41, 46, 48; compared with
  Sophocles, 22; and Du Laurens, 74,
  75; on madness, 9, 135; in medieval
  universities, 45; on melancholy and
  genius, 55, 134, 248; neoclassical
  revival of, 133, 134; on passions, 41;
  and Tasso, 69–70; and *Thirtieth
  Problem,* 13, 134, 248

Armida, 70, 71
Arrowsmith, William, 25
Artaud, Antonin, 250, 268–71, 272, 276, 280, 322
asthenia, 159–60, 176, 196
astrology, 53, 55, 60, 62
asylums. *See* insane asylums
Athena, 22, 23, 24, 36
Athenian theater and philosophy. *See* Greeks
Augustans, 100, 102, 103, 113–22, 126, 162
Augustine, 95, 174
Aurélia (Nerval), 207–9
autism, 261
Autobiographical Study, An (Freud), 245–48
Avicenna, 60, 105

Bacchae, The (Euripides), 27–30
Bachelard, Gaston, 59, 329n. 5
Bad-Tempered Man, The (Menander), 37
Bakhtin, Mikhail, 88
Balzac, Honoré de, 154
Bataille, Georges, 129–30
Bateson, Gregory, 139, 283–89, 293, 294, 334n. 4
Battie, William, 111–13, 119
Battle of the Books, The (Swift), 115
Baudelaire, Charles, 189, 190, 198, 200, 205, 209–13, 221, 228
Bayle, Antoine, 195
beat generation, 214, 221
Beckett, Samuel, 295–98, 300, 302, 313, 320
Bedlam, 113, 114, 116, 118, 120, 125. *See also* insane asylums
behaviorism, 285
Bellerophon, 13, 14, 157, 161
Bell Jar, The (Plath), 272
Benn, Gottfried, 252, 253
Bergson, Henri-Louis, 113
Bernard, Claude, 164, 197, 332n. 6
Berryman, John, 250
bestiality, 47, 56, 74, 109–10, 113
Beyond the Pleasure Principle (Freud), 236

Bible, 46–47, 62
Bicêtre asylum, 131
Bichat, Marie-François-Xavier, 111, 133, 196
biochemistry, 206
biology, 201, 204, 214, 216, 225, 226, 237, 240–41, 285, 316–18, 320
Birds, The (Aristophanes), 36
Blake, William, 60
Blanche, Emile, 207
Blanchot, Maurice, 206
Bleuler, Eugen, 227, 232, 233, 261
"Blonde Eckbert, Der" (Tieck), 187–89
blood circulation, 8, 9, 99, 106
body: Artaud on, 269; Baudelaire's poetry on, 210, 212–13; Descartes on separation of mind and, 93, 95, 97–99; Du Laurens and fear of, 74–75; Galen on, 42; in Homer, 15; Hyvrard on, 314–15; as machine, 98, 99; as political allegorical figure for state, 29, 76; Sade on, 127–30; social body, 29; somatic-psychic distinction, 15–16, 17; somatic unity of, 15–16
"body politick," 76
Boerhaave, Hermann, 107, 108–9, 122, 226
Böhme, Jakob, 168
Boileau, Nicolas, 118, 227
Bordeu, Théophile de, 123, 124
Borel, Jacques, 330n. 4
Borelli, Giovanni Alfonso, 107
Borges, Jorge Luis, 5, 59, 174
Bowie, Malcolm, 245, 333n. 14
brain: compared with computer, 282; Griesinger on, 202; Kraepelin on involvement of cerebral cortex in dementia praecox, 230; Magendie's experiments on spinal fluid, 196–97; pre-Socratic view of, 19, 21. *See also* mind
Brant, Sebastian, 51, 53
Breton, André, 217, 250, 259–64
Breuer, Josef, 236
Broussais, François, 195–96
Brown, John, 159–60, 176, 196
Brownianismus, 159, 176
Buffon, Georges-Louis Leclerc de, 160

Bunney, B. B., 317
Burton, Robert, 45–46
Byrd, Max, 329n. 11

Calchas, 23
Canguilhem, George, 133, 330n. 1
"Caractères de l'hérédité dans les mal-
    adies nervreuses" (Morel), 204
Carlson, Erec T., 233
Cartesian dualism, 93–101, 103
Castle, The (Kafka), 295
Castro, Americo, 327n. 7
catatonia, 232
causality, 17, 21, 46, 112, 196, 202,
    228–30
Cavalcanti, Guido, 56
Céline, Louis-Ferdinand, 250
Cellular Pathology (Virchow), 205
Celsus, 54
Cervantes, Miguel de, 72, 77, 85–95,
    97, 100, 101, 115–16, 127, 179
Chambers, Ross, 209
Chamfort, Sébastien-Roch Nicolas, 154
chants de Maldoror, Les (Lautréa-
    mont), 214–18
Charcot, Jean-Martin, 201, 229, 230,
    233, 236, 321
Chesler, Phyllis, 294
Cheyne, George, 143
Chiarugi, Vincenzo 146
"chose freudienne, La" (Lacan), 290
Christianity: and Aristotelianism,
    40–41, 46, 48; breakdown of master
    allegory in, 49–50; Christian consen-
    sus of Middle Ages, 44–49; and
    Counter Reformation, 68–72, 75; of
    Erasmus, 53; and Galen, 41–43, 45,
    50; and Heinroth, 173–77; and origi-
    nal sin, 40, 47; and Reformation, 70;
    response of, to Descartes, 104–7; and
    Stoics, 40–41, 52, 174
Cicero, 39–41, 46, 52, 132, 146, 147,
    149, 150, 174, 180
Civilization and Its Discontents
    (Freud), 236
Cixous, Hélène, 303
classification. See taxonomy
Clérambault, Gaëtan Gatian de, 259

Clinical Psychiatry (Kraepelin), 230,
    233
Clouds, The (Aristophanes), 34–35
Cocteau, Jean, 163, 242
cogito, 96
Coleridge, Samuel Taylor, 210
coma, 108
comedy: compared with tragedy,
    21–22, 31; dance in, 36–37; dialectic
    of, 31; and double deviance, 34–36;
    Greek comedy, 30–38, 113; and
    laughter, 33–34; and madness,
    30–33, 113; in Middle Ages, 31; and
    nature of the comic, 32–34; in
    Renaissance, 31, 32; Roman comedy,
    31; romantic comedy, 37–38. See
    also specific works
"Complaint" (Hoccleve), 47–48
complexity theory, 134
Comte, Auguste, 201, 219
Condillac, Étienne Bonnot de, 134, 136
Confessions (Rousseau), 141–42,
    144–45
consciousness: Bateson on, 289; Den-
    nett on, 319; drug-induced alterna-
    tions in, 198–200, 206, 209–10;
    hermeneutics of, 178; history of, 174;
    Ideler on, 178, 181; Lacan on,
    287–90; Moreau on, 198–200. See
    also mind
Consciousness Explained (Dennett),
    319
Cornford, Donald, 39
corporis humani fabrica, De (Vesalius),
    64
correlation principle, 196–97, 208,
    209, 316–17
"Correspondances" (Baudelaire), 200,
    210–11
Counter Reformation, 51, 68–72, 75
Cowper, William, 115
crasis (equilibrium), 29
Creon, 25
Crying of Lot 49, The (Pynchon),
    299
Cullen, William, 147, 159, 176, 231
Curtius, Ernst Robert, 39
Cuvier, Georges, 207, 209

cybernetics, 161, 164–65, 166, 282–85, 300, 309, 315, 318–20

"Daddy" (Plath), 272–73
Daedalus, 242–43
dance, 36–37
Dante, 5, 10, 48–49
Daphne, 313
Daquin, Joseph, 149, 330n. 10
Darius, 14
Darwin, Charles, 160, 204, 205, 232
"Dead Heart, The" (Sexton), 279
death instinct, 247
Death Notebooks, The (Sexton), 276
deconstruction, 17, 209, 267
degeneracy doctrine, 204
Delille, Jacques, 134
delirium, 108, 263
Delumeau, Jean, 51
dementia, 123, 150, 209–10
dementia praecox, 227, 230, 231–33, 263
Demeny, Paul, 218–19
Democritus, 325n. 1
Demole, Victor, 142
Dennett, Daniel C., 6, 319
depression, 209–14, 244–45, 318. See also melancholy
De Quincey, Thomas, 210
Derrida, Jacques, 96
Descartes, René, 4, 72, 77, 92–105, 107, 109, 112, 117, 153, 173
devil worship trials, 47
diabolic possession, 46, 50, 68
Diagnostic and Statistical Manual of Mental Disorders (DSM), 151, 225, 227, 234, 321
Dialogues (Rousseau), 141, 144
Dicaeopolis, 36
Dickinson, Emily, 303, 307, 324
Dictionnaire universel de Medecine (James), 122
Diderot, Denis, 103, 109, 114, 115, 122–27, 190, 330n. 1
Diefendorf, A. Ross, 230
Ding an sich ("thing in itself"), 170
Dionysus, 27, 28, 30

Discours de la conservation de la veue (Du Laurens), 73
Discourse Concerning the Mechanical Operation of the Spirit (Swift), 115
Discourse on Method (Descartes), 77, 94
"disease of the state," 29, 76
divided self myth, 208–9
Divine Comedy, The (Dante), 48–49
Doob, Penelope, 46–47
"Don Giovanni" (Hoffmann), 193, 194
Don Juan, 114, 193
Don Quixote (Cervantes), 77, 85–92, 93, 95, 115–16, 192
dopamine, 317
Doppelgänger, 190. See also doubles
Dostoyevsky, Fyodor, 190
double bind, 285–87, 295, 298, 299–300
Double, The (Dostoyevsky), 190
doubles, 188–89, 190, 192–94, 220, 256–57, 274–75
"Dream and Derangement" (Trakl), 258
dream hypothesis, 95–96
dreams: Breton on, 259; Diderot on, 124; Freud on, 186, 244, 248, 259; German Romantics and madness as, 186–89; Ideler on, 181; in Novalis's Heinrich von Ofterdingen, 186; Reil on, 172; and romantics, 172; in Tieck's "Der Blonde Eckbert," 187–89
drives, conflict between passions and, 179–82
drugs, 198–200, 206, 209–10, 269, 316–17, 322
"Drunken Boat, The" (Rimbaud), 222–23
DSM. See Diagnostic and Statistical Manual of Mental Disorders (DSM)
dualism. See Cartesian dualism
Du Laurens, André, 73–77, 80, 83
Dunciad, The (Pope), 119–22
Duns Scotus, John, 64, 65
Duras, Marguerite, 304–8, 313
Dyskolos (Menander), 37

ecology, 302, 315
Ecrits (Lacan), 288
Ecriture et folie (Plaza), 322
Edelman, Gerald, 4–5, 286
Edschmid, Kasimir, 254
ego: Freud on, 4, 241–42, 244–45, 247; Lacan on, 288, 289–91
Ego and the Id, The (Freud), 236, 244–45
Eichendorff, Joseph, 183–86, 187
Electra, 243
Eliot, George, 302
Elixiere des Teufels, Die (Hoffmann), 193
"Elm" (Plath), 275
Eluard, Paul, 262–63, 266
Emile (Rousseau), 144
Emily L. (Duras), 306–7
Empedocles, 155
Emperor's New Mind, The (Penrose), 319
empiricism, 167, 168, 170, 181
"Enchantment in Autumn" (Eichendorff), 183–85
Encyclopédie (Diderot), 122–23
English empiricism, 103
English Malady, The (Cheyne), 143–44
Enlightenment, 102, 103, 105–7, 113–32, 142, 143, 147–52, 159–61
Entwurf einer Psychologie (*Project for a Scientific Psychology;* Freud), 236–37
Epictetus, 147
Epicurus, 117
epilepsy, 7, 9, 11, 21, 105, 225, 320, 325n. 1, 326n. 3
equilibrium and madness, 18–20, 29, 30, 38
Erasmus, Desiderius, 44, 51–53, 54, 68, 70, 88, 126, 127
Eros and Civilization (Marcuse), 52
eros as madness, 54–57, 63, 74, 75, 82, 321
Esquirol, Jean-Étienne-Dominique, 153, 201
"Essai de simulation du délire d'interprétation" (Breton), 264
Essay on Man, An (Pope), 119, 121

Eumenides, 14, 15
Eumenides (Aeschylus), 15
euphoria, 210–11
Euripides, 18, 22, 24–30
Every Man in His Humor (Jonson), 32
evil, 178
evolution, 160
Examen de ingenios para las ciencias (Huartes), 86
expressionism, 214, 251–58, 267

fairies, 65, 67
fantastic tales, 183–89
fantasy, 181–82, 194, 242, 247
fate, 22–23
father's role: Lacan on, 291–93. *See also* Oedipal complex
Faust, 59
Feder, Lilliane, 326n. 7
feminism, 127–28, 165, 293, 294, 302–4. *See also* gender and madness; women and insanity
Ficino, Marsilio, 54–57, 59, 60, 71, 74, 75, 327n. 7
First Discourse (Rousseau), 142
Fischbach, Gerald D., 316
Fitzgerald, Edward, 13
Flaubert, Gustave, 205
Flowers of Evil, The (Baudelaire), 205, 211–12
folie circulaire, 213
Folscia, Arnolida, 68
"For the Year of the Insane" (Sexton), 279–80
Foucault, Michel, 6, 9, 86, 94, 95, 111, 232–33, 277, 325nn. 3–4, 328n. 5
Fourteen Books of Paragraphs, The (Paracelsus), 62–63
French Revolution, 130, 132, 141–42
Freud, Sigmund: Breton on, 259; and causality, 229; on death instinct, 247; on desires, 189; on dreams, 186, 244, 248, 259; on eros, 55; and Ficino, 55, 56, 57; on Hoffmann, 190; on id, ego, and superego, 4, 56, 241–42, 244–45, 247; on incest, 189; literature used by, 226, 234–35, 237–43, 246–49; on lust and duty, 180; and

Freud, Sigmund (*continued*)
  neurology, 224–25, 234–35, 237; on
  Oedipal complex, 67, 241–44, 277,
  286; on poetry, 248, 251; as pop
  icon, 164; precursors of, 124, 174,
  181–82, 201; and psychoanalysis,
  161, 224–26, 234–49; on psychosis,
  67, 174, 243–48, 277; on repression,
  57, 224–25, 236; on self, 177, 236,
  241–42, 244–45, 247, 263–64; on
  stress and mental illness, 229–30; on
  sublimation, 57; on transference,
  279; Woolfs' editing of, 333n. 17;
  writings by, 236
Furies, 15
furor poeticus, 176

Galen: challenges to generally, 54, 58;
  Christianity's acceptance of, 41–43,
  45, 50; debate between Cicero and,
  149; Du Laurens and continuing
  Galenic orthodoxy, 73–77; end of
  inclusion of significance of, 160,
  226; followers of, 87; Garzoni's displacement of, 63–65; and humors
  theory, 5, 18; on madness, 41–43,
  55; orthodoxy of, in seventeenth
  century, 73; Paracelsus's rejection
  of, 59–61, 63; on soul, 20; translation of, 44
Galileo, 77, 93, 95, 102, 327n. 7
Gall, Franz Joseph, 196
Ganzheit, 167
Garzoni, Tommaso, 54, 55, 63–68, 82,
  85, 328n. 15
gastroenteritis, 196
Gautier, Theophile, 200
gender and madness: feminist visions of
  rupture with (male) logos, 302–4;
  introduction to, 293–95; Lacan on
  "phallic signifier," 291–93; male
  postmodern madness, 295–301;
  mother's role in madness, 293–94;
  psychotic defenses of madness by
  women, 308–15. *See also* women and
  insanity
general paralysis, 11, 195, 196, 209,
  225, 263, 320

genetic determinism, 204, 205, 229,
  260
Georget, Etienne Jean, 153, 154
German expressionism, 251–58
German romantics: and Diderot's
  Rameau's Nephew, 125; fantastic
  tales by, 183–89; Heinroth and theological dimension of romantic
  madness, 173–77; Hoffmann and
  need for critical irony, 189–94;
  Ideler and allegories of drives and
  instincts, 177–82; and madness as
  dream, 186–89; and Nerval, 206;
  and psychiatry, 111, 133, 164,
  167–68; Reil and rhapsodies about
  madness, 169–73; significance of,
  163–64; text as allegory for psyche,
  182–85
Getsi, Lucia, 255
ghosts, 80–81, 82
gnostic tradition, 60
God: Descartes on, 96, 97; Freud on,
  258, 277; Lautréamont on, 215–16;
  Sexton on, 276–77, 280; Trakl on,
  258; "twilight of the gods," 252–53,
  258
Gödel's theorem, 300, 319
Goethe, Johann Wolfgang von: on
  empathetic sensibility, 146; and
  Faust, 59; and Freud, 247; on Hoffmann, 190; and Ideler, 179; and
  rational self, 153; significance of generally, 5; singular mad voices created
  by, 115, 135–41, 144, 152; translation of Diderot's *Rameau's Nephew*
  by, 125
Goldman-Rakic, Patricia S., 322, 323
Gravity's Rainbow (Pynchon), 299,
  300–301
Greeks: Athenian theater, 2, 11, 14–15;
  comedy and madness, 30–38, 113;
  Hippocrates and rationalist world of
  pre-Socratics, 15–22, 24, 29, 33, 38,
  39, 42, 45; logos and madness in
  early Greek literature, 2, 11, 12,
  13–15, 161; Platonic view of madness, 38–39; tragedy's depiction of
  madness, 18, 21–30

Griesinger, Wilhelm, 200–204, 206, 213–14, 226, 227, 228, 248
Grundriss der Seelenheilkunde (Outline of mental therapy; Ideler), 178, 179
guilt, 169, 174
Gulliver's Travels (Swift), 116
Guyénot, Emile, 104–5

hagiography, 8
Haller, Albrecht von, 123, 132, 133, 329–30n. 1
Hamburger, Michael, 143
Hamlet (Shakespeare), 80–84, 85, 162, 194
"Hanging Man, The" (Plath), 275–76
happiness, Rousseau on, 144
harmony, in Greek art, 29–30
Harvey, William, 8, 9, 99, 102, 106
Hashish and Mental Illness (Moreau), 198–200
Hecker, Ewald, 232
Hegel, G. W. F., 8, 12, 148, 175, 277, 300
Heidegger, Martin, 253
"Heilige Serapion, Der" ("The Hermit Serapion"; Hoffmann), 191–92
Heinrich von Ofterdingen (Novalis), 186
Heinroth, J. C. A., 169, 173–78, 190
"Helian" (Trakl), 256–58
Henry IV, 73
Hera, 25, 26
Heracles (Euripides), 25–26
Heraclitus, 15, 166
hereditary influences on madness, 204, 205, 229, 241, 251–54, 260
hermeneutics: of consciousness, 178; of Freud, 240; of madness in Shakespeare, 77–85, 178–79; modern hermeneutics, 209; and psychoanalysis, 179, 194
hermeticism, 255
Heym, Georg, 252
Hippocrates and "Hippocratic corpus": biographical information on Hippocrates, 325n. 1; challenges to, 54, 58; compared with Athenian literary genre, 33; and Descartes, 99; end of inclusion of, in medical curriculum, 160; on epilepsy, 9; and Galen, 42; hope in beneficent power of nature, 113; and Kraepelin, 228; Littré's edition of, 226; on madness, 11, 15–20, 24, 38, 149; on medicine as knowledge of mankind, 7; neoclassical revival of Hippocratic medicine, 102, 131, 132, 133, 146, 148, 149; Pinel on, 148; and Plato's *Timaeus*, 39; printed editions of, in Middle Ages, 45; on *psyche*, 15–16, 18–20; rephrasing of, in *Don Quixote*, 88; on *thymos*, 17–18; translations of, 326n. 3
Hippolytus, 25, 239
Histoire de la folie (Foucault), 6, 94
Histoire du traitement de la mélancholie (Starobinksi), 42
Histoire naturelle (Buffon), 160
Histoire naturelle de l'âme (La Mettrie), 109
history, 7–12, 142, 144, 174
History of the Psychoanalytic Movement (Freud), 235–36
Hoccleve, Thomas, 47–48, 49, 71
Hoffmann, E. T. A., 125, 183, 190–94, 205, 220, 244
Hoffmann, Heinrich, 107–8
Hölderlin, Friedrich, 12, 115, 142–43, 154–58, 253, 254
Homer, 2, 4, 5, 13, 14, 157, 161
Homme machine (La Mettrie), 108, 109–10
homosexuality, 142
Horace, 118
hormone imbalance, 318
Hospitale de' pazzi incurabili (Garzoni), 63
How It Is (Beckett), 297
Huartes, Juan, 86
Huart, Marie-José-Imbault, 44
hubris, 22, 24, 27
Hume, David, 112, 252
humors theory, 5, 18–21, 32, 37, 41–42, 46, 56, 149
hypochondria, 42, 63, 107

hysteria, 67, 107, 209, 233–34, 236, 321
hysteriform obsessions and reactions, 142
Hyvrard, Jeanne, 304, 311–15

"I": in Beckett, 296; Descartes on, 96; Griesinger on, 213–14; Jakobson's definition of, 4; Lacan on, 290; of Lautréamont, 217–18; in linguistics, 310; of Rimbaud, 218, 220. See also self
iatro-chemical medicine, 104–7, 168
iatro-mechanical era: Augustans' derision of madness, 113–22; exemplary iatro-chemical understanding of madness, 104–7, 168; iatro-mechanical consensus on machine man's madness, 107–10, 123, 159–60; literary materialists and machine man's madness, 122–30; science of insanity in, 111–13
iatro-mechanical medicine, 107–10, 123, 159–60
Ibsen, Henrik, 204
Icarus, 243
id, 30, 56, 241, 244–45
Ideler, Karl Wilhelm, 169, 178–82, 185, 190, 194
idiocy, 150
idiolect, 267
"idiopathic phrenesy," 108
Iliad (Homer), 13, 14
Illuminations (Rimbaud), 214, 219, 222
imagination, 154, 181, 247, 287–88
L'Immaculée Conception (Breton and Eluard), 263
imperial self, 132, 142
incertitudine, De (Agrippa), 58
incest, 187, 189
inflammations, 196
information theory, 284, 310. See also cybernetics
insane asylums, 63–68, 113–16, 118, 120, 125, 131, 136, 150, 260, 265, 294, 296–97, 312
insanity. See psychiatry; psychoanalysis; psychosis; specific categories, such as melancholy; specific writers in literature and medicine
International Classification of Diseases (World Health Organization), 225
Interpretation of Dreams (Freud), 236
Introductory Lectures (Freud), 237–39
introspection, 199
Irigaray, Luce, 303
Irish families, 320
irony: allegories used with, 51; in Baudelaire, 210; in Breton and Eluard, 263; in Cervantes, 92; in Enlightenment writers generally, 118; in Erasmus, 51–53; in Hoffmann, 189–94, 205; in Lacan, 227–28; in Lautréamont, 217; in New Criticism, 267; in Plath, 274; in Pope, 120; in Rimbaud, 219; in Swift, 115, 116
"Irren, Die" (The mad; Heym), 252
"Irrenhaus" (Stadler), 253
isonomia (equality of rights of bodily qualities), 29, 30

Jakobson, Roman, 4
James, Robert, 122
Janet, Pierre-Marie-Félix, 142, 259
Jerusalem Delivered (Tasso), 69–70, 72
Jerusalem Liberated, 70–71
"Johnny Panic and the Bible of Dreams" (Plath), 272
Johnson, Samuel, 114
Johnson, Stanley, 20–21
Jonson, Ben, 32
Joyce, James, 163, 240, 242–43, 277, 279
Julian of Norwich, 327n. 3
Juliette ou les prospérités du Vice (Juliette or the prosperity of vice; Sade), 128

Kafka, Franz, 80, 242, 243, 275, 277, 279, 295, 302
Kahlbaum, Karl, 232
Kant, Immanuel, 136, 147, 163, 168–73, 179–81, 183, 191, 192, 320
Kekulé, Friedrich August, 300
Kempe, Margery, 327n. 3

Kepler, Johannes, 77
King Lear (Shakespeare), 83, 84–85, 140
"Klage" (Lament; Trakl), 255–56
"Knight Gluck" (Hoffmann), 190–91
Koyré, A., 57
Kraepelin, Emil, 176, 213, 224, 225, 227–34, 236
Kristeller, Paul Oskar, 55
Kuhn, Thomas, 10, 325n. 4

La Bruyère, Jean de, 154
Lacan, Jacques: Bowie's work on, 333n. 14; compared with Kant, 181–82; on consciousness, 287–90; and Duras, 304, 307–8; on ego, 288, 289–91; on human subject, 4, 287–88; on hysteria, 321; on imagination, 247, 287–88; irony in, 227–28; and linguistics, 284–85, 288–92; on mind, 287–88; on mirror stage in human development, 173, 290; on "phallic signifier," 291–93; on psychosis, 291–93; on the "real," 291; on self, 287–91, 294; on signifier, 291, 292, 295, 298; and tragedies in logos, 287–93; on unconscious, 289
"Lady Lazarus" (Plath), 275
la folie, De (Georget), 153
Laforgue, René 142
Lamarck, Jean, 150, 204
"Lament" (Trakl), 255–56
La Mettrie, Julien Offroy, 108, 109–12, 128, 160
language: Beckett on, 297–98; deconstructive theories of, 17; Descartes on, 96–97; in *Don Quixote,* 87; Edelman on self and, 4–5; and Garzoni's types of madness, 66–67; and human community, 161; imaginative use of, and madness, 281; Lacan on, 284–85, 288–92; La Mettrie on, 110; madness and rejection of, 310–11; shared language and rationality, 16; structuralist reductionism of, 4; Wittgenstein on, 3, 6, 86, 202. *See also* linguistics; logos

language games, 3–4, 6, 33–34, 86, 87, 202, 226, 234, 267
Laszlo, Ervin, 318
Latour, Bruno, 226
Lautréamont, 205, 214–18, 258
Lavoisier, Antoine-Laurent, 133
layered self, 207
Le Camus, Antoine, 111
Lectures on Clinical Psychiatry (Kraepelin), 230–31
Leda, 264
leeches, 196
Lehrbuch (Kraepelin), 225, 227, 230, 231
Lehrbuch der Störungen des Seelen-lebens (Textbook on the disturbances of soul life; Heinroth), 174
Leibniz, Gottfried Wilhelm, 107, 114, 129, 171
Leonardo da Vinci, 246
Lersch, Philippe, 172
Lettre sur les aveugles (Letter on the blind; Diderot), 123
Lévi-Strauss, Claude, 284
Libation Bearers, The (Aeschylus), 14–15
Lindenberger, Herbert, 258
linguistics, 161, 165, 282–85, 288–92, 308–9, 310. *See also* language
Linnaeus, Carolus, 145, 231
literature: categories for periodization in, 6–7; compared with medicine generally, 6–7, 161–62; compared with science, 5; Freud's use of, 226, 234–35, 237–43, 246–49; history of, 7; and madness generally, 152–53, 162, 321–24; modernity in generally, 163, 205–6, 250–51. *See also* specific authors and works
Littré, Maximilien Paul Emile, 226
Locke, John, 4, 99, 112, 134
logos: "applied logos," 308; Bateson, schizophrenia, and theory of double bind, 285–87; Christian view of, 40, 42–43; and cybernetic theories of psyche, 282–85; feminist visions of rupture with (male) logos, 302–4; Greek view of, 11, 13–19, 29, 30, 31,

logos (*continued*)
  38, 161, 165, 166, 282–83; Heraclitus on, 166; and human community, 161; Lacanian tragedies in, 287–93; and linguistic theory of psyche, 282–85; and Pope, 118; postmodern view of, 165–66. *See also* language
Lol V. Stein (Duras), 305–6
Lombardo, Marco, 48–49
Loméchuse, La (Santos), 309–11
"Loss of Reality in Neurosis, The" (Freud), 247
Lucretius, 5
Luther, Martin, 53
Lycus, 25

Macbeth (Shakespeare), 62, 80, 83
Mach-Duhem-Poincaré hypothesis, 318
Machiavelli, Niccolò, 53–54, 87
machine man: Battie on, 111–13; demise of, and neoclassicism, 132–35; Descartes on, 98, 99; and Diderot, 103, 123, 125–26; iatro-mechanical consensus on madness of, 107–10, 123; literary materialists and madness of, 122–30; and Pope, 121; and Sade, 103, 127–30, 136; Van Helmont on, 104–7
Madame Bovary (Flaubert), 205
madness. *See* psychiatry; psychoanalysis; psychosis; specific categories, such as melancholy; specific writers in literature and medicine
Magendie, François, 111, 133, 168, 196–97, 213
magic, 53, 58, 65–66, 71, 89, 98
magnetism, 196
Malherbe, François de, 227
mania, 21, 39, 149, 150, 213, 263
manic-depressive syndrome, 321
Manifesto of Surrealism, 260
Manson, Charles, 262
Marcuse, Herbert, 52
Marxism, 52, 285
materialism, 196–200
materialist monism, 198–201, 203, 204, 210–11, 228
mechanical model. *See* machine man

Médecin d l'esprit, Le (The Mind Doctor; Le Camus), 111
Medical-Philosophical Treatise on Mental Alienation, or Mania (Pinel), 131, 148–53
Medici, Lorenzo de', 55
medicine: Broussais on disease as matter of inflammations, 195–96; categories for periodization in, 6–7; compared with literature generally, 6–7, 161–62; correlation principle in, 196; in *Don Quixote*, 87–88; Du Laurens on madness and continuing Galenic orthodoxy, 73–77; Galen and Greco-Roman medicine, 5, 18, 20, 41–44, 45, 50; Hippocrates and rationalist world of pre-Socratics, 15–22, 29, 33, 38, 39, 42, 45; history of, 7–12; iatro-chemical understanding of madness, 104–7; iatro-mechanical consensus on machine man's madness, 107–10; on madness during Renaissance, 54–68; in Middle Ages, 44–46; modernity in generally, 162–63, 226; in Molière's *Don Juan*, 114; neoclassical revival of Hippocratic medicine, 102, 131, 132, 133, 146, 148, 149; Nerval on police function of doctors, 207; in Plato's *Timaeus*, 38–39; in Pope's *Dunciad*, 119–22; in Renaissance, 32, 44; Roman view of, 39–40; Rousseau on, 145, 146; in Shakespeare's *All's Well That Ends Well*, 78–80; transformation of medicine of symptoms to medicine of lesions, 195–96; and Vesalius, 50; and vitalism, 123, 132–33, 146. *See also* pathological anatomy; psychiatry; psychoanalysis; specific doctors
medieval period. *See* Middle Ages
Meditations on First Philosophy (Descartes), 77, 94–98
Megara, 25
Melancholia metamorphosis, 176
Melancholie amoureuse, 75
melancholy: Aristotle on genius and, 55, 134, 248; and Baudelaire, 209–14; Burton on, 45–46; Cheyne

on, 143–44; Delille on, 134; in *Don Quixote,* 88; faddish affectation of, in late seventeenth century, 134; Griesinger on, 213; history of, 321; humors theory of, 20–21; Pinel on, 150, 153; of Rousseau, 142; vapors theory of, 42

Menander, 31, 32, 37–38

meningitis, 195

mental hospitals. *See* insane asylums

Mental Illness and Psychology (Foucault), 277

Mental Pathology and Therapeutics (Griesinger), 200–203

Mère la mort (Hyvrard), 312–15

mesmerism, 146

metamorphosis, 56, 65–66

Meynert, Theodore, 235

microbiology, 152, 226

Middle Ages: breakdown of Christian master allegory in, 49–50; Christian consensus of, 44–49; comedy in, 31; defense of rationality in Renaissance literary discourse, 50–54; madness as described in, 46–49; medical thought on madness during Renaissance, 54–68; medicine in, 44–46; and Reformation, 70; Tasso and madness of Counter Reformation, 68–72, 75

Midsummer Night's Dream, A (Shakespeare), 321

Mill on the Floss (Eliot), 302

mimesis, 193, 194, 248

mind: Anaxagoras on, 16–17; Bateson on, 285, 288; compared with computer, 282; Dante on, 49; Dennett on, 319; Descartes on separation of body and, 93, 95, 97–99; Heinroth on, 174; Heraclitus on, 166; Lacan on, 287–88; as locus of actualization of linguistic system, 282; and logos, 17; Moreau on, 198–200; Penrose on, 318–19; postmodern view of, 165, 282; rejection of mechanistic model of, 133–34; Rimbaud's somatic view of, 221; and vitalism, 133–34

mirror analogy, 173, 290

"Mirror" (Plath), 275

"Mnemosyne" (Hölderlin), 155–58

modernity: definition of *modern,* 162–63; Du Laurens and continuing Galenic orthodoxy, 73–77; introduction to, 159, 162–66; in literature generally, 163, 205–6, 250–51; in medicine generally, 162–63, 226; and romantic irony, 189–90; "symbolists," 205–23. *See also* specific authors and works

molecular biology, 320

Molière, 35, 88, 114

monarchia (dominance of one quality), 29

monomania, 213

Montaigne, Michel de, 59, 94

monumental history, 8

moon, as cause of insanity, 149

moral treatment, 147, 149

Moreau, Jacques-Joseph, 198–200, 203, 206, 210, 221, 228

Morel, Benedict, 142, 204, 231

Morgani, 331n. 1

Moriae Encomium (Praise of Folly; Erasmus), 51–53

"Mothers" (Sexton), 277–78

mother's role, 293–94. *See also* Oedipal complex

Murphy (Beckett), 296–97

myths, 10, 14, 60, 239–40, 264, 313

Nabokov, Vladimir, 250

Nadja (Breton), 260–62

Narcissus, 194

National Socialism, 253–54, 258

natural causality axiom, 17, 21

Natural History of the Soul (La Mettrie), 109

naturalism, 72, 204

Natural Method of Curing the Diseases of the Body (Cheyne), 143

nature, 61–62, 71–72, 93

Navratil, Leo, 265, 266

Nazi movement, 253–54, 258

Nebuchadnezzar's Children (Doob), 47

neoclassicism: and demise of machine man, 132–34; and Diderot's *Rameau's Nephew*, 126; and Hippocratic revival, 102, 131, 132, 146, 148, 149; and Hölderlin, 154–58; and imperial self, 132; and myth of madness as epiphanic vision, 131, 132, 134–46; Pinel and philanthropic psychiatry, 131, 135, 146–54; of Pope, 118–22; and singular literary voices speaking of their madness, 134–46
Neoplatonism, 54–57, 60, 82, 83, 104–5
Nerval, Gerard de, 205, 206–9, 300
neurobiology, 323
neuroleptics, 317
neurological subject, 4
neurology, 11, 161, 200–201, 224–25, 227, 235, 237, 287, 316
neurosis, 243, 247, 260
New Criticism, 267
New Introductory Lectures on Psychoanalysis (Freud), 244, 246
Newton, Sir Isaac, 8, 100, 108, 119, 146
Nietzsche, Friedrich, 8, 24, 29–30, 277
Nosographie philosophique (Pinel), 146–47
nostalgia, 176, 182, 213
noumenal world, 168, 170, 173
Nous (mind or intelligence), 17
Novalis, 183, 186, 244

O'Brien-Moore, Ainsworth, 22, 326n. 7
obsessions, 142
Occleve, Thomas. *See* Hoccleve, Thomas
occult and hermetic sciences, 58, 59
Odysseus, 243
Oedipal complex, 67, 241, 242, 243, 244, 270–71, 277, 286
Oedipus, 12, 23, 24, 29, 36, 194, 241, 243
Oedipus (Sophocles), 29
Oedipus Rex (Cocteau), 163, 242
On Ancient Medicine, 20

One Hundred Years of Psychiatry (Kraepelin), 227
On Human Nature, 18
On Regimen, 18–19
On the Nature of Man, 18, 20
opposites, 18–20
oratio (speech), 40
Orestes, 14–15
original sin, 40, 47, 204
Origin of Species (Darwin), 205
Orlando Furioso (Ariosto), 65
otherness, 28
Outline of Psycho-Analysis, An (Freud), 236
Ovid, 56

Pagel, Walter, 60
paleontology, 207
Pamela (Richardson), 127
Panofsky, Erwin, 55
Paracelsus, 8, 54, 55, 59–63, 73, 75, 104, 117, 155, 168
Paradoxe sur le comédien (Paradox about the actor; Diderot), 123–24
paralysis. *See* general paralysis
paranoia, 66, 269, 274, 295, 317
paranoia catholica, 176
paresis, 196
Parkinson's disease, 11
Pascal, Blaise, 145
passions: Aquinas on, 41; Aristotle on, 41; Cicero and Stoics on, 40, 41, 46, 76, 82; Descartes on, 93, 98, 99–100; Heinroth on, as sin, 174–75; Ideler on conflict between drives and, 169, 179–82; and madness, 40, 41, 46, 76, 82, 149, 242; Pinel on, 153; Rousseau on, 144
Pasteur, Louis, 226
pathological anatomy: background to positivist psychiatry, 195–98; Griesinger and positivist view of madness, 26, 200–204; Moreau and materialist poetics of madness, 198–200
Pathologie und Therapie der psychischen Krankheiten (Griesinger), 200–203

Paul, Jean, 190
Penrose, Roger, 318–19
Pentheus, 27–28, 30
Peripatetics, 41
Persians, The (Aeschylus), 14
person. *See* self
Pèse-nerfs (Artaud), 269–70
Phaedra, 24–25, 239
Phaedra (Plato), 38
"phallic signifier," 291–93
Phantasiestücke (Hoffmann), 193
phenomena (making present of being through vision), 17
philanthropic psychiatry, 131, 135, 146–54, 169
Philocleon, 36
philosophe movement, 102
philosophers, Rousseau on, 145
Philosophia occulta (Agripppa), 58
Philosophie de la folie (Daquin), 149
phrenitis, 21
phrenology, 196
physiology, 161, 197–98, 206, 213
Piazza universale di tutte le professione del monde, La (Garzoni), 63
Pinel, Philippe: and *anima*, 133; compared with romantic psychiatrists, 168; and Daquin, 330n. 10; and Griesinger, 201; and Heinroth, 176; on Hippocrates and "Hippocratic corpus," 148; Hoffmann's reading of, 190, 191; on imagination, 154; Kraepelin on, 227; on Locke and Condillac, 134; on melancholy, 150, 153; and moral treatment, 147, 149; on passions, 153; and philanthropic psychiatry, 12, 131, 135, 146–54, 164; and Platonism, 147; precursor of, 141; on Rousseau's melancholy, 142; taxonomy of, 147–48, 231
Plath, Sylvia, 216, 250, 271–76, 280
Plato and Platonism: and Christian logos, 40; compared with cybernetics, 319–20; and Ficino, 55–56; on healthy self, 18, 38; and Hippocrates, 15; on madness, 38–39, 83; and *Phaedra*, 38; Pinel on, 147; rationality of, 16; and *The Republic*, 30, 38,

83; and Socrates, 35; on soul, 20; and *Symposium*, 55; and *Timaeus*, 38–39. *See also* Neoplatonism
Platonic love, 55
Plautus, 31
Plaza, Monique, 322
Plotinus, 40, 56
Plutarch, 147
Poe, Edgar Allan, 187, 189, 190
poetry: American confessional poetry, 271–81; Freud on, 248, 251; German expressionism, 251–58; insane poetic text, 265–71; introduction to modernist writers, 250–51; surrealism, 259–64, 267–71; "symbolists," 205–23; Trakl and experience of psychiatric determinations of madness, 254–58. *See also* specific poets
polis, 30, 36
Pomme, Pierre, 159
Pope, Alexander, 103, 114, 115, 118–26, 129, 162
positivism, 153, 160–61, 164, 167, 195, 205, 245, 247
positivist psychiatry, 195–98, 200–206, 223
postmodernism: Duras and silence of madness, 304–8; feminist visions of rupture with (male) logos, 302–4; gender and madness generally, 293–95; introduction to, 161, 162, 165–66; male postmodern madness, 295–301; metaphors of, 283; postmodern mind, 165, 282; psychotic defenses of madness by women, 308–15
Pound, Ezra, 250
Praise of Folly (Erasmus), 51–53
"prescientific mind," 329n. 5
pre-Socratics, 15–22, 29, 38, 76
pride, 22, 24, 27
Prince, The (Machiavelli), 53–54
progress, Rousseau on, 142, 144
projection, 72, 193–94
Prost, P. A., 149, 330n. 10
Proust, Marcel, 240, 242, 243, 277
Prussians, 179–80

psyche: as concept generally, 3–4; cybernetic theory of, 282–85; Freud on, 236, 241–42, 244–45, 247; German Romantics and text as allegory for, 182–85; Hippocratic writings on, 15–16, 18–20; linguistic theory of, 282–85; Reil on, 171; somatic-psychic distinction, 15–16, 17; translations of, 18. *See also* self

psychiatry: Artaud on, 268–69; beginnings of, 111–12; Breton on, 259, 261; coinage of term, 111, 133, 164, 167–68; compared with psychoanalysis, 223, 241, 249, 251; and cybernetic and linguistic theories, 282–85; as enemy to modern artists and writers, 249, 251, 268–69; Foucault's critique of "essentialism" in, 232–33; Griesinger and positivist view of madness, 200–204; Heinroth and theological dimension of romantic madness, 173–77; history of, 10–11, 226–27; Ideler and allegories of drives and instincts, 177–82; Kraepelin's classifications of madness, 213, 224, 227–34; Nerval on police function of doctors, 207; nineteenth-century history of, 111; Pinel and philanthropic psychiatry, 131, 135, 146–54, 164; and Plath, 272; positivist psychiatry, 195–98, 200–206, 223; Reil and rhapsodies about madness, 169–73; romantic psychiatry, 167–82, 185; and Sexton, 278–79; and Trakl, 254–59

psychic depth, 170

psychoanalysis: compared with judicial procedure, 240–41; compared with psychiatry, 223, 241, 249, 251; and dreams, 186; and expressionist view of artist, 251–52; foundations of, 234–43; and Freud, 161, 224–26, 234–49; and Heinroth, 176–77; hermeneutics developed by, 179, 194; and Ideler, 180; introduction to, 161, 163–66; literary mode of explanation in, 226, 234–35, 237–43, 246–49; and Sexton, 276

psychosis: cybernetic explanation of, 284; and fantasy, 242; feminist view of, 165; Foucault on, 277; Freud on, 67, 174, 243–48, 277; Lacan on, 291–93; and mimesis, 194; psychiatric theory of, 227; women writers' defenses of, 308–15. *See also* Psychiatry; Schizophrenia

psychosomatic, 174

Purgatory (Dante), 48–49

Pynchon, Thomas, 295, 298–302, 314

Queneau, Raymond, 334n. 14

Rabelais, François, 44, 51, 58, 68, 92, 190

Rameau's Nephew (Diderot), 124–27, 190

rationalism: of Descartes, 92–101; of Kant, 168–69; of Pope, 118–22. *See also* rationality; reason

rationality: of Dante, 48–49; of Erasmus, 53; of Machiavelli, 53–54; of Plato, 16; of pre-Socratics, 15–22; in Renaissance literary discourse, 50–54; and shared language, 16. *See also* logos; rationalism; reason

ratio (reason), 40

Ravissement de Lol V. Stein, Le (Duras), 305–6

reality: Lacan on the "real," 291; Mach-Duhem-Poincaré hypothesis on, 318; versus madness in *Don Quixote*, 85–92

reason: and French Revolution, 130; Lautréamont on, 215–16; Rousseau's attack on, 142; Van Helmont on, 105. *See also* rationalism; rationality

reason in madness: Diderot on, 123–24; in *Don Quixote*, 89–92; in *Hamlet*, 80–84; in Hoffmann's works, 191–92

Reformation, 70

Reil, J. C., 133, 146, 167, 169–73, 190, 191

Relativism, 117–18

Renaissance: and breakdown of Christ-

ian master allegory, 49–50; comedy in, 31, 32; creativity of, 50–51; defense of rationality in literary discourse of, 50–54; definition of, 50; fear of madness during, 51, 68–72; madness as interest of, 45–46, 49–51, 68–72; medical thought on madness during, 54–68; medicine in, 32, 44, 54–68; and Reformation, 70; Tasso and madness of Counter Reformation, 68–72, 75
Renan, Joseph-Ernest, 219
repression, 224–25, 236, 242, 260
Republic, The (Plato), 30, 38, 83
Rêve de d'Alembert (D'Alembert's dream; Diderot), 124
"Rêve parisien" (Baudelaire), 211–12
Rêveries (Rousseau), 141
Rhapsodieen über die Anwendung der psychischen Curmethode auf Geisteszerrüttungen (Rhapsodies upon the Use of the Psychic Cure Method for Mental Disturbances; Reil), 169–73
Richardson, Samuel, 127
Richard the Third (Shakespeare), 178
Rimbaud, Arthur, 203, 205, 214, 218–23, 258
Rinaldo, 70, 71
"Ritter Gluck" (Hoffmann), 190–91
Rogers, Benjamin Bickley, 35
Romans, 31, 39–40
romantic comedy, 37–38
romantic psychiatry, 167–82, 185
romantics. *See* German romantics
"Rot" (Red; Alexander), 265–66
Rousseau, Jean-Jacques, 55, 115, 135, 141–46, 148, 150–53, 157, 185, 330n. 4
"Rousseau" (Hölderlin), 143, 157
Royal College of Physicians, 118
Ruesch, Jurgen, 283, 285

Sacred Disease, The, 19, 21, 26
Sade, Marquis de, 103, 114, 115, 122, 127–31, 136, 162
Sandman, 194
Santos, Emma, 304, 309–11, 314–15
Sartre, Jean-Paul, 285, 334n. 3

satire, 115–18, 120, 124–26
Schelling, Friedrich, 174, 175
schismogenesis, 334n. 4
schizophrenia, 139, 142, 227, 230, 232, 265–67, 285–87, 293, 297–300, 317, 318, 320, 323
Schizophrenie und Sprache (Navratil), 265
Schlegel, Friedrich von, 182
Schubert, G. H. v., 172
science: compared with literature, 5; history of, 7–9; Rimbaud on, 218–19. *See also* specific scientific disciplines, such as biology
Season in Hell, A (Rimbaud), 218–22
Second Discourse (Rousseau), 144
secularization of madness, 77–78
Seele (spirit, soul, or self), 175
Sein und Schein (being and appearance), 173
self: Agrippa on, 59; and allegory, 72; Baudelaire, on, 213; centered self, 38; as concept generally, 3–4; Dante on, 48–49; Descartes on dualism of world and, 77; Edelman on self and language, 4–5; Erasmus on, 53; in Euripides, 24–30; Freud on, 177, 236, 241–42, 244–45, 247, 263–64; German Romantics and text as allegory for, 182–85; Griesinger on, 213–14; Heinroth on, 175, 177; historical development of, 10, 12; imperial self, 132, 142; and irony, 52; Lacan on, 287–91, 294; in Lautréamont, 217–18; layered self, 207; Lockean person, 4; myth of divided self, 208–9; and neoclassicism, 132; new concept of, in seventeenth century, 76; Plato on healthy self, 18, 38; Reil on, 170–71; Rimbaud on, 218, 220; Schlegel on metaphors for, 182; as series of boxes, 263–64; in Sophocles, 18, 22–24; speculum view of, 188–89; surrealist view of, 263–64
self-knowledge, 38
self-objectification, 217–18
self-referentiality, 91–92, 120–21, 295

self-reflexivity, 295, 296, 300, 319
Seneca, 147
Serapionsbrüder, Der (The Serapion
  Brethren; Hoffmann), 191
Serraglio degli stupori del mondo, Il
  (Garzoni), 63
Sexton, Anne, 276–80
Shakespeare, William: antecedents of,
  59; compared with Rousseau, 145;
  madness in plays by, 29, 53, 72,
  77–85, 94, 97, 101, 145, 178–79;
  madness stripped of allegorical
  dimensions in Shakespeare, 76, 77,
  79; medicine in *All's Well That Ends
  Well,* 78–80; and Paracelsus, 60;
  significance of generally, 5, 100; and
  Stoic will, 152–53
Shannon, Claude Elwood, 284
Ship of Fools, The (Brant), 51, 53
Simon, Bennett, 36
sin, 174–75, 176, 178. *See also* original
  sin
Singer, Charles, 147–48, 172
singular mad heroes, 134–46
Smart, Christopher, 115
social body, 29
social order, 27–30
Socrates, 33, 34–35, 56
Sokel, Walter, 252
somatic unity, 15–16
Sophocles, 18, 22–24, 29, 326n. 7
Sorrows of Young Werther, The
  (Goethe), 135–40
soul: as concept generally, 3, 4;
  Descartes on, 93, 94, 97–100, 102;
  Galen on, 20; German psychiatrists
  on, 197; medical view of, 102–3;
  Plato on, 20; theological view of,
  103; Van Helmont on, 104–6. *See
  also* self
speculum view: of madness, 173,
  174–75; of self, 188–89
spirit. *See* self
Spurzheim, Johann Christoph, 196
"Stade du mirroir" (Lacan), 290
Stadler, Ernst, 253
Stahl, George Ernst, 132–33, 168
Starobinksi, Jean, 42, 142

Stendhal, 154
Steps to an Ecology of Mind (Bateson),
  285–86, 288
sthenia, 159–60, 176, 196
Stoics, 39–41, 52, 70, 76, 82, 124, 147,
  149, 150, 152, 174
Stone Age, 1
Strepsiades, 34–35
stress, 229–30
Studies on Hysteria (Freud), 236
stupore, 63, 65, 67–68, 82
Sturm und Drang, 134
subject: Cartesian thinking subject, 4;
  as concept generally, 3; Lacanian
  subject, 4, 287–88; neurological subject, 4. *See also* self
sublimation, 277
suicide, 135–36, 139, 155, 258, 268,
  271, 276
Suite de l'entretien (Diderot), 124
superego, 30, 241–42, 244–45, 260,
  270
surrealism, 127–28, 214, 215, 221,
  259–64, 267–71
Swift, Jonathan, 103, 114–20, 122–24,
  126, 162, 190
Sydenham, Thomas, 107
Sylvius, Franciscus, 106
"symbolists," 205–23
"sympathetic phrenesy," 108
Symposium (Plato), 55
syphilis, 59, 195

Tale of a Tub, A (Swift), 115–18,
  120
Tasso (Goethe), 135, 136, 138–41
Tasso, Torquato, 68–72, 75, 92,
  138–41, 153, 157
taxonomy: in biology, 231, 232; of
  Garzoni, 55, 63–68; of Griesinger,
  213; of Heinroth, 176; of Kraepelin,
  227–34; as language game, 234; of
  Pinel, 147–48
Tecmessa, 23–24
Telemachus, 240
teleological history, 8
telos (final cause), 46
temperaments theory, 42, 86

Terence, 31
"theater of brains," 63, 64
theatricalization of madness, 63–68, 113, 125, 126, 169, 172–73, 180, 220–21, 230–31, 233
theatrical therapy, 172–73
Theatro de' varii e diversi cervelli mondani (Garzoni), 63, 65
Theologiae platonicae de immortalitate animorum (Ficino), 55
Theophrastus, 154
Theseus, 25–26
Thirtieth Problem (Aristotle), 13, 134, 248
Three Essays on Sexuality (Freud), 236, 240–41
thymos, 3, 4, 17–18. *See also* self
Tieck, Ludwig, 183, 187–89
Timaeus (Plato), 38–39
Tiresias, 27
totality theory, 186
tragedy: compared with comedy, 21–22, 31; Greek tragedy's depiction of madness, 18, 21–30; Shakespeare's tragedies, 80–85, 140, 162, 194. *See also* specific authors and works
Traité de l'homme (Descartes), 98
Traité des affections vaporeuses des deux sexes (Pomme), 159
Traité des passions (Descartes), 98
Traité médico-philosophique sur l'aliénation mentale ou la manie (Pinel), 131, 148–53
Trakl, Georg, 254–59, 272, 280
transference, 279
Traumdeutung, Die (*The Interpretation of Dreams;* Freud), 236
"Traum und Umnachtung" ("Dream and Derangement"; Trakl), 258
Treatise on Madness (Battie), 111–13
trephinations, 1
Trial, The (Kafka), 295
Trieb der Menschheit (drive to love and love of humanity), 179
Triebe (drives), 179–81
truth-value, 88–89, 93, 100, 105
Tuke, William, 146
"Tulips" (Plath), 273–74

Tusculan Disputations, The (Cicero), 39–40
"twilight of the gods," 252–53, 258
typology. *See* taxonomy

Ulysses, 22, 240
Ulysses (Joyce), 163, 240, 243, 279
unconscious: and art, 246; Breton on, 262; as concept generally, 3; Freud on, 242, 246; Heinroth on, 175, 177–78; Ideler on, 178; Lacan on, 289; Reil on, 171–72; surrealist view of, 263–64
Underwood, E. Ashworth, 148, 172
Unendlich (infinite), 174
Unkindest Cut, The (Menander), 38
Unnameable, The (Beckett), 298
utopia, 222, 259–60, 262

van Gogh, Vincent, 268–69
Van Gogh le suicidé de la société (Artaud), 268–69
Van Helmont, Jan Baptist, 104–7, 127
vapors theory of madness and melancholy, 42
Verlaine, Paul, 220
Vesalius, Andreas, 50, 64, 112
Virchow, Rudolf, 111, 205
vitalism, 123, 132–34, 146, 168
Voltaire, 114
Von der Lebenskraft (On the life force; Reil), 170

Wasps, The (Aristophanes), 36
Whitman, Cedric H., 34
Wiener, Norbert, 284
Willis, Thomas, 9, 107, 112, 118, 331n. 1
Winkelmann, Johann Joachim, 29–30
witchcraft trials, 47, 54, 67, 68
Wittgenstein, Ludwig, 3, 6, 86, 92, 202
Woman and Madness (Chesler), 294
Women and insanity: Chesler on, 294; Duras and silence of madness, 304–8; in Euripides' *Bacchae*, 27–30; feminist visions of rupture with (male) logos, 302–4; Garzoni on, 67–68; hysteria, 67, 107; postmodern view

Women and insanity (*continued*)
   of, 165; psychotic defenses of mad-
   ness by women, 308–15
Woolf, Leonard, 333n. 17
Woolf, Virginia, 333n. 17
Words for Doctor Y. (Sexton), 278–79
World Health Organization, 225
World War I, 229–30, 255, 259
World War II, 300
"Writers and Day-Dreaming" (Freud), 248

Xeres, 14

Yeux bleus, cheveux noirs (Duras),
   306

"Zauberei im Herbst" (Enchantment
   in autumn; Eichendorff), 183–
   85
Zeus, 25, 26
Zola, Émile, 204